Attention, Development, and Psychopathology

Attention, Development, and Psychopathology

Edited by
Jacob A. Burack
James T. Enns

THE GUILFORD PRESS
New York   London

© 1997 The Guilford Press
A Division of Guilford Publications, Inc.
72 Spring Street, New York, NY 10012

Printed in the United States of America

This book is printed on acid-free paper.

Last digit is print number: 9   8   7   6   5   4   3   2   1

Library of Congress Cataloging-in-Publication Data

Attention, development, and psychopathology / edited by Jacob
   A. Burack, James T. Enns.
     p. cm.
   Includes bibliographical references and index.
   ISBN 1-57230-198-8
   1. Attention. 2. Psychology, Pathological. I. Burack,
Jacob A. II. Enns, James T.
   RC455.4.A85A88 1997
   616.89′071–dc21   97-9198
                                                CIP

Contributors

Janette Atkinson, PhD, Visual Developmental Unit, Department of Psychology, University College London, London, England

Marc H. Bornstein, PhD, National Institute of Child Health and Human Development, Bethesda, Maryland

Darlene A. Brodeur, PhD, Department of Psychology, Acadia University, Wolfeville, Nova Scotia, Canada

Susan E. Bryson, PhD, Department of Psychology, York University, North York, Ontario, Canada

Jacob A. Burack, PhD, Department of Educational and Counseling Psychology, McGill University, Montreal, Quebec, Canada; Department of Psychology, Hebrew University of Jerusalem, Mount Scopus, Jerusalem, Israel

Jeffrey T. Coldren, PhD, Department of Psychology, Youngstown State University, Youngstown, Ohio

Kris Corradetti, BS, Department of Psychology, Youngstown State University, Youngstown, Ohio

James T. Enns, PhD, Department of Psychology, University of British Columbia, Vancouver, British Columbia, Canada

Joseph F. Fagan III, PhD, Department of Psychology, Case Western Reserve University, Cleveland, Ohio

Ellen C. Farwell, BA, Center for Human Development Research, Department of Psychiatry and Behavioral Sciences, University of Texas Medical School at Houston, Houston, Texas

Michael S. Gazzaniga, PhD, Dartmouth College, Hanover, New Hampshire

Ian H. Gotlib, PhD, Department of Psychology, Stanford University, Stanford, California

Marcia Grabowecky, PhD, Department of Psychology, Northwestern University, Evanston, Illinois

Pamela M. Greenwood, PhD, Cognitive Science Laboratory, The Catholic University of America, Washington, DC

Jodi Haiken-Vasen, PhD, Department of Psychology, Case Western Reserve University, Cleveland, Ohio

Timothy J. Harpur, PhD, University of Wisconsin Medical School, Madison, Wisconsin

Bruce Hood, PhD, Visual Development Unit, Department of Psychology, University College London, London, England

Alan Kingstone, PhD, Department of Psychology, University of Alberta, Edmonton, Alberta, Canada

Karen Kopera-Frye, PhD, Fetal Alcohol and Drug Unit, Department of Psychiatry and Behavioral Sciences, University of Washington Medical School, Seattle, Washington

David S. Kosson, PhD, Department of Psychology, Finch University of Health Sciences, The Chicago Medical School, North Chicago, Illinois

Reginald Landry, MA, Department of Psychology, York University, North York, Ontario, Canada

Colin MacLeod, PhD, Department of Psychology, University of Western Australia, Nedlands, Perth, Western Australia

George R. Mangun, PhD, University of California at Davis, Davis, California

Linda C. Mayes, MD, Yale Child Study Center, New Haven, Connecticut

Amy M. Norton, M.A., Center for Human Development Research, Department of Psychiatry and Behavioral Sciences, University of Texas Medical School at Houston, Houston, Texas

Jonathan M. Oakman, PhD, Department of Psychology, University of Waterloo, Waterloo, Ontario, Canada

Heather Carmichael Olson, PhD, Fetal Alcohol and Drug Unit, Department of Psychiatry and Behavioral Sciences, University of Washington School of Medicine, Seattle, Washington

Raja Parasuraman, PhD, Cognitive Science Laboratory, The Catholic University of America, Washington, DC

Deborah A. Pearson, PhD, Center for Human Development Research, Department of Psychiatry and Behavioral Sciences, University of Texas Medical School at Houston, Houston, Texas

Dale M. Stack, PhD, Department of Psychology, Concordia University, Montreal; Montreal Children's Hospital, Montreal, Quebec, Canada

Richard A. Steffy, PhD, Department of Psychology, University of Waterloo, Waterloo, Ontario, Canada

Ann P. Streissguth, PhD, Fetal Alcohol and Drug Unit, Department of Psychiatry and Behavioral Sciences, University of Washington School of Medicine, Seattle, Washington

Lana M. Trick, PhD, Kwantlen University College, Vancouver, British Columbia

Monica A. Valsangkar, BS, Department of Psychology, University of Alberta, Edmonton, Alberta, Canada

J. Ann Wainwright, MA, Department of Psychology, York University, North York, Ontario, Canada

Philip R. Zelazo, PhD, Departments of Psychology and Pediatrics, McGill University, Montreal; Montreal Children's Hospital, Montreal, Quebec, Canada

Preface

In the past decade, the emerging discipline of developmental psychopathology has begun to bridge traditional divisions between the areas of developmental and abnormal psychology (Cicchetti, 1989, 1990). The foundation of developmental psychopathology is based on the premise that typical developmental processes provide information about atypical processes and that knowledge of atypical processes is essential to understanding typical development. Although still in its formative years, the development of this discipline has given rise to a journal, *Development and Psychopathology,* and several volumes edited by prominent researchers in a variety of related fields.

The focus of the edited volumes within developmental psychopathology has typically centered around either (1) specific atypical populations or (2) general issues in the development of psychopathology. Examples of the former include edited volumes on developmental issues among persons with Down syndrome (Cicchetti & Beeghly, 1990), and other types of mental retardation (Burack, Hodapp, & Zigler, in press; Hodapp, Burack, & Zigler, 1990), children with autism (Baron-Cohen, Tager-Flusberg, & Cohen, 1993), maltreated children (Cicchetti & Carlson, 1989), and psychiatric patients (Cicchetti & Toth, 1992; Zigler & Glick, 1986). Examples of the latter include edited volumes on risk and protective factors (Rolf, Masten, Cicchetti, Neuchterlein, & Weintraub, 1990), various handbooks (Cicchetti & Cohen, 1995a, 1995b; Lewis & Miller, 1990; Luthar, Burack, Cicchetti, & Weisz, 1997; Lenzenweger & Haugaard, 1996), and products of symposia on general empirical and theoretical issues (e.g., Cicchetti, 1989, 1990; Cicchetti & Toth, 1991, 1994, 1995; Keating & Rosen, 1991).

There have been few attempts, however, to provide a forum for work within specific areas of development (i.e., attention, memory) as they relate to development and various types of psychopathology (for an exception, see Cicchetti & Beeghly, 1987). As a result, relatively large bodies of related research activities are spread across a wide range of disparate journals, books, and edited volumes.

The development of attention in atypical populations is an example of a specific aspect of development that is widely studied but that has not emerged as a cohesive area of empirical and theoretical work. Researchers in psychiatry; developmental, abnormal, clinical, and educational psychology; and special education study attention and attentional impairments from a variety of perspectives, methodologies, and orientations. However, the lack of a single forum for researchers of attention from these areas has prevented the effective integration of knowledge regarding the relationship between the typical development of attention and examples of impaired attention in various atypical groups. Two influential books on the development of attention, Hale and Lewis's (1979) *Attention and Cognitive Development* and Enns's (1990) *The Development of Attention: Theory and Research,* include a few selected chapters on atypical populations but do not focus primarily on the wide range of issues related to attention and developmental psychopathology.

The lack of connectedness among the researchers in this area was highlighted for us by our initial conversations about the work in our respective areas. We were both interested in similar issues related to the development of typical attention and occurrences of atypical attentional functioning. Yet, we were continuously struck by the extent to which each of us was unaware of the works and researchers cited by the other. Assuming that we are somewhat typical of our colleagues (no disrespect intended), it was apparent that there was a need for awareness and connectedness among the researchers of attention, development, and psychopathology.

Thus, our primary goal in organizing this volume was to provide an initial forum for researchers in these areas. Although we were unable to include many important researchers or all relevant topics, we attempted to involve contributors with diverse approaches and interests in populations with a variety of disorders throughout the lifespan. As with many other initial forums, this volume is not meant as a comprehensive text but rather as a catalyst for more collaborative work in this emerging discipline. To this end, we are particularly appreciative of the commitment, hard work, good nature, and originality of all the contributors. We thank Seymour Weingarten, editor in chief of The Guilford Press, for his initial encouragement in the project and continued patience throughout. We are indebted to Julie Brennan for organizing the flow of chapters among the contributors, editors, and the publisher.

During the preparation of this volume, the "family" of contributors was saddened by the death of Nancy Burl Zelazo, wife and longtime friend of Philip R. Zelazo. To Nancy, we dedicate this volume. She was a graduate-level RN in maternal and child health, and a full collaborator with Phil on several influential experiments on early neuromotor development. These studies have had important implications for children with early neuromotor disabilities, including children with Down syndrome—the population reported on in Phil's chapter with Dale Stack. Nancy had a burning commitment to serve persons with disabilities and those who are disadvantaged. We hope that in Nancy's spirit the research reported here will eventually help to improve the lives of some children and adults with developmental difficulties such as those discussed in this volume.

JACOB A. BURACK
JAMES T. ENNS

REFERENCES

Baron-Cohen, S., Tager-Flusberg, H., & Cohen, D. J. (Eds.). (1993). *Understanding other minds: Perspectives from autism*. New York: Oxford University Press.

Burack, J. A., Hodapp, R. M., & Zigler, E. (Eds.). (in press). *Handbook of mental retardation and development*. New York: Cambridge University Press.

Cicchetti, D. (Ed.) (1989). *The emergence of a discipline: Rochester Symposium on Developmental Psychopathology*. Hillsdale, NJ: Erlbaum.

Cicchetti, D. (1990). A historical perspective on the discipline of developmental psychopathology. In J. Rolf, A. Masten, D. Cicchetti, K. H. Neuchterlein, & S. Weintraub (Eds.), *Risk and protective factors in the development of psychopathology*. Cambridge, England: Cambridge University Press.

Cicchetti, D., & Beeghly, M. (Eds.). (1987). *Atypical symbolic development* (pp. 47–68). San Francisco: Jossey-Bass.

Cicchetti, D., & Beeghly, M. (Eds.). (1990). *Children with Down syndrome: A developmental perspective*. New York: Cambridge University Press.

Cicchetti, D., & Carlson, V. (Eds.). (1989). *Child maltreatment: Theory and research on the causes and consequences of child abuse and neglect*. Cambridge, England: Cambridge University Press.

Cicchetti, D., & Cohen, D. J. (Eds.). (1995a). *Developmental psychopathology: Vol. 1. Theory and methods*. New York: Wiley.

Cicchetti, D., & Cohen, D. J. (Eds.). (1995b). *Developmental psychopathology: Vol. 2. Risk, disorder and adaptation*. New York: Wiley.

Cicchetti, D. & Toth, S. L. (Eds.). (1991). *Models and integrations: Rochester Symposium on Developmental Psychopathology*. Rochester, NY: University of Rochester Press.

Cicchetti, D., & Toth, S. L. (Eds.). (1992). *Developmental perspectives on depression: Rochester Symposium on Developmental Psychopathology*. Rochester, NY: University of Rochester Press.

Cicchetti, D., & Toth, S. L. (Eds.). (1994). *Disorders and dysfunctions of the self: Rochester Symposium on Developmental Psychopathology*. Rochester, NY: University of Rochester Press.

Cicchetti, D., & Toth, S. L. (Eds.). (1995). *Emotion, cognition, and representa-*

tion: Rochester Symposium on Developmental Psychopathology. Rochester, NY: University of Rochester Press.

Enns, J. T. (Ed.). (1990). *The development of attention: Research and theory.* Amsterdam: North Holland Elsevier.

Hale, G. A., & Lewis, M. (Eds.). (1979). *Attention and cognitive development.* New York: Plenum Press.

Hodapp, R. M., Burack, J. A., & Zigler, E. (1990). Summing up and going forward: New directions in the developmental approach to mental retardation. In R. M. Hodapp, J. A. Burack, & E. Zigler (Eds.), *Issues in the developmental approach to mental retardation.* New York: Cambridge University Press.

Keating, D. P., & Rosen, H. (Eds.). (1991). *Constructivist perspectives on developmental psychopathology and atypical development.* Hillsdale, NJ: Lawrence Erlbaum Associates.

Lenzenweger, M. F., & Haugaard, J. J. (Eds). (1996). *Frontiers of developmental psychopathology.* New York: Oxford University Press.

Lewis, M., & Miller, S. M. (Eds.). (1990). *Handbook of developmental psychopathology.* New York: Plenum Press.

Luthar, S., Burack, J. A., Cicchetti, D., & Weisz, J. R. (Eds.). (1997). *Developmental psychopathology: Perspectives on risk and disorder: Essays in honor of Edward Zigler.* Cambridge, England: Cambridge University Press.

Rolf, J., Masten, A., Cicchetti, D., Neuchterlein, K. H., & Weintraub, S. (Eds.). (1990). *Risk and protective factors in the development of psychopathology.* Cambridge, England: Cambridge University Press.

Zigler, E., & Glick, M. (1986). *A developmental approach to adult psychopathology.* New York: Wiley.

Contents

SECTION I

INTRODUCTION

1. Attention, Development, and Psychopathology: 3
   Bridging Disciplines
   James T. Enns and Jacob A. Burack

SECTION II

**DEVELOPMENT OF ATTENTION
ACROSS THE LIFESPAN**

2. Development of Visual Attention   31
   Janette Atkinson and Bruce Hood

3. Selective Attention to Novelty as a Measure   55
   of Information Processing across the Lifespan
   Joseph F. Fagan, III and Jodi Haikan-Vasen

4. Selective Attention over the Lifespan   74
   *Darlene A. Brodeur, Lana M. Trick, and
   James T. Enns*

SECTION III

**INFANCY, ATTENTION,
AND PSYCHOPHARMACOLOGY**

5. Attention Regulation in Infants Born at Risk: 97
   Prematurity and Prenatal Cocaine Exposure
   Linda C. Mayes and Marc H. Bornstein

6. Attention and Information Processing in Infants   123
   with Down Syndrome
   Philip R. Zelazo and Dale M. Stack

7. Conceptual Relations between Attention Processes 147
in Infants and Children with Attention-Deficit/
Hyperactivity Disorder: A Problem-Solving Approach
Jeffrey T. Colren and Kris Corradetti

SECTION IV
CHILDHOOD, ATTENTION,
AND PSYCHOPATHOLOGY

8. Teratogenic Effects of Alcohol on Attention 171
*Karen Kopera-Frye, Heather Carmichael Olson,
and Ann P. Streissguth*

9. Attention-Deficit/Hyperactivity Disorder 205
in Mental Retardation: Nature of Attention Deficits
*Deborah A. Pearson, Amy M. Norton,
and Ellen C. Farwell*

10. A Componential View of Executive Dysfunction 232
in Autism: Review of Recent Evidence
*Susan E. Bryson, Reginald Landry, and
J. Ann Wainwright*

11. Paying Attention to the Brain: The Study 263
of Selective Visual Attention
in Cognitive Neuroscience
*Alan Kingstone, Marcia Grabowecky, George R.
Mangun, Monica A. Valsangkar, and Michael
S. Gazzaniga*

12. Attention in Aging and Alzheimer's Disease: 288
Behavior and Neural Systems
Pamela M. Greenwood and Raja Parasuraman

13. Attentional Functioning in Individuals 318
Diagnosed and at Risk for Schizophrenia
Richard A. Steffy and Jonathan M. Oakman

14. Information Processing in Anxiety and Depression: 350
A Cognitive-Developmental Perspective
Ian H. Gotlib and Colin MacLeod

15. Attentional Functioning of Psychopathic 379
Individuals: Current Evidence and Developmental
Implications
David S. Kosson and Timothy J. Harpur

Index 403

Attention, Development, and Psychopathology

SECTION I
INTRODUCTION

Attention, Development, and Psychopathology

BRIDGING DISCIPLINES

James T. Enns
Jacob A. Burack

The discipline of developmental psychopathology was formally introduced with the publication of a special edition of *Child Development* (Cicchetti, 1984) and the inauguration of a specialized journal 5 years later (Cicchetti, 1989a). As evidenced in the name, the conceptual frameworks for this field evolved primarily from the areas of development and psychopathology, although its roots are also in child psychiatry, neurology, biology, and genetics (Sroufe & Rutter, 1984). As is typical with fledgling fields of study, the formalization period did not so much mark the beginning of work in the field but rather served as a forum to delineate the goals, theoretical frameworks, and empirical guidelines that were already in place. In these endeavors, developmental psychopathology was differentiated from the related fields of developmental and abnormal psychology, and child psychiatry and child clinical psychology.

The emergence of a discipline that incorporates aspects of development and psychopathology was, paradoxically, both unlikely and inevitable. It was unlikely because researchers in each of these two fields had little interest in the other, apparently disparate discipline. Traditionally, the academic study of human development was focused on the identification and "construction" of universal laws that are common to all people, whereas the investigation of psychopathology was essentially one of deconstruction that entailed the search for specific defects that could account for given disorders at a certain moment in the lifespan. In keeping with this bifurcation, developmentalists examined developmental processes in typical children from usual backgrounds and ignored examples of discrepancies from atypical persons or situations. Conversely, the psychopathologists limited their research to specific areas of functioning among persons with certain disorders and were only interested in typical persons to the extent that they could be used as comparison subjects in the study of persons with disorders.

Yet, the advent of a discipline that incorporates development and psychopathology was also inevitable since knowledge in each of these areas is instructive to the other. Typical developmental processes provide a context and the basic principles for understanding the onset, course, and eventual outcome of atypical behaviors (e.g., Sroufe & Rutter, 1984; Zigler & Glick, 1986). Rather than being viewed simply as a behavioral anomaly at a given moment in time, psychopathology can be considered one of many aspects of the continuing development of affected individuals within their environments. Concordantly, the investigation of psychopathology is informative about the limits and potential sources of deviations of basic developmental processes and mechanisms (Hodapp & Burack, 1990). Borrowing from other fields of study, Cicchetti (1984) elegantly articulated the inherent relationship between the two disciplines with a statement that became the battlecry of developmental psychopathologists: "We can learn more about the general functioning of an organism by studying its pathology and, likewise, more about its pathology by studying its normal condition" (p. 1).

THE DEVELOPMENTAL INFLUENCE

The traditional theories of developmental psychology (i.e., those of Jean Piaget and Heinz Werner) view the organism as a dynamic and organized whole that develops according to universal laws and processes. Within the orthogenetic framework articulated by Werner (1957), this organization is portrayed as proceeding from a state of relative undifferentiation to one that is increasingly differentiated and hierarchically integrated. The organized whole is a system of parts that transact, such that they continuously affect each other. Development, therefore, encompasses change both among the various components and in the internal reorganization of the hierarchically structured organism. Developmental inquiry is directed toward understanding principles of organization and the evolving relationships among the parts and whole (e.g., Reese & Overton, 1970).

The scope of developmental research is typically limited due to the inherent intricacies in studying a developing organism that comprises numerous interrelated components within an integrated system that is continuously in the process of change. Thus, the early developmentalists primarily studied the maturing organism independent of the variations in the surrounding environments, pathologies or impairments, social influences, and other factors that might be related to individual differences. Development was conceptualized within a framework in which the processes of change and transformation (i.e., assimilation and accommodation) were the same for all children as they progressed through similar sequences of development within each of several interrelated domains of cognitive functioning. Similarly, discrepancies in the rate and/or quality of development across individuals was rarely examined (for exceptions, see Inhelder, 1968; Werner, 1957).

The narrow focus of mainstream developmental psychology was expanded in the 1960s and 1970s as emerging influences from other realms of psychology and related areas began to permeate the field (Kaplan, 1967; Cicchetti & Wagner, 1990). Consistent with Western societies' heightened interest in social issues and the roles of individuals and individuality within society, these changes reflected a shift in emphasis from the study of cognition and universals to that of social and biological development with a focus on individual differences. Thus, variables such as gender, motivation, personality, parenting history, physiological integrity, emotions, temperament, and communal, cultural, and societal background were increasingly studied by developmentalists. The importance of these factors was further highlighted with the shift toward lifespan development and the consideration of development in adolescence and beyond, when rate of cognitive growth was thought to diminish considerably and emerging aspects of social functioning were considered primary.

As these issues were introduced into the mainstream, the nature of the field's theoretical questions and, subsequently, the empirical paradigms changed significantly. Piagetian-type qualitative analyses of cognitive processes, functions, and structures were abandoned in favor of models and analyses that were more characteristic of the behaviorist approach. These changes allowed for quantitative assessments of the effects of numerous extracognitive factors (e.g., social, emotional, and personality). Despite its organismic holistic roots, the study of developmental psychology became increasingly mechanistic and deconstructivist, such that researchers became increasingly compartmentalized and had little in common with each other. This transformation represented so marked a change in orientation and conceptualization that the most prominent of developmental theorists declared that the "king [Piaget] was dead" (Kessen, 1984) and considered whether the age of development had come to an end (e.g., Bronfenbrenner, Kessel, Kessen, & White, 1986; Frye, 1991; Kessen, 1984).

Despite the increased prominence of mechanistic-like models, there was a recognition that such an approach to theoretical and empirical work was not sufficient for understanding individual differences related to the complexity of the environment, extracognitive factors, atypical developmental paths, and the relationship among all these variables and the developing individual. This led to the growth of theoretical schools whose adherents attempted to incorporate issues of individual differences and the environment within traditional principles of development. For example, the neo-Piagetians integrated traditional cognitive-developmental notions with other less monolithic frameworks such as those of information processing (e.g., Case, 1992) and Skinnerian behaviorism (e.g., Fischer, 1980). Similarly, complexities within environments were increasingly considered by Bronfenbrenner (1979) and others who proposed models that included various layers of social systems in which children develop and interrelate. With emerging interest in individual and environmental differences, post-Piagetians were more willing than their predecessors to consider the role of psychopathology, impaired functioning, and deleterious behavior.

As interest grew in atypical development, there was a particular focus on anomalous biological, social, and environmental histories that appeared to put children at risk for less than optimal outcomes. At first, with the use of post hoc analyses, impaired performance was seen as the inevitable outcome of a wide variety of pre -, neo -, and postnatal problems including low birthweight, anoxia at birth, and history of childhood abuse. However, in a landmark review, Sameroff and Chandler (1975) demonstrated that most children, except those who suffer severe biological insult, appear relatively resilient and develop typically if raised in reasonably intact environments. This work led to the increased application of the transactional world view (Sameroff, 1990) to the field of development, as it provided a framework for conceptualizing the complex transactions among the many aspects of the individual's genotype, phenotype, and environment. Unfortunately, its inherent complexity has precluded a systematic increase in empirically rigorous studies within this framework.

THE PSYCHOPATHOLOGY CONTRIBUTION

The prevailing principles of psychopathology are typically diametric to those of developmental psychology. Whereas the latter is historically a constructivist science that is focused on identifying and documenting universal laws for a holistically organized organism, psychopathology is primarily a deconstructionist and mechanistic discipline. Psychopathological research is typically directed at ascertaining impairments in specific processes or mechanisms that are associated with certain disorders or with identifiable biological, psychological, or environmental risk factors. Indeed, the very notion of a discipline of psychopathology might well be considered a misnomer, since researchers in this area share only a common interest in understanding atypical functioning along with some methodological considerations. Otherwise, they vary greatly among themselves with regard to the populations and aspects of functioning that they study.

The study of psychopathology has largely been devoid of developmental influences, as the typical focus is on specific disorders at given moments in persons' lives. The principle exception is the study of familial, genetic, physiological, and environmental variables that increase the risk for later psychopathology. The examination of these variables, alone and in tandem, provide psychopathologists with their own version of the nature–nurture debate in which they examine the long-term outcomes of factors that fit into both categories. This emphasis on risk variables served as a precursor to the work on resilience, vulnerability, and risk and protective factors that is a hallmark of research in developmental psychopathology (for discussions of this topic, see Robbins & Rutter, 1990; Rolf, Masten, Cicchetti, Neuchterlein, & Weintraub, 1990).

THE HISTORICAL PRECURSORS

Despite the historical differences between the disciplines of development and psychopathology, some prominent workers combined the study of both and laid the groundwork for the field's formalization. Sigmund Freud was an original—and maybe the best example of a theorist of developmental psychopathology. He initially used information from his observations of patients with neuroses and other disorders to build a model of development, and subsequently applied this model to the study and treatment of various types of psychopathology. The inherent role of development in the onset of psychopathology was explicit as he stressed that adult psychopathology was the outcome of both internal and interpersonal conflicts in childhood. Paradoxically, Freud rarely observed or interacted with children (his one time meeting with Little Hans being a notable exception) and therefore his developmental formulations were deduced from his patients' reconstructions of their childhoods. This post hoc analysis was historically the source of much criticism by detractors of the psychoanalytic approach and the primary reason that Freud's work was, for the most part, abandoned by academic psychologists within the mainstreams of developmental and abnormal psychology. Yet, with the renewed interest in the relation between the two fields, issues originally introduced by Freud and his disciples were reintroduced into the empirical literature.

In this century, Heinz Werner was the clinician/researcher most influential in formulating the relationship between development and psychopathology. In formulating the orthogenetic principle of development, Werner (1957) argued that cognitive styles displayed by persons with different types of psychopathology allowed for a developmental ordering that mirrored typical developmental progression. For example, on developmental evaluations of responses to Rorschach blots, Werner found that persons with hebephrenic–catatonic schizophrenia (most severely impaired) resembled children between 3 and 5 years old, persons with paranoid schizophrenia (moderate impairment) scored similar to children between 6 and 10 years old, and persons with psychoneuroses displayed responses that were comparable to those of persons between 10 years of age and adulthood.

This legacy was continued into the 1960s and 1970s by workers such as Edward Zigler, Norman Garmezy, and Michael Rutter, who shared common interests in the interplay between development and psychopathology (see the preface to Cicchetti, 1989b). They emphasized the value of this combined approach because of its implications for better understanding of disorders and its role in implementing intervention programs, as well as an informational guide to typical developmental processes. Within a single theoretical framework, they were able to examine populations that varied greatly with regard to type, severity, and proneness to psychopathology. Accordingly, the study of developmental psychopathology includes persons manifesting traditional psychiatric pathology, problem behaviors, or developmental disorders, as well as those who are at risk for later pathology due to any number of reasons related to community, environmental, and/or familial situations, personal experiences, and/or biological anomalies. The universal utility of this approach is especially evident in the diversity of populations studied by these researchers and their many students. Since the formalization of the discipline in the 1980s (Cicchetti, 1984, 1989a, 1989b), numerous psychological disorders and risk factors have been considered within this framework.

ATTENTION AND DEVELOPMENTAL PSYCHOPATHOLOGY

Attention is one cognitive component that is often cited in the functioning of a wide range of atypical populations. Although a single definition is elusive and the term actually refers to several aspects of functioning, the notion that the inability to "attend" efficiently is a source of behavioral, intellectual, and/or emotional problems is intuitively appealing. Attentional processes are considered basic to all aspects of functioning and are therefore a source of interest in the study of certain atypical populations.

As these processes emerge early in life and continue to evolve, specific instances of inefficiency or deficits throughout the lifespan are implicated in the development of individual and group differences (see Enns, 1990; Hale & Lewis, 1979). Of course, the specific nature and consequences of the attentional deficits differ with regard to type of disorder, age of the person, and the particular manifestation of the attentional deficit.

The study of attention among atypical populations can be framed within several, often overlapping perspectives. First, among infants and children, it is examined as a predictor of later problems including low IQ, acting-out behaviors, and psychiatric disorders. Within the orthogenic perspective, the cumulative effects of early problems may be profound and far reaching. Second, in persons with identified biological disorders such as Down syndrome, attentional problems can be viewed as a consequence of biological anomalies related to the disorder. In turn, attentional problems can impede development in a variety of domains of functioning or exacerbate other problems arising from the biological insult. Third, among persons with behavioral and/or academic problems, attentional problems can be seen as the outcome, cause of, or even in transactional relationship with, cognitive styles that arise from lifetime histories of frustration and feelings of failure or inadequacy. Similarly, among persons with psychopathology, these problems can be viewed as causing, coexisting with, or resulting from the disorder. For many populations, any one or more of these perspectives may be relevant.

WHY IS ATTENTION NECESSARY?

Within modern psychology, it is safe to say that attention has now attained the status of a natural category (Wittgenstein, 1953). That is, the concept is conceded by everyone to be essential to an understanding of behavior; yet a definition that would pass the ideal muster involving "necessary" and "sufficient" attributes has proven to be extremely elusive. Whether the concept will ever achieve this status will depend largely on its usefulness to such disciplines as development and psychopathology. Within the framework of these other fields, the validity of attentional theories will be tested in a variety of ways, as attempts are made to extend and expand the constructs to changes that occur over the lifespan and to differences among individuals.

The necessity of the concept of attention can be glimpsed if one imagines what would happen if it should suddenly cease to exist. A good case can be made that it would have to be reinvented immediately by anyone seriously interested in the study of behavior. Ironically, something close to this has already occurred at least once in the history of psychology.

Over a hundred years ago William James (1890) declared: "Every one knows what attention is. It is the taking possession by the mind . . . of one of . . . several simultaneously possible objects or trains of thought. . . . It implies withdrawal from some things in order to deal effectively with others" (pp. 403–404). Yet, almost 60 years later Donald O. Hebb (1949) felt compelled to defend himself against the behaviorist mainstream by arguing that "attention is not mystical . . . nor anthropomorphic, animistic, or undefinable" (p. 4). In his words, all discussion of attention had in common the "recognition that responses are determined by something else besides the immediately preceding sensory stimulation" (p. 5).

Why is this elusive, ill-defined concept so difficult to purge from our theories? The answer seems to be that some sort of selectivity (i.e., attention, in the words of James) is inherent and necessary to the notion that brains use sensory information to guide action. This is hardly a controversial starting point, although it leads relentlessly to the often-controversial concept of attention. Historically, the connection between information processing and processing selectivity has been made within three different and mutually insightful perspectives.

One perspective is that of ecological psychologists who view attention as naturally essential for two reasons: (1) the behaving organism is faced at every moment by an infinitely large barrage of available information by which its actions may be controlled, and (2) for an action to occur within finite time, some information must be chosen as relevant to the behavior while other information is disregarded. Although the postulation of selectivity in information processing is generally accepted, this position is controversial for some because of questions concerning what determines the selection procedure. For James J. Gibson (1966), the father of this movement, the answer was that "the available stimulation surrounding an organism has structure, both simultaneous and successive, and this structure depends on sources in the outer environment. If the invariants of this structure can be registered by a perceptual system, the constants of the neural input will correspond to the constants of the stimulus energy" (p. 663). In other words, the problem of attention was one of "tuning," that is, a tuning of the brain of an organism by forces of evolution, development, and learning to select, or "resonate" with, the appropriate information in the environment.

A second line of reasoning that leads to attention begins with a consideration of the perceiver, the one who does the information processing. It is an inescapable fact that the sensory and perceptual systems of the brain are limited in many ways. Each has spatial and temporal limitations in its function, along with very real biological limits in its structure. Thus, some mechanism is required to ensure that the system is not overloaded by the environmental stimulation. Donald E. Broadbent's (1958) notion of a filter (a mechanism to switch the flow of information from one processing channel to the other) is an example of such a mechanism and has been cited in much of cognitive research during the past two decades. A direct descendant of this idea that holds current sway is Anne Treisman's feature integration theory (Treisman & Gelade, 1980; Treisman, 1988; Treisman & Sato, 1990). The "filter" has now become a "spotlight of attention" that can be directed across the visual field by salient stimuli in a reflexive fashion or by the voluntary control of the observer in a strategic fashion.

The third argument for selectivity begins with consideration of the tasks that brains must perform (Marr, 1982; Ullman, 1984). Even the most mundane of tasks require that some information be processed before other information (i.e., a problem of selection in space and time). For example, the seemingly trivial problem of determining whether a dot on a page lies within or outside of the bounds of a closed-line drawing on the same page cannot be solved without first being broken down into a sequence of steps (Ullman, 1984). Researchers who have disregarded this point have been deceived by "the apparent immediateness and ease of perceiving spatial relations . . . [which] conceals in fact a complex array of processes that have evolved to establish certain spatial relations with considerable efficiency" (Ullman, 1984, p. 99).

THE MANY FACES OF ATTENTION

It is admittedly easier to establish the necessity of attention than to define it, localize it in the brain, or even to make behavioral predictions about when and where it will exert its influence. The first modern functional taxonomy of attention was given by James (1890), who identified no fewer than six possible varieties by considering the combinations of three polar constructs: Attention could be focused on either sensory objects (perception) or intellectual objects (ideas and memories); it could be immediate (directed to the object itself) or derived (directed by an object's signal value to an associated object of real interest); and it could be passive (reflexively driven by the stimulus) or active (voluntarily initiated by the observer).

This early taxonomy has been broad enough to encompass many subsequent ones (see, e.g., Kinchla, 1980, 1992; Parasuraman & Davies, 1984). We will focus primarily on only two here because, seen together, they nicely illustrate how the definition and utility of attention can differ dramatically, depending on whether one begins by focusing on the stimulus (the sensory environment) or the perceiver (the biological machinery).

Werner's (1948, 1957) discussion of selectivity in perception is rooted in the observation that the sensory systems are bombarded by environmental stimulation. Consistent with his orthogenetic principle of development, Werner's notion of "perceiving" an event is the appreciation that the event has both a highly differentiated set of components (parts) and a hierarchically organized structure (whole) in which those parts are related. Werner's (1957) subdivision of perception into three "stages" illustrates this principle. In stage 1, perception is dominated by global attributes of the event. Perceiving, acting, feeling, and imagining are not differentiated. In stage 2, perception is analytic, focused on the parts. Perception can be differentiated from action. In stage 3, perception is integrated, in that the parts are at the same time highly differentiated and synthetically related to one another.

This dialectical approach to attention was also used by James J. Gibson (1966) and Eleanor J. Gibson (1969). For them, attention was synonymous with the selective "gathering" or "extraction" of information. The factors determining which information was gathered included those of human nature (e.g., humans, and especially children, are inherently both active and curious), goals and motivations (e.g., walkers and mountain climbers base their behavior on different pieces of information), and ecology (e.g., the possible actions on an object determines its perceptual value). The heart of this approach was summarized in the principle "seek and ye shall find," meaning that there was no need for a perceiver to "go beyond" the information in the stimulus array or to "construct" a mental representation of the stimulus (E. J. Gibson, 1977, p. 157).

A very different starting point, namely, a consideration of the machinery of perception, led Hebb (1949, 1966) to a very different definition. He began by noting that even simple behaviors such as a manual reaction to the onset of light led inevitably to talk of attention. At the same time that he lamented the absence of a clear definition of attention, Hebb argued vigorously that researchers could not afford "to sit around with hands folded, waiting for the physiologist to solve [the problem of attention] . . . the problem requires a knowledge of the psychological as well as the physiological evidence for its solution" (1949, p. 11). He proposed that, as a working hypothesis, attention should be associated with specific patterns of neural firing in the brain.

Continuing in this tradition, Michael I. Posner and colleagues (see, e.g., Posner, 1980; Posner & Boies, 1971) provided behavioral evidence for three different attentional systems: arousal, limited-capacity attention, and selectivity. Arousal referred to the momentary level of excitation of the whole organism, a level that could be manipulated by varying such factors as general alertness and cognitive readiness. Limited-capacity attention referred to all the cognitive resources that were available to perform a given task. If a subject was given two tasks and these tasks involved the same resources (e.g., short-term memory, the visual sensory system), then maintaining a given level of performance on one task meant that performance on the other task must suffer. Thus, selective attention referred to the specificity with which resources were allocated to task demands. For example, choosing to focus the "mind's eye" on a particular location in visual space was shown to facilitate the perception of subsequent stimuli in that location but at the expense of impaired perception of stimuli that occurred at other locations.

This approach to the definition of attention was extended in the 1980s and 1990s largely on the basis of evidence from brain imaging techniques (Posner & Raichle, 1994). Attention is used as an overarching term to refer to several quite different and widely distributed systems of coordinated brain activity. Two such systems that have been investigated extensively are one for visual orienting and one for the conscious awareness of objects. The visual orienting system involves (1) a thalamic brain structure known as the pulvinar, which acts to block neural inputs to the cortex from sensory systems that are currently unattended; (2) a midbrain structure known as the superior colliculus, which serves to move attention from one region of visual space to another; and (3) a cortical structure, the parietal lobe, which permits processing of a given stimulus to completion so that another stimulus can be processed. The system for the conscious detection of objects is sometimes called the executive function, because it appears to be critical in the conscious execution of instructions (e.g., "I must press a key"; "I must name the color of the ink but not read the word out loud"). It has tentatively been associated with a forebrain structure called the anterior cingulate gyrus.

WHAT IS IT THAT DEVELOPS?

Armed with this range of definitions for attention, it is possible to explore the views of development that are both explicit and implicit in them. Werner's (1957) orthogenetic principle provides a seamless framework in which principles of biological development become the metaphor for both perceptual development (changes in perception over age) and the development of a perception (changes in perception over a microtime scale). Just as the biological development of a human progresses from that of a single-cell organism to that of a multicell fetus to that of a multiorgan individual, the perception of an infant is at first undifferentiated, only becoming more analytic and organized with development. This progression from global to local to integration can even be seen when adults view an object for the first time.

Like Werner, Eleanor J. Gibson (1969) described perceptual development in terms of twin forces of increasing differentiation and integration.

However, unlike Werner, she placed more emphasis on the role of experience (learning) than on physiology (maturation), to the extent that perceptual learning was for all practical purposes synonymous with attentional development. A major emphasis in her writing was on the optimization of attention. By this she meant the exploratory behaviors of eye movements, the head and body movements used to orient sensory systems with the important sources of information, as well as the nonobservable processes involved in attending to the shape of an object rather than to its color. With experience, children become less captive to the aspects of the stimulus made salient by the sensory systems (e.g., bright lights, sudden movements) and better able to guide these behaviors on the basis of longer term goals.

For stimulus-inspired theorists, then, changes in the development of attention are essentially changes in the skills used to analyze, synthesize, and coordinate the sensory experiences that bombard the eye and ear. The biological equipment required to perform these skills, to the extent it is even considered, is assumed to be relatively constant across development. This is quite different from the notion of attention as brain structure, in which what changes in development is the machinery itself. Hebb (1949), like E. J. Gibson, viewed perceptual learning and development as involving many of the same processes. However, Hebb differed radically from Gibson in his view that these experiences altered the very nature of the perceptual machinery. Considering perception of a triangle, Hebb argued strongly for the case that a human infant did not "see" a triangle without a great deal of learning. Furthermore, "learning to see" a triangle changed the pattern of neural activity in the brain in an irreversible way.

This theme is continued and elaborated in the extension of Posner's ideas to perceptual development. In the distributed systems approach, development is associated with increasingly complex neural circuitry that permits the organism increasing control over the way in which information available to the sensory systems is processed. In this view, perceptual development changes the way in which the higher regions of the brain, especially those involved in consciousness, take control of these sensory areas. It does relatively little to change the functioning of the lower level brain centers that are specialized for each sense. For example, in the case of visual exploration, Posner and Raichle (1994) describe infants under 6 months of age as "looking machines" (p. 193). The lowest levels of the visual system are eager to perform their built-in functions, which include fixating on contours and orienting to novel stimuli. In very young infants, this results in such well-known phenomena as obligatory looking (i.e., infants are sometimes distressingly unable to remove their gaze from a contour) and orienting biases to the temporal visual fields (i.e., faced with a competition of new objects in each visual field, infants will orient to the temporal side). Development involves bringing these primary functions under higher level control. Intentions can be used to overcome obligatory looking, and orienting to novel objects becomes more symmetric, presumably because of improved communication between the parietal cortex and the superior colliculus.

A second example begins with the everyday observation that infants that are hungry or in pain can sometimes be distracted by drawing their attention to a novel toy. However, when distress levels were measured in a controlled way, researchers observed that the loss of overt signs of distress were not necessarily accompanied by a loss of distress in all areas of the brain (Posner & Raichle, 1994). When a series of novel toys were presented and removed, overt distress levels always returned to the same level, regardless of the size of the reduction in the presence of the toy. This suggests that attention does not involve changes to the sensory systems themselves but rather has to do with whether the information there is permitted to gain control of consciousness.

How Is Attention Measured?

With such a diversity of views on attention and development, it should come as no surprise that there is considerable debate regarding how best to measure attention. One of the keys to finding a path through this diversity is the insight that attention as skill, represented in this review by Werner and E. J. Gibson, leads naturally to different methodologies than atten-tion as brain structure, as represented by Hebb and Posner.

Werner (1957) analyzed the content of subjects' verbal responses in order to draw inferences about the content of subjects' attention. For ex-ample, he noted that verbal responses to Rorschach pictures consisted almost entirely of "whole" responses in 3-year-olds, more "details" among 6- to 8-year-olds, and a much larger proportion of "integrated whole" responses in older children. Although modern researchers look askance at such practices, it is notable that Werner was able to draw parallels be-tween the developmental progression of responses (ontogenesis), the responses of adults viewing the same pictures under increasingly long ex-posure durations (microgenesis), and the pattern of responses from in-dividuals diagnosed with schizophrenia (psychopathology).

E. J. Gibson (1969) also examined the content of behavior in order to make inferences about attention. One of her most celebrated methods involved observing the behavior of infants of various ages in the visual cliff apparatus. The finding of greatest theoretical significance was that visual sensitivity to the cliff coincided with the onset of crawling. That is, the information afforded by the cliff was only used when it was rele-vant to the infant's goals and possible actions.

Notably, there was no specific manipulation of attention in each of the two foregoing examples. Attention only played the role of a theoretical construct—one that was useful in explaining differences in behavior caused by events and stimuli that are not immediately evident in the stimulus situation.

Wendell Garner (1962, 1974) developed a more direct way to study attention (for other examples, see Lockhead & Pomerantz, 1991) that was based on an approach that began with a careful definition of an n-dimensional stimulus space (usually $n = 2$). Stimuli in this space can vary in two or more attributes. They are presented, usually in a random order, to subjects who are asked to perform several different tasks with them. For example, in a speeded classification task, they may be told to sort all the stimuli into two groups on the basis of only one of the two dimensions. By comparing performance on this task with control tasks in which the values of the second (task-irrelevant) dimension are fixed, a measure of selective attention is obtained (e.g., no difference would indicate perfect selection). Similar sets of speeded classification tasks have been designed to measure divided attention. This methodology is used to examine such issues as whether perception begins with the part or the whole, how perception changes with development, and how perception differs between species.

Quite naturally, the links between a theoretical construct of attention and specific behavioral manipulations can be seen more clearly when attention is viewed as brain structure. In an early example, Hebb (1966) suggested an elegant method for distinguishing empirically between perceptual selectivity (which he preferred to call "attention") and response selectivity (which he preferred to call "set"). Imagine a stimulus consisting of two horizontally arrayed digits, a 6 and a 3. A manipulation of perceptual selectivity might involve the instruction "name the rightmost digit" versus "name the leftmost digit." Contrast this with two conditions involving the same stimulus but where the task is now either to "name the result of subtracting the right digit from the left digit" or "name the result of adding the two digits." The first two conditions differ in their demands for perceptual selectivity; the second two in their demands for response selectivity. In both cases, an internal event caused by events long removed from the sensory systems determines selection among a set of possible processing events.

By far the most systematic work on the measurement of attention has come from Posner's (1980) cost–benefit methodology. In a typical visual orienting task, the subject is given the simple task of pressing a key whenever a predefined target is presented (the onset of a light or a simple shape). Observers' eye movements are usually controlled, either by presenting cue–target sequences that are less than 200 milliseconds in duration or by instructing observers not to move their eyes and then monitoring their behavior. The critical manipulation is the presentation of a stimulus (called a cue) immediately preceding the target event. If the cue indicates a location that is the same as that of the subsequent target, the trial is called valid; if it indicates a different location from the subsequent target, the trial is called invalid. If the cue provides no location-specific information, the trial is called neutral. The specific measure of attention is a subtractive comparison of invalid and valid response times (RT) to the target, where neutral RT versus valid RTs are interpreted as the benefit of precuing and invalid RT versus neutral RT are interpreted as the cost of having been miscued. Increasingly, these behavioral measures are being collected concurrently with physiological measures (e.g., positron emission tomography scans, event-related brain potentials, functional magnetic resonance imaging) in order to permit imaging of the brain during various attentional states (see Posner & Raichle, 1994).

Response Time as an Index of Attention

The widespread use of RT by Posner and others necessitates some consideration of issues that might qualify conclusions based on them, especially in the context of studies involving different developmental or psychopathological populations. The first issue concerns the separability of the mean and the variance of an RT distribution. Most statistical comparisons are based on means, under the assumption that variances are homogeneous. Yet, the data show that these two measures are invariably related. Thus, researchers of development and psychopathology need to address the appropriateness of entering nontransformed RT into statistical analyses when age and/or psychopathology may be associated with changes in the duration of the so-called psychological moment (Birren, 1965; Kail, 1990; Salthouse, 1991; Welford, 1965).

A second issue concerns the interpretation given to differences in RT. It is traditional to interpret these as pure measures of attention, since the experimental conditions are assumed to be equated with regard to sensory and motor processes. How then is a larger difference for group to be interpreted? If the concomitant change in variability is ignored or independent effects are assumed, interpretation is unhindered—the attention effect is larger for the group with the larger difference. Also, if one takes an ecological view of RT—organisms of all ages escape predation and find food in the same functional time units—then direct comparisons of RT differences seem warranted. However, if RT is interpreted as a relative and indirect measure, more caution should be exercised.

A final issue concerns the importance of collecting coordinated RT and accuracy data. This is particularly important in studies of development and psychopathology because there is always the possibility that an age or group difference in RT may be attributable to an underlying speed–accuracy trade-off (Pachella, 1974; Wickelgren, 1977). The slower responding of very young children, elderly adults, or persons with a handicap or disorder when compared to that of typical young adults may be symptomatic of a heightened emphasis on accuracy. As such, interpretations based upon RT alone will be misinformed. In most cases where speed–accuracy trade-offs have been examined (e.g., Cerella, 1990; Enns, 1990; Kail, 1990; Plude & Doussard-Roosevelt, 1990), they have not been found to account for the age effects obtained. Nonetheless, it is important to examine coordinated RT and accuracy data because even small changes in error rate may be associated with large differences in RT.

METHODOLOGICAL ISSUES

Researchers intent on interdisciplinary study are sometimes rightfully said to be gluttons for punishment. This is simply because it is more difficult to meet two different sets of research standards than only one. For new research to be accepted by more than one discipline, it must not only achieve the standards established for one discipline but must also achieve the standards of the others. In the present case, for example, this means that any examination of attention in a developing cross section of psychopathological individuals must not only reflect theory and methodology appropriate to each of the fields of attention (e.g., measures of attention must be acceptable to attention researchers in the mainstream), development (e.g., the study must consider changes over time in the life of the individual), or psychopathology (e.g., the study must examine issues of diagnostic classification, group differences, or treatment effectiveness) considered individually; indeed, it must reflect theory and methodology acceptable to all three realms collectively. This is no undertaking to be considered lightly; at the same time we believe that the chapters in this book demonstrate that it is an undertaking that promises to reap large rewards.

The most common of the studies regarding attention and developmental psychopathology are studies of group comparisons. The primary purpose of this type of research is the identification of specific markers of deviance in a group (or groups) or as in indicator of at-risk status for later problems. Thus, this type of research includes studies of genetic, neurological, or other psychophysiological phenomena, behavioral functioning, and/or social conditions. For all these areas of research, there is the evident need to identify the target group(s) that is (are) the central focus of the study and to establish some kind of standard against which find ings from the target group(s) can be compared. The latter goal is typically accomplished by including one or more other groups as comparison. Although this strategy is routinely used, insufficient attention is paid to its precise utilization. At the most semantic level, there is even considerable confusion regarding the depiction of the nontarget subjects. These participants are often inappropriately referred to as control rather than comparison subjects. The former term is, of course, relevant to clinical studies that include intervention and control conditions, each with subjects from the same population, but not to studies where persons from different populations are compared on the same conditions.

The efficacy of the comparison groups is contingent upon (1) precise classificatory criteria and homogeneity of subject groups; (2) the choice and use of comparison populations; (3) the matching of persons in the target and comparison groups; and (4) the consideration of the developmental level of the subject groups.

Precision in Defining Populations

Precise definitions of both the target and comparison groups is necessary to tell a specific story. In the case of measuring behavior, the typical story is that members of the target population perform in a certain manner, and this may be similar to or dissimilar from the comparison population(s). When the subjects are carefully defined, comparisons across studies are more informative, as questions regarding concordance in criteria for subject inclusion can be readily evaluated. High concordance should result in a greater chance of replicating the findings. And even in cases where concordance is low, precise specifications alert readers and researchers to a likely source of the differences among studies. In particular, researchers need to specify the exact diagnostic or classification systems utilized for both the target and comparison subjects; the number of persons in each of the specific etiological or diagnostic groups and subgroups; the severity, duration, and extent of the disability or problematic social situation; and the precise levels of functioning.

With groups of persons homogeneous with regard to precise etiology and/or diagnosis, precise comparison statements can be enunciated. However, although such precision is always methodologically preferable, it can lead to the exclusion of potential subjects (who are often difficult both to find and to recruit) and precludes conceptual generalizations. The solution for both these problems is typically the utilization of groups that are more heterogeneous with regard to etiology and/or classification. Yet, this solution is problematic for two related and insurmountable reasons: No specific comparisons statements can be made can be made among groups, and there may be little reliability among studies due to the inconsistency in the makeup of the groups. For example, in study 1 group g may be comprised of X number of people with problem A, Y people with problem B, and Z people with problem C, but in study 2 group g is made up of Z people with problem A, X people with problem B, and Y people with problem C. In this case, groups g do not represent an actual population or even a specific amalgam. Therefore, groups g are not adequate target or comparison groups, as no conclusions can be drawn about the characteristics of population G (which group g was supposed to represent). Performance of group g in either study would artifactually be related to the specific group membership.

Choosing the Comparison Groups

The choice of comparison group depends largely on the main story line. If the intent is to assess whether the target group is typical or atypical, then the target group is compared to the general population. However, if the primary questions revolve around the uniqueness of certain characteristics to the target group, then the target group is ideally compared to other groups that are similar with regard to all characteristics except for the one under consideration (for a review of issues related to comparison strategies, see Wagner, Ganiban, & Cicchetti, 1990). For example, persons with Down syndrome are often compared to other persons with mental retardation to ensure that the specific deficit is not a function of their lower IQ, and they are compared to others with organic etiologies to ensure that certain characteristics are not simply the general consequents of organic insult. With all the differences among the various etiological groups of persons with mental retardation, comparison groups are ideally composed only of persons with a single etiology, such as fragile X and Williams syndromes. At a more precise level, differentiation is useful even among the trisomy 21, translocated, and mosaic subtypes of Down syndrome (Burack, Hodapp, & Zigler, 1988).

Issues of Matching

The comparisons between target and comparison subjects are only informative to the extent that discrepancies between the groups can be attributed to the specified level of differentiation between the groups (e.g., diagnosis, history of abuse) and not to other factors that may initially be dissimilar among the groups. Typically, the primary goal of matching in developmental psychopathology involves equating groups by level of development (functioning). As is stated in reference to studies of adults with schizophrenia (Chapman & Chapman, 1973) and children with autism (Yule, 1978; Frith & Baron-Cohen, 1987) little is learned when persons functioning at lower levels perform worse than those at higher levels. Thus, simple matching by chronological age is usually not sufficient in studies of persons with disorders. Although apparently obvious, this issue was long overlooked by researchers studying pathological groups and led to the common acceptance of "truths" that are not supported by empirical data. Currently prominent among such truths is that mental retardation is inherently associated with attentional deficit (e.g., Melnyk & Das, 1992), although there is little evidence of a relation between low intelligence and attentional functioning especially when mental age (MA) and organicity are accounted for (see Iarocci & Burack, in press).

Choosing the measure of functioning that is the basis for matching is a complex task. Typically, general measures of MA based on standardized IQ tests are used for this task, although several problems have been cited. First, the tests, the value of which has generally been decried by skeptics, are of especially questionable utility with persons with certain impairments (e.g., sensory, motor, or intellectual), persons from the nonmajority cultures and backgrounds, or persons with behavior problems/styles that may impede test performance. Second, measures of general functioning may be inappropriate for atypical groups with specific profiles of strengths and weaknesses across domains, since they may either overcompensate for or undervalue levels of functioning in areas specifically related to the task at hand. Third, as the nature of questions change with age, the continuity of MA measures across the lifespan is problematic. In an attempt to account for these issues, researchers increasingly employ tests for matching that are least prejudicial to background, abilities, and age and that are most relevant to the areas of functioning that are being tested. Although varying strategies may be appropriate given differences in subjects' ages, the populations studied, and the focus of research, choices of matching strategies and measures are central methodological concerns.

Other factors that are often potentially confounding include socioeconomic status, residential status (home, community setting, or institution), gender, language abilities, and ethnic background. As specific atypical groups often vary from each other as well as from the typical population on one or more of these variables, appropriate matching is necessary but difficult.

Developmental Issues and Implications

Consideration of the precise developmental level is important for making sense of group differences. It is possible, and not that uncommon, for persons with a certain disorder to show an apparent deficit in a given area at a specific age/level of functioning but not later on. This is indicative of a developmental lag among persons in the target group that can only be ascertained by the study of persons with a given disorder at different levels of functioning. Without longitudinal studies, or series of cross-sectional studies in which level of functioning and/or age are considered, the evidence regarding deficits and developmental lag is often hard to assess (see Burack, 1992) and may be inconsistent across studies.

A common reason for inconsistencies in research is that a defect or delay in a specific area of behavior may be manifested in different ways throughout development. Thus, the long-term or cumulative effects of an early attentional problem may be profound in several domains of functioning, including those not obviously related to attentional functioning per se. For example, attentional impairments in infancy or childhood may be the antecedents for academic, cognitive, or social problems throughout the lifespan (e.g., Douglas & Peters, 1979).

CONCLUSION

In keeping with the general orientation of the discipline of developmental psychopathology, the chapters that follow are informative for understanding both typical developmental processes and atypical ones in persons with specific disorders. The issues vary by age group and by disorder.

In the study of infants, attention and related aspects of information processing are less well differentiated than they are in the study of older children and adults. This is consistent with the orthogenetic principle espoused by Werner (1957). Atkinson and Hood (Chapter 2) lead the reader through a careful progression of ideas, beginning with a consideration of central nervous system development, leading eventually to a detailed analysis of looking behavior in the first year of life. Fagan and Haiken-Vasen (Chapter 3) discuss a basic attentional process that is evident in infancy and continues to be central to functioning throughout the lifespan. This processing is related to intellectual functioning at all ages and is said to be less biased than most tests of intellectual functioning. Accordingly, infant attention is viewed as the best predictor of future intelligence and later in life continues to be highly correlated with efficiency of attentional functioning. Beginning in childhood, the different aspects of attention become more differentiated, as examined by Brodeur, Trick, and Enns (Chapter 4). Therefore, it is necessary to look at individual components of attention since there may be considerable differences among groups with regard to specific areas of developmental delay and deviance.

The value of infant attention as a predictor of later functioning applies to several different types of populations. Mayes and Bornstein (Chapter 5) study attention as an indicator of underlying neurological and cognitive deficits that are thought to be the sequelae of pre- and perinatal occurrences that predispose the infant to risk (substance-abusing mothers and premature birth). Also interested in at-risk children, Coldren and Corradetti (Chapter 7) attempt to identify infants that are most likely to develop attention-deficit/hyperactivity disorder (ADHD). For both groups, indices of early functioning should help practitioners identify children that need to be targeted for early intervention programs. Conversely, Zelazo and Stack (Chapter 6) study attention as one aspect of the sequelae of Down syndrome, an easily identified organic disorder associated with mental retardation. Information regarding attentional functioning in these infants provides information regarding the wide-ranging consequences of Down syndrome. In all these groups, following the development of attentional and related processes from infancy through childhood and into adolescence and adulthood allows for insight into the charting of typical development.

As with infants, attention in children is also of interest, both as an index of underlying neurological delays and deficits and in populations that are at risk in these areas due to environmental factors. Kopera-Frye, Olson, and Streissguth (Chapter 8) argue that attentional difficulties from infancy through adolescence are manifestations of teratogenic effects of alcohol on central nervous system (CNS) dysfunction among children exposed prenatally to alcohol. The study of attention is also informative in childhood disorders, many of which are diagnosed on the basis of behavioral symptomatology. Attentional difficulties, dysfunctions, and peculiarities are central to some diagnoses (e.g., ADHD), secondary to others (e.g., autism), and only tangentially related to others (e.g., mental retardation). Pearson, Norton, and Farwell (Chapter 9) provide initial evidence of attentional functioning in persons who are diagnosed with ADHD from within a larger population that is diagnosed as mentally retarded. Thus, they specify a group of children who display severe attentional difficulties in conjunction with their impaired intellectual ability. Their work has implications for drug treatments for children who, previous to the diagnosis of ADHD, would not have been considered candidates for this type of therapy. Bryson, Landry, and Wainwright (Chapter 10) highlight the role of attentional research in understanding neurological development and specific sources of deficit among persons with autism. By merging the research on executive and attentional functioning they plot the strategies undertaken in the search to highlight the source(s) of autism.

The role of attentional deficits in the different adult groups varies considerably according to the type of disorder. In the examples of patients with brain lesions, Kingstone, Grabowecky, Mangun, Valsangkar, and Gazzaniga (Chapter 11) demonstrate the unique problems experienced by persons as a function of damage to specific parts of the brain. By studying various lesion sites and split-brain patients, researchers are able to identify brain sites that are integral to both functional and dysfunctional attentional processes. The issue of identifying neural sources of attention is further highlighted by Greenwood and Parasuraman (Chapter 12) in their analysis of attention in aging persons and those with Alzheimer's disease. They examine attentional deficits in relation to brain changes that occur in normal aging and with the onset of Alzheimer's.

The other general grouping of adults include those with psychiatric disorders that are based on behavioral diagnoses, such as schizophrenia, depression, anxiety, and psychopathy. Schizophrenia, depression, and anxiety disorders are primary adult psychiatric problems in the DSM-IV (American Psychiatric Association, 1994). Although there is considerable variation among individuals within each of these disorders with regard to levels of functioning and developmental course and outcome of the disorders, faulty attentional processing is identified and implicated as central to all of these disorders. Steffy and Oakman (Chapter 13) review clinical signs, empirical evidence, and theoretical models of attentional anomalies that are related to the atypical development and behaviors of persons with schizophrenia. Gotlib and MacLeod (Chapter 14) assess the relative impact of different aspects of information processing in the development of depression as compared to that of anxiety disorders. They argue that depressive disorders are characterized by biases in memory functioning whereas the anxiety disorders are characterized by attentional deficits.

Psychopathy is not included in DSM-IV, as there is considerable disagreement regarding specific diagnostic criteria. Although research efforts are limited by diagnostic inconsistencies, Kosson and Harpur (Chapter 15) identify attentional and related cognitive and neurological characteristics that appear common to groups of persons with psychopathy. They demonstrate links between unsocialized aggressive conduct, adolescent psychopathy, and adult psychopathy that are indicative of identifiable developmental progressions of attention/cognition.

Finally, we acknowledge that one of the least developed of the bridges represented in this book is that between attention in psychopathological populations and typical populations. The chapters found here focus primarily on the bridges between attention and psychopathology and between attention and development. With the exception of the chapter by Kingstone et al., who examine the effects of pathology that is largely environmental in nature (e.g., brain lesions and surgery), there is almost no emphasis given to the insight that abnormal attentional functioning may provide for attentional functioning in typical individuals. It is our long-term hope that such a bridge may yet emerge, perhaps sparked in part by some subset of the rich range of ideas presented in this book.

ACKNOWLEDGMENTS

Work on this chapter was supported by a Social Sciences and Humanities Research Council New Researcher Grant awarded to Jake Burack and to a Natural Sciences and Engineering Research Council (Canada) Operating Grant to Jim Enns. We thank Beth Randolph for her comments on various drafts and Julie Brennan for her help in transmitting the drafts between the authors, editing, and preparing of the final manuscript.

REFERENCES

American Psychiatric Association. (1994). *Diagnostic and statistical manual of mental disorders* (4th ed.). Washington, DC: Authors.

Birren, J. E. (1965). Age changes in speed of behavior: Its central nature and physiological correlates. In A. T. Welford & J. E. Birren (Eds.), *Behavior, aging and the nervous system* (pp. 191–216). Springfield, IL: Charles C Thomas.

Broadbent, D. E. (1958). *Perception and communication.* London: Pergamon.

Bronfenbrenner, U. (1979). *The ecology of human development.* Cambridge, MA: Harvard University Press.

Bronfenbrenner, U., Kessel, F., Kessen, W., & White, S. (1986). Toward a critical social history of developmental psychology. *American Psychologist, 41,* 1218–1230.

Burack, J. A. (1992). Debate and argument: Clarifying developmental issues in the study of autism. *Journal of Child Psychology and Psychiatry, 33,* 617–622.

Burack, J. A., Hodapp, R. M., & Zigler, E. (1988). Issues in the classification of mental retardation: Differentiating among organic etiologies. *Journal of Child Psychology and Psychiatry, 29,* 765–779.

Case, R. (1992). Neo-Piagetian theories of intellectual development. In H. Beilin & P. B. Pufall (Eds.), *Piaget's theory: Prospects and possibilities* (pp. 61–104). Hillsdale, NJ: Erlbaum.

Cerella, J. (1990). Aging and information processing rate. In J. E. Birren & K. W. Schaie (Eds.), *Handbook of the psychology of aging* (3rd ed., pp. 201–221). New York: Academic Press.

Chapman, L. J., & Chapman, J. P. (1973). *Disordered thoughts in schizophrenia.* New York: Appleton-Century-Crofts.

Cicchetti, D. (1984). The emergence of developmental psychopathology. *Child Development, 55*(1), 1–6.

Cicchetti, D. (1989a). Developmental psychopathology: Some thoughts on its evolution. *Development and Psychopathology, 1*(1), 1–4.

Cicchetti, D. (Ed.). (1989b). *The emergence of a discipline: Rochester Symposium on Developmental Psychopathology.* Hillsdale, NJ: Erlbaum.

Cicchetti, D., & Wagner, S. (1990). Alternative assessment strategies for the evaluation of infants and toddlers: An organizational perspective. In S. J. Meisels & J. P. Shonkoff (Eds.), *Handbook of early childhood intervention* (pp. 246–277). New York: Cambridge University Press.

Douglas, V. I., & Peters, K. G. (1979). Towards a clearer definition of attention deficit of hyperactive children. In G. A. Hale & M. Lewis (Eds.), *Attention and cognitive development*. New York: Plenum Press.

Enns, J. T. (1990). Relations between components of attention. In J. T. Enns (Ed.), *The development of attention: Research and theory* (pp. 139–158). Amsterdam: Elsevier.

Fischer, K. (1980). A theory of cognitive development: The control and construction of a hierarchy of skills. *Psychological Review, 87,* 477–531.

Frith, U., & Baron-Cohen, S. (1987). Perception in autistic children. In D. J. Cohen & A. Donnelan (Eds.), *Handbook of autism and pervasive developmental disorders* (pp. 85–102). Silver Spring, MD: Winston.

Frye, D. (1991). The end of development. In F. S. Kessel, M. H. Bornstein, & A. J. Sameroff (Eds.), *Contemporary constructions of the child: Essays in honor of William Kessen* (pp. 265–278). Hillsdale, NJ: Erlbaum.

Garner, W. R. (1962). *Uncertainty and structure as psychological concepts*. New York: Wiley.

Garner, W. R. (1974). *The processing of information and structure*. Potomac, MD: Erlbaum.

Gibson, E. J. (1969). *Principles of perceptual learning and development*. New York: Appleton-Century-Croft.

Gibson, E. J. (1977). How perception really develops: A view from outside the network. In D. LaBerge & S. J. Samuels (Eds.), *Basic processes in reading: Perception and comprehension* (pp. 155–173). Hillsdale, NJ: Erlbaum.

Gibson, J. J. (1966). *The senses considered as perceptual systems*. Boston: Houghton Mifflin.

Hale, G. A., & Lewis, M. (Eds.). (1979). *Attention and cognitive development*. New York: Plenum Press.

Hebb, D. O. (1949). *The organization of behavior*. New York: Wiley.

Hebb, D. O. (1966). *A textbook of psychology*. Philadelphia: Saunders.

Hodapp, R. M., & Burack, J. A. (1990). What mental retardation teaches us about typical development: The examples of sequences, rates, and cross-domain relations. *Development and Psychopathology, 2,* 213–225.

Iarocci, G., & Burack, J. A. (in press). Understanding the development of selective attention in persons with mental retardation: Challenging the myths. In J. A. Burack, R. M. Hodapp, & E. Zigler (Eds.), *Handbook of mental retardation and development*. New York: Cambridge University Press.

Inhelder, B. (1968). *The diagnosis of reasoning in the mentally retarded*. New York: Day.

James, W. (1890). *Principles of psychology*. New York: Holt.

Kail, R. (1990). More evidence for a common, central constraint on speed of processing. In J. T. Enns (Ed.), *The development of attention: Research and theory* (pp. 159–173). Amsterdam: Elsevier.

Kaplan, B. (1967). Meditations on genesis. *Human Development, 10,* 65–87.

Kessen, W. (1984). Introduction: The end of the age of development. In R. Sternberg (Ed.), *Mechanisms of cognitive development* (pp. 1–17). San Francisco: Freeman.

Kinchla, R. A. (1980). The measurement of attention. In R. S. Nickerson (Ed.), *Attention and performance VIII* (pp. 213–238). Hillsdale, NJ: Erlbaum.

Kinchla, R. A. (1992). Attention. *Annual Review of Psychology, 43,* 711–742.

Lockhead, G. R., & Pomerantz, J. R. (1991). *The perception of structure.* Washington, DC: American Psychological Association.

Marr, D. (1982). *Vision.* San Francisco: Freeman.

Melnyk, L., & Das, J. P. (1992). Measurement of attention deficit: Correspondence between rating scales and tests of sustained and selective attention. *American Journal of Mental Retardation, 96*(6), 599–606.

Pachella, R. G. (1974). The interpretation of reaction time in information processing research. In B. H. Kantowitz (Ed.), *Human information processing: Tutorials in performance and cognition* (pp. 41–82). Hillsdale, NJ: Erlbaum.

Parasuraman, R., & Davies, D. R. (1984). *Varieties of attention.* New York: Academic Press.

Plude, D. J., & Doussard-Roosevelt, J. A. (1990). Aging and attention: Selectivity, capacity, and arousal. In E. A. Lovelace (Ed.), *Cognition and aging* (pp. 97–133). Amsterdam: Elsevier.

Posner, M. I. (1980). Orienting of attention. *Quarterly Journal of Experimental Psychology, 32,* 3–25.

Posner, M. I., & Boies, S. E. (1971). Components of attention. *Psychological Review, 78,* 391–408.

Posner, M. I., & Raichle, M. E. (1994). *Images of mind.* New York: Freeman.

Reese, H., & Overton, W. (1970). Models of development and theories of development. In L. R. Goulet & P. Baltes (Eds.), *Life span developmental psychology: Research and theories* (pp. 115–145). New York: Academic Press.

Robbins, L., & Rutter, M. (1990). *Straight and devious pathways from childhood to adulthood.* Cambridge, England: Cambridge University Press.

Rolf, J., Masten, A., Cicchetti, D., Neuchterlein, K. H., & Weintraub, S. (Eds.). (1990). *Risk and protective factors in the development of psychopathology.* Cambridge, England: Cambridge University Press.

Salthouse, T. A. (1991). *Theoretical perspectives on cognitive aging.* Hillsdale, NJ: Erlbaum.

Sameroff, A. J. (1990). Neo-environmental perspectives on developmental theory. In R. M. Hodapp, J. A. Burack, & E. Zigler (Eds.), *Issues in the developmental approach to mental retardation* (pp. 93–113). New York: Cambridge University Press.

Sameroff, A. J., & Chandler, M. J. (1975). Reproductive risk and the continuum of caretaking casualty. In F. D. Horowitz (Ed.), *Review of child development research* (pp. 187–244).

Sroufe, L. A., & Rutter, M. (1984). The domain of developmental psychopathology. *Child Development, 55,* 17–29.

Treisman, A. (1988). Features and objects: The fourteenth Bartlett memorial lecture. *Quarterly Journal of Experimental Psychology, 40A,* 201–237.

Treisman, A., & Gelade, G. (1980). A feature integration theory of attention. *Cognitive Psychology, 12,* 97–136.

Treisman, A., & Sato, S. (1990). Conjunction search revisited. *Journal of Experimental Psychology: Human Perception and Performance, 16,* 459–478.

Ullman, S. (1984). Visual routines. *Cognition, 18,* 97–159.

Wagner, S., Ganiban, J. M., & Cicchetti, D. (1990). Attention, memory, and perception in infants with Down syndrome: A review and commentary. In

D. Cicchetti & M. Beeghly (Eds.), *Children with Down syndrome: A developmental perspective* (pp. 147–179). New York: Cambridge University Press.

Welford, A. T. (1965). Performance, biological mechanisms and age: A theoretical sketch. In A. T. Welford & J. E. Birren (Eds.), *Behavior, aging and the nervous system* (pp. 3–20). Springfield, IL: Charles C Thomas.

Werner, H. (1948). *Comparative psychology of mental development.* New York: International Universities Press.

Werner, H. (1957). The concept of development from a comparative and organismic point of view. In D. B. Harris (Ed.), *The concept of development* (pp. 125–148). Minneapolis: University of Minnesota Press.

Wickelgren, W. A. (1977). Speed–accuracy tradeoff and information processing dynamics. *Acta Psychologica, 41,* 67–85.

Wittgenstein, L. (1953). *Philosophical investigations* (G. E. M. Anscombe, Trans.). New York: Macmillan.

Yule, W. (1978). Research methodology: What are the "correct controls?" In M. Rutter & E. Schopler (Eds.), *Autism: A reappraisal of concepts and treatments* (pp. 155–162). New York: Plenum Press.

Zigler, E., & Glick, M. (1986). *A developmental approach to adult psychopathology.* New York: Wiley.

SECTION II

DEVELOPMENT OF ATTENTION ACROSS THE LIFESPAN

T W O

Development of Visual Attention

Janette Atkinson
Bruce Hood

I n everyday vision we normally look directly at objects to which
we are attending. This is called "foveation" or "fixation"—we
image the object on the center of the retina. The underlying
mechanisms that allow us to select a particular part of the visual
array for scrutiny are usually referred to as those of "selective attention."
Shifts of attention often coincide with eye movements; these eye movements either can occur as a response to the sudden appearance of a visual
target or may be driven by an internal searching process. The former is
said to be under *exogenous* control, whereas the latter is under *endogenous*
control. Saccades under exogenous control are called "reflexive," largely
because they cannot easily be inhibited and have very short latencies. Saccades under endogenous control are said to be "intentional" or "voluntary" and in general have longer latencies than reflexive saccades do. Adults
switch between endogenous and exogenous modes depending upon the
particular stimulus conditions.

Many paradigms and approaches to the study of the development of
attention have been put forward over the last 25 years. Because the field
is so vast this short chapter will of necessity be a little ideosyncratic, considering some areas more fully than others. In addition to studies of normal development, several recent studies on abnormal development of
attention will also be included. The paradigms used to gauge development
of attention discussed in this chapter are as follows:

1. Measures of changes in saccadic eye movements used to select an
   object for scrutiny in visual orienting
2. Measures of changes in spontaneous eye movements in scanning
   visual patterns

3. Measures of changes in the length of repeated fixations in visual habituation studies
4. Measures of changes in focusing accuracy or accommodation to targets at different distances

However, before we discuss these paradigms, a brief outline of current neurobiological theories of infant development, including attentional development will be considered. These models will then be used in discussing some of the developmental results.

CURRENT NEUROBIOLOGICAL MODELS
OF VISUAL DEVELOPMENT

Many recent theories of visual development are based on the idea of two visual systems: the subcortical systems define crudely "where" an object is located, while cortical mechanisms define "what" is being scrutinized. Bronson (1974) suggested that newborn vision is totally subcortically controlled, with the cortex maturing at around 2 months postnatally. One of us (Atkinson, 1984) put forward a modified model in which the newborn visual system is *largely* subcortically controlled, with a sequence of specific cortical streams starting to function at different times postnatally. For example, those subserving stereoscopic discriminations do not start to operate until around 4 months postnatally. There is elaborate interaction between the infant's developing sensitivity to certain pattern parameters and maturation of eye movement and attentional systems. Based on studies in our laboratory of saccadic shifts to fixate peripherally presented salient visual targets, we have suggested that increasing ability with age to make these attentional shifts might reflect a changeover from subcortical to cortical control (Atkinson, 1984; Braddick & Atkinson, 1988). Johnson's (1990) model reiterates the subcortical–cortical transition in attentional development and suggests that changes in oculomotor behavior reflect progressive maturation of layers within the primary visual cortex. His idea is that as there is some evidence that the visual cortex matures in a serial fashion, with the deeper layers maturing before more superficial ones; this developmental sequence may allow certain cortical circuits to become functional before others.

Two related models of adult vision have influenced these theoretical ideas on infant development. The first model of the adult visual system is based largely on primate studies, which have dissociated a "where" and a "what" system *within* the cortical pathways. Zeki (1973, 1977; Zeki & Shipp, 1988) and his coworkers first defined an area selective for motion information (V5 or MT) and a color-specific area (V4). Ungerleider and Mishkin (1982) suggested that the two streams are associated with different visual capacities: a largely parietal module is involved in localizing objects within a spatial array, while the temporal lobe contains mechanisms tuned to "what" aspects such as form and color. Clinical observations of patients with specific focal lesions have shown a dissociation between loss of position or movement perception and deficits of object recognition (e.g., Damasio & Benton, 1979; Zihl, von Cramon, & Mai, 1983).

The second model of the adult system arises out of the first and is based the idea of parvocellular and magnocellular streams. The two streams are distinct at ganglion cell and lateral geniculate nucleus levels and project to different parts of primary visual cortex, V1, and continue within independent cortical streams to V4 and V5 (Livingstone & Hubel, 1988; Van Essen & Maunsell, 1983; Maunsell & Newsome, 1987). The parvocellular-based system is thought to subserve detailed form vision and color whereas the magnocellular system subserves movement perception and some aspects of stereoscopic vision. Comparisons have been made between psychophysical data on adults and the functioning of the parvo-based and magno-based pathways. Similar comparisons have been made in modeling the development of vision in human infants over the first 6 months postnatally, to delineate the developmental time course of various cortical streams, each subserving different aspects of spatial vision (Atkinson, 1992).

Several different cortical and subcortical circuits have been proposed for controlling saccadic eye movements of adult humans and primates (Schiller, Malpeli, & Schein, 1979; Schiller, 1985), but as yet there is very little known about the development of these systems in the human infant. Schiller has suggested that in the adult primate brain the cortical pathway controlling saccades projects directly to a number of striate and extrastriate visual areas as well as indirectly to areas in the temporal lobe, parietal lobes, and frontal eye fields. The subcortical pathway projects to the superior colliculus in the brainstem, which then project to the saccadic mechanisms. This pathway only conveys information about the location and brightness of objects and would therefore be suitable for use in simple orienting responses or reflexive saccades. The cortical pathways convey much more detailed pattern information and may therefore be the pathway responsible for goal-directed or voluntary saccades.

In addition to these excitatory channels, in Schiller's model the superior colliculus is inhibited by certain cortical areas via the basal ganglia and substantia nigra (see Hikosaka & Wurtz, 1983a, 1983b, 1983c, 1983d). The purpose of this inhibitory pathway is to keep the system clamped down by inhibition to prevent stimulus-bound eye movements. Using Schiller's model, Johnson has suggested that much of the newborn infant's oculomotor behavior is controlled by a functioning subcortical pathway operating without the influence of the cortical inhibitory pathway, as this is mediated via cortical layers that are late to mature (Johnson, 1990).

In general these models of differential developmental functioning of subcortical and cortical pathways are used to explain many of the findings on attentional saccadic shifts made by infants at different stages of development. Less detailed links between physiology, neuroanatomy, and behavior can be made when other infant paradigms are considered as discussed below.

MEASURES OF CHANGES IN SACCADIC EYE MOVEMENTS USED TO SELECT AN OBJECT FOR SCRUTINY IN VISUAL ORIENTING

One approach to attention is to consider it a mechanism that enables "selection for action," the action being either a saccade to fixate the object or a direct motor movement such as a reach toward the object of interest. Such motor acts have been taken as indicators of a shift of *overt* attention, in contrast to *covert* attention when we attend to certain parts of the visual array without fixating or foveating the object of interest. Allport's (1989) theory of overt selective attention proposes that this mechanism has evolved to enable the organism to prepare to engage in a pattern of motor actions selected from a range of potential actions, which may compete for the same underlying or limited resource (Posner, 1978; Shallice, 1972). The role of the selective attentional mechanism is to select a particular set of stimulus parameters and link them to a specific action pattern, avoiding or preventing the intrusion of other stimuli.

Hence, one goal in looking at the development of selective attention is to identify changes in the properties of stimuli that are selected to drive particular motor actions. One such motor action called *visual orienting* consists of rapid conjugate saccadic eye movements in combination with head and body posture changes, to foveate and scrutinize an initially eccentric target. In adults the latency to execute a saccade in orienting is around 200 milliseconds (Schiller, 1985). But a saccade planned to the left can be replaced by one to the right, provided that the new target to the right appears not later than 50–80 milliseconds before the beginning of the first saccade (Becker & Jürgens, 1979). This suggests that much of the time involved in generating a saccade in orienting must be taken up with some process other than determining the onset and coordinates of the target. These computations are thought to reflect the activity of selective attention. Many of the studies discussed below involve attempts to measure changes in these computations for exogenously and endogenously controlled shifts. Models will be presented that assume differential development of these two control systems, each being related to different underlying neural circuitry.

Both endogenously controlled and exogenously controlled overt attentional shifts have been measured in infants by monitoring saccades made from the central field into the peripheral visual field to foveate an object of interest. The spatial limitations of foveation have been called the "extent of the visual field," and the clinical term for making such measures is called "perimetry." Changes in effective field size has been found to increase over the first year of life (e.g., van Hof-van Duin & Mohn, 1986) and in particular over the first few months. The newborn or 1-month-old's attentional field appears to be relatively limited in lateral extent to an angle somewhere between 20° to 30°, this being the visual angle of the area over which a stimulus can elicit a foveating saccade. A number of early studies have addressed this issue (e.g., Tronick, 1972; Harris & MacFarlane, 1974; MacFarlane, Harris, & Barnes, 1976, reviewed in Salapatek, 1975, pp. 179–186). The role of attentional factors at this early age is highlighted by the finding that the field appears to be restricted when a central fixation target remains visible at the time of the second target appearance (Harris & MacFarlane, 1974; Finlay & Ivinski, 1984). However, the effect of a competing central target would also seem to decrease with age. From this result, it would seem likely that as well as increased sensitivity with age, a second process is developing. This process es is needed to relinquish attention from the central target and shift attention to the peripheral target. Hence, changes in covert attention have been studied by modifying the simple foveation paradigm to include a distracting or competing stimulus ("probe" or "mask") that captures visual attention and prevents or delays saccadic shifts of attention to other targets. This "competition effect," where the most recently appearing target, has to compete with the already attended target has been extensively investigated in a series of studies in our own laboratory (Atkinson & Braddick, 1985; Braddick & Atkinson, 1988; Atkinson, Hood, Braddick, & Wattam-Bell, 1988; Hood, 1991).

The general apparent increase with age in effective field size could be in part due to increased sensitivity (acuity and contrast sensitivity) with age. In one of our studies we have attempted to dissociate the effects of improved contrast sensitivity and acuity with age, from improved ability to disengage from a central fixated target and make a saccade to a newly appearing peripheral target. The direction and latency of saccadic eye movements exogenously triggered by the onset of peripherally located visual targets were measured. The stimuli used as fixation and orienting targets were relatively large patterned patches consisting of one cycle of square wave grating (12° wide and 32° high). These patches phase-reversed at 6 hertz and could appear in the left or right visual field (the inner edge being at 23° eccentricity). The mean luminance of these targets was matched to the background. The contrast of the grating could be adjusted either up or down to make the target more or less visible. In addition to peripheral targets, there was also a central target that acted as a fixation stimulus prior to the onset of the peripheral target and also as a competition stimulus when presented in addition to a peripheral target. The observer, who was unaware of the location of the peripheral target, recorded the direction and time of the first horizontal saccade using a hand-operated switch to give an estimate of the saccadic latency. By use of a psychophysical staircase procedure, it was estimated that the average threshold contrast that would reliably produce orienting eye movements to a single peripheral target was 35% for the 1-month-olds and 16% for 3-month-olds. Below these thresholds, infants would not refixate the targets above chance.

The effect of competition from a second identical target in central vision on the detection rate and latency to refixate a peripheral target was examined using the thresholds estimated for a noncompetition target. Noncompetition and competition conditions were examined in the same infants. In terms of correct latencies, 1-month-olds averaged 1.62 seconds (SD = 1.48 seconds) in the noncompetition condition and 3.89 seconds (SD = 1.82 seconds) in the competition condition. Latencies for 3-month-olds were 1.26 seconds (SD = 5.6 seconds) for the noncompetition condition and 1.91 seconds (SD = 1.58 seconds) for the competition condition. The latencies of 1-month-olds were significantly more affected by this type of competition than were those of 3-month-olds; 1-month-olds showed considerable difficulty in disengaging from the central target if it remained visible when the peripheral target appeared. However, because this study involved equating the two age groups for sensory detectability, the residual significant differences between age groups appeared to be due to an additional factor, namely, the disengage mechanism.

The general findings from this study are consistent with earlier studies (e.g., Atkinson & Braddick, 1985; Schwartz, Dobson, Sandstrom, & van Hof-van Duin, 1987) and have been replicated in one recent study of infants in this age range using rather different targets (Johnson, Posner, & Rothbart, 1991). However, in Johnson and colleagues' study no attempt was made to match the age groups on detection sensitivity, so the competition effect is likely to be due to both differences in sensitivity with age and differences in the ability to disengage. Additional conditions used in our own studies have also shown that in competition the disengage differences between 1- and 3-month-olds are also found if two peripheral targets (one on each side of fixation) simultaneously appear (Atkinson, Hood,

Wattam-Bell, & Braddick, 1992). This result further confirms the involvement of a switching mechanism to enable attention to move from one location to another, but this need not necessarily be from the fovea to the periphery; it can be between one location in the periphery to a second peripheral location.

If very young infants have difficulty in disengaging/shifting visual attention from a central stimulus, then this has implications for estimating their effective fields. This problem may also arise in clinical subjects who have suffered damage to those mechanisms that are responsible for disengagement. In one of our studies (Hood & Atkinson, 1990a) we identified a group of neurologically impaired children and tested them with the same competition/noncompetition paradigm. Some of this group showed behavior similar to the 1-month-olds in that they refixated in noncompetition but failed to refixate if the central stimulus remained visible in competition. Nevertheless some of these same children showed a significant visual evoked potential (VEP) to this peripheral target while fixating the central target. This result suggests that the sensory detection mechanism responsible for generating the VEP was operating normally while the attentional disengage processes were not.

Recently we have studied two infants who underwent complete hemispherectomy to relieve intractible focal epilepsy (Braddick et al., 1992). Study of vision in these infants provided the rare opportunity to investigate the activity of the subcortical pathway in isolation from cortical influence, allowing a direct test of the two-visual-systems theory of visual orienting, as well as the role of cortical mechanisms in the competition effect.

Magnetic resonance images of the two infants showed morphological changes consisting of absence of gyri, thickening of the cortex, and marked signal abnormality in the remaining white matter. These abnormalities were predominant in the right hemisphere for one child and in the left hemisphere for the other, indicating congenital unilateral megalencephaly. This condition is associated with intractable epilepsy, which does not respond well to drug treatment. Hemispherectomy was carried out on one child at 5 months and on the other at 8 months of age. Removal of the cortical hemisphere obliterates the cortical representation of the contralateral visual field. However, as the surgery involves the removal of tissue from above the level of the thalamus, this leaves the retinocollicular pathways intact.

Both infants were seen preoperatively and showed very poor visual behavior, with no consistent shifts of visual attention in informal testing. This was probably in part due to a combination of epilepsy and the heavy medication regime used to attempt to control their seizures. However, in postoperative testing, both children were visually alert with a full range of eye movements. Both infants had hemiparesis contralateral to the removed hemisphere but were capable of reaching across the midline when they foveated an object of interest. However, this did not occur spontaneously and each child appeared to completely ignore toys presented in the affected hemifield, although they promptly reached for the same toys in the ipsilateral "good" half-field. This behavior is consistent with a loss of visual input from the contralateral visual field. Each infant was tested on the same fixation shift procedure described for our earlier studies.

The computer controlling the experiment was interfaced with a video recorder so that an independent record of eye movements, type of condition, and the frame code for stimulus onset could be logged for analysis at a later date (described in detail in Hood, 1991). Both infants oriented to the peripheral target in either half-field in the noncompetition condition; thus both showed performance considerably above chance for orienting to a target that did not have a cortical representation. One of the infants showed shorter latencies to respond to the target in his "good" field (the right) compared to his "bad" field. For one child we tested orienting using each eye alone. She could respond above chance to both the left and right with one eye (the right eye, the left cortex having been removed). With the left eye she could only make saccades into the left half field but not to the right. This result suggests that no uncrossed pathway capable of transmitting information from the left eye to the damaged left side of the brain can elicit saccadic eye movements. Under competition conditions one child showed reduced saccadic shifts when the peripheral target appeared on his bad side, but he showed rapid shifts into his good field. He often blinked and nodded his head when the target appeared in his bad field, as though to unlock his attention from the central stimulus. The important finding from this study is to show that both infants are capable of producing saccadic eye movements to stimuli presented in the "blind" field, which would support the idea that subcortical pathways can subserve this orienting under noncompetition conditions. The other important finding is that the child tested monocularly could not initiate a saccade in a nasal-ward direction with the left eye. These findings are consistent with studies of monocular target detection in infants demonstrating that infants younger than 2 months are much more likely to detect and make an eye movement to a visual target presented in their temporal visual field compared to their nasal visual field (Lewis, Maurer, & Blackburn, 1985; Lewis & Maurer, 1992). This asymmetry between the temporal and nasal visual fields are believed to reflect the neuroanatomic distribution of retinocollicular fibers. It has been claimed that there is very little input from the temporal retina (nasal visual field) via the direct retinocollicular pathway (Hubel, LeVay, & Wiesel, 1975; Pollack & Hickey, 1979). Instead, the temporal retina influences the superior colliculus via the geniculostriate pathway and, as this pathway may not be mature in young infants, this accounts for their temporal field bias. Given that this pathway is absent in the hemispherectomized child for stimuli presented in the nasal field of the left eye, this would explain the results of the monocular study. We suggest that nasal-ward as opposed to temporal-ward eye movements require cortical input. Exactly how and why the cortical areas influence these movements is not clear, and of course it is always possible that the routing of these pathways is abnormal in these infants compared to normal development.

Adult hemispherectomized patients maintain the ability to make visual discriminations using a forced choice paradigm in the hemianopic visual field, although they do not experience any conscious appraisal of the stimuli in the so-called blind field (Perenin, 1978; Perenin & Jeannerod, 1978; Ptito, Lassonde, Leporé, & Ptito, 1987). It seems that this "blindsight" (Pöppel, Held, & Frost, 1973; Weiskrantz, 1986) may provide some information, albeit unconscious, to guide the orienting system.

A number of researchers measuring adult eye movements have also demonstrated that the presence of a foveal stimulus overlapping in time with the onset of a peripheral target inhibits saccades (e.g., Fischer, 1986). However, if a temporal gap is introduced between the offset of a central stimulus and the onset of a peripheral target, saccadic latencies are substantially shorter than in conditions in which there is an overlap in time with the center stimulus (e.g., Saslow, 1967). The disappearance of the object during the temporal gap is thought to produce an automatic disengagement of attention, thereby bypassing one of the computational processes that contribute to the latency (Posner & Petersen, 1990; Fischer, 1986).

As different subcortical and cortical modules are in differential states of maturation early in life, it seems likely that different properties of the disengage and engage processes might be discernible by use of different paradigms that vary the temporal parameters between one stimulus for fixation and another. In particular, the gap paradigm should produce the shortest latencies compared to the overlap condition from the earliest age, as the retinocollicular pathway, thought to subserve rapid saccades, is relatively mature compared to cortical structures in the newborn. However, the overlap paradigm should produce the longest latencies in younger infants compared to older ones, as the structures responsible for disengaging attention are predominantly extrastriate cortical areas that continue to develop over at least the first year of life. We (Hood, 1991; Hood & Atkinson, 1991a, 1991b) have carried out extensive tests of infants between 6 weeks and 6 months of age, varying the gap interval between the disappearance of the central target and appearance of the peripheral target, including an overlap condition when the central target remained on for 2 seconds following the onset of the peripheral target; 6-week-olds showed slower responses (longer latencies) on all conditions than those of older infants. All age groups showed longer latencies for the overlap condition, with the effect of overlapping being greatest for the youngest infants. In general the "gap" condition produced the shortest latencies for all infants. We also found similar results for adults, although adults overall were faster.

The data presented so far have been concerned with overt shifts of visual attention (saccadic) that are triggered by exogenous events (peripheral targets). Although visual attention and direction of gaze often coincide, this is not necessarily the case. The phenomenon of covert attention has been studied extensively by M. I. Posner and his colleagues, where detection of a target is facilitated by informative cues (an arrow pointing in the direction of the ensuing target) before the event. If subjects are precued to the spatial location of an impending visual target, their reaction times to that target are shorter relative to reaction times to targets appearing at other spatial locations. This can be achieved in the absence of eye movements during the cuing phase and has led Posner to describe attention as a spotlight that can move independently of eye movements to a spatial location, facilitating all information processing of stimuli that appear within this spotlighted are. This *facilitation* is reflected in various manual reaction time tasks (Maylor, 1985; Posner & Cohen, 1980) and in the latency to make a subsequent saccadic eye movement toward the target (Posner, Rafal, Choate, & Vaughan, 1985). Symbolic cues can be used such as arrows presented at the point of fixation or peripheral cues such as a change in luminance at one of the target locations.

According to the Posner model (Posner, Inhoff, Friedrich, & Cohen, 1987), the act of shifting attention to a peripheral cue is achieved by a sequence of partially overlapping yet separate mental operations. First, the cue produces a general alerting state that interrupts ongoing activity, is not spatially selective, and works to potentiate all targets following the cue. The coordinates of the cue are then fed into the orienting system prior to the shift of attention. The shift of attention is achieved by first disengaging from the current task, next moving the spotlight, and then engaging attention at the new spatial location. However, if the spotlight of attention moves back to the direction of gaze or to another location, processing of subsequent stimuli appearing at the cued location is inhibited relative to targets appearing at other spatial locations. This effect has been termed "inhibition of return" (IOR) and is thought to last for about 2 seconds following the shift of attention away from the cued location (Posner & Cohen, 1980). The IOR effect is believed to reflect an evolutionary adaptive mechanism that biases an organism against returning attention to a spatial location already processed so that preferential attention is given to information presented at novel locations. According to the Posner model, with short stimulus onset asynchronies (SOAs) peripheral cues initially produce facilitation; however, with longer SOAs the spotlight of attention moves away from the cued location producing subsequent inhibition at that location.

Posner and Petersen (1990) have proposed that a number of different neural structures underlie shifts of attention and, in particular, that orienting attention in space is mediated by the posterior attention system (the posterior parietal cortex, associated thalamic areas of the pulvinar, reticular nucleus, and superior colliculus). Specifically, several lines of evidence indicate that the superior colliculus plays a major role in the IOR phenomenon. Progressive supranuclear palsy, which causes damage to the superior colliculus, has been found to interfere with the IOR effect (Posner et al., 1985). Secondly, under monocular viewing, an asymmetry of the IOR effect has been demonstrated with stimuli presented in the nasal compared to the temporal hemifield, and this is believed to reflect the temporal-nasal asymmetry of retinal projections to the superior colliculus (Rafal, Calabresi, Brennan, & Sciolto, 1989; Rafal, Henik, & Smith, 1991). Several recent studies have reported that IOR develops in infants after 3 months of age (Hood & Atkinson, 1990a, 1990b, 1991a, 1991b; Clohessy, Posner, Rothbart, & Vecera, 1991; Johnson & Tucker, 1993). Clohessy et al. (1991) looked at overt shifts of attention in which the infants make head and eye movements to the peripheral locations. In their paradigm, the infant oriented to a single peripheral target followed by a return of attention to the center. To test for IOR, the infant was then presented with two targets bilaterally and any bias in orienting noted (i.e., to the cued or noncued side). Typically, infants older than 6 months oriented to the target at the new location rather than returning to the side in the unilateral trial, whereas 3-month-olds did not show a significant bias.

We (Hood & Atkinson, 1990a, 1990b, 1991a, 1991b) tested with both short and long SOAs in 3- and 6-month-olds and in a group of adults. The idea was to attempt to measure both facilitation and inhibition of return according to the Posner model. Typically, covert shifts of attention are achieved by instructing subjects to fixate a central point while visual cues and targets are presented in the periphery. However, as infants do not understand instructions, they might direct their eye movements toward the cue and not the target. Therefore, to produce covert shifts of attention and prevent overt orienting to the cue, the competition effect was exploited, namely, that high contrast stimuli in foveal vision inhibit refixations to peripheral targets. Four cue conditions were tested. In the short SOA condition, the cue appeared for 100 milliseconds and was immediately followed by the offset of the central stimulus and the onset of a peripheral target, either at the same spatial location as the cue or on the opposite side. In the long SOA condition, the cue appeared for

100 milliseconds, followed by a 500-millisecond gap in which the central stimulus remained visible. After this SOA of 600 milliseconds, the central stimulus disappeared and a peripheral target appeared at either the same or opposite location to the cue. There was no significant evidence of facilitation or IOR in the 3-month-olds. However, the 6-month-olds showed both a facilitation and an IOR effect as predicted. The adults showed no evidence of facilitation but did show an IOR effect. A similar result has been found by Johnson and Tucker (1993) using stimuli somewhat different than those in the Hood and Atkinson studies (above). Johnson and Tucker found IOR in slightly younger infants (4-month-olds rather than 6-month-olds), and no effect in 2-month-olds. Of course, it seems quite possible that the IOR effect is not an "all-or-nothing" phenomenon, becoming functional at a given age, but is rather the interplay between the relative salience of two mechanisms—one controlling facilitation and one inhibition. Different stimulus parameters, such as eccentricity, may favor one mechanism rather than another, just as one combination of stimulus and temporal parameters might yield facilitation while another might yield inhibition in the same infant. Indeed, with certain stimulus parameters it may be possible to demonstrate IOR at any age, and a recent publication by Valenza and his colleagues has suggested that IOR can be demonstrated in healthy newborns (Valenza, Simion, & Umilta, in press).

In conclusion, from all these studies of attentional shifts, we have suggested that, by analogy with adult modeling, the change in attentional control between 1 and 3 months of age is likely to be related to the onset of function at around 3 months of attentional mechanisms involving superior colliculus, striate and extrastriate connections. The 1-month-old's behavior is usually largely under subcortical control (Atkinson & Braddick, 1985; Braddick & Atkinson, 1988), although there may be certain limited conditions where cortical functioning can be demonstrated. The inability of 1-month-olds to shift fixation to a peripheral target if a central target is already fixated is very similar to what is called "sticky fixation" in a neurological condition called Balint syndrome. The patient does not suffer from "neglect" or optic apraxia but rather lacks the coordination of mechanisms controlling saccadic eye movements and selective attention to provide accurate spatial localizing. Balint syndrome involves bilateral lesions in parieto-occipital areas but may also involve the circuitry between the superior colliculus and parietal lobes for controlling shifts of attention (see the review by De Renzi, 1982). Very similar behavior to that of patients with Balint syndrome has been seen in primates with bilateral parietal damage (Mountcastle, 1978). Schiller (1985) has reported similar deficits with damage to the superior colliculus and frontal eye fields. Again, the evidence for development of cortical streams lends support to the idea that crude localizing of single targets can be carried out by sub-

cortical collicular mechanisms, whereas more elaborate selective processes to shift attention from one object to another require executive control
from the striate and extrastriate cortex. These latter networks are also
likely to involve the functioning of the pulvinar for linking subcortical and
cortical areas.

CHANGES IN THE PATTERN
OF SCANNING EYE MOVEMENTS WITH AGE

Inferences about development of attention have been made by investigators monitoring changes in eye scanning patterns, varying age and the type
of stimulus used. A number of studies have reported changes in spontaneous eye scanning patterns with age (Maurer & Salapatek, 1976; Bronson, 1990; Hainline 1993). Bronson has claimed that newborns in the
first 6 weeks of life make many unguided scanning movements, that is,
the eye movements are often unrelated to the stimulus parameters, with
long periods when a single target is fixated. Older infants scan between
the features of targets in static displays and make more accurate target-
elicited saccades than newborns. Bronson has also claimed that if the target is dynamic or flickering, the amount of scanning between features is
reduced; the infant tends to fixate a single flickering target for relatively
long periods of time in a manner similar to the scanning patterns of newborns. From these results Bronson (1990) proposed an older system phylo-
genically, the subcortex, for flickering stimuli and a cortical mechanism
that can inhibit eye movement control by the older system to allow targets to be selected for attention. Hainline (1993) found no consistent
changes in scanning patterns either in type or latency in the first 3 months
of life and suggested that many of the earlier findings were related to
posture and "state." If newborns were in a somewhat more drowsy state
for much of the time compared to 3-month-olds, then they might show
reduced eye scanning patterns in spontaneous looking.

   Of course another significant factor affecting attention in the first few
weeks of life may be the infant's level of arousal, and this has been measured by Richards and his colleagues (see Casey & Richards, 1988;
Richards, 1985, 1987, 1989). Measuring heart rate they demonstrated
several distinct phases of physiological reaction to the presentation of a
novel stimulus. One phase has been called "reactive" attention and the
other "sustained." Reactive attention is the physiological orienting response
that coincides with stimulus onset and is marked by initial acceleration
of heart rate. Sustained attention begins after the orienting response and
is characterised by lowered heart rate.

   This change in physiological state is believed to facilitate information processing by inhibiting ongoing behavior and allowing attention to be focused. As information is taken in about the stimulus, the heart rate returns to its prestimulus level. If a second visual stimulus is introduced when the heart rate has returned to prestimulus levels, fixation shifts to this target are significantly faster compared to trials when the second stimulus is introduced during the sustained attention phase. As infants grow older they can maintain longer periods of sustained attention, allowing a more detailed and thorough analysis of information input. Although these studies have demonstrated a correlation between levels of arousal and shifts of visual attention, it is unlikely that these physiological changes alone account for the age differences in shifts of visual attention to a second visual target. In a study of infants between 3 and 6 months of age, Richards (1989) found, like many other researchers, that the older infants took less time to refixate toward a peripheral target. However, these changes in rate of attentional shift with age were not paralleled by the same changes in physiological response, suggesting that either some other mechanism or an additional one, as yet unidentified, must be underpinning shifts of visual attention.

One set of interesting studies, where the results suggest a dissociation between reactive and sustained attention, are those of Foreman and his colleagues (Foreman, Flelder, Price, & Bowler, 1991). They compared full-term infants with preterm infants on their latency to turn toward checkered stimuli (reactive) and the duration of the initial fixation (sustained). Initial fixation time was found to follow a similar developmental function for both infant groups, but an acceleration of development was found for the preterm group from latency measures over the first 30 postnatal days. This result is similar to a finding from our own studies on very-low-birth weight preterm infants, who showed shorter latencies at 4–5 weeks postterm than did their postterm age-matched controls for refixating a peripheral target (Atkinson et al., 1991). Such demonstrations of independence of developmental functions for different parts of the attentional response may be taken as weak evidence of separate physiological mechanisms, but as yet the data is only suggestive.

MEASURES OF THE LENGTH
OF REPEATED FIXATIONS IN VISUAL
HABITUATION/DISHABITUATION STUDIES

In visual habituation we assume there is a direct link between scanning the visual display and attending to its content. When the infant looks away from the pattern we assume that the infant is no longer "attending" to it or processing information from it. In general the more familiar the infant becomes with a certain pattern, the less time is spent scanning it. Hence a particular time criterion (usually a very brief look) can be set when we "believe" the infant has completed processing the pattern and is "familiar" with it. Of course, this time limit is arbitrarily set depending on the age and the stimulus used, but it can be adjusted in "infant controlled habituation" where the point of habituation is related to the average fixation time of the individual infant (Horowitz, Paden, Bhana, & Self, 1972). When the child has reached the predetermined criterion for habituation, that is, there has been a certain decrease in looking time, we test for discrimination between patterns by measuring "dishabituation"—an increase in looking time when a novel pattern is displayed. In all studies where the basic measure is the duration and number of fixations, we assume a relationship with underlying attentional processes. However, this relationship is by no means simple, nor is there an accepted theoretical account. Sometimes short fixation times are regarded as an indicator of an efficient rapid attentional processor in adults and infants (e.g., in comparisons made between fast and slow infant habituators whose respective short and long inspection times have been related to later IQ scores), whereas in other circumstances individuals with short fixation times are said to have "fleeting" visual attention or "poor" attention.

The eye scanning patterns in newborns are under certain circumstances concentrated in the external contour of the pattern. If the new pattern has an identical outer contour to that of the pattern to which the infant is habituated, then we may see no dishabituation when the new pattern is displayed. This tendency to fail to discriminate patterns with identical outer contours has been called the "externality effect" (e.g., Milewski, 1976; Bushnell, 1979). The circumstances under which this effect is manifest may tell us something about the relative attentional salience of the outer and inner contours of the pattern, namely, the features of the pattern that have been selectively attended in the process of habituation. Bushnell (1979) and Girton (1979) found that the externality effect could be nulled if the inner contours were made dynamic while the outer ones stayed stationary. Once again this result is similar to those found by Bronson (1990), considered earlier in this chapter.

In a number of studies it has been claimed that infants at 1 month of age tend to scan only the external contours of the pattern whereas older infants scan both external and internal contours (Haith et al., 1977; Maurer & Salapatek, 1976). Haith and colleagues suggested that this "capturing" of attention by the outer contours is a built-in mechanism to provide maximum neural firing (the outer contour being of higher overall contrast than the inner contours by virtue of its extensive high-contrast edges). This argument could also be applied to the relatively higher salience of dynamic contours in overcoming the externality effect, in that it seems quite reasonable to assume that a flickering or moving contour will cause a higher overall rate of neuronal firing than a stationary one.

An effect possibly related to the externality effect is called "lateral masking" or "visual crowding" and has been studied in preschool children rather than infants (Atkinson, Pimm-Smith, Evans, Harding, & Braddick, 1986; Atkinson, Anker, Evans, & McIntyre, 1987; Atkinson, Anker, Hall, & Pimm-Smith, 1988; Anker, Atkinson, & McIntyre, 1989; Atkinson, 1991, 1993). In a typical "crowded" display a single letter has a ring of different letters surrounding it laterally and the child is asked to select and attend to the letter in the center of the display and ignore the letters surrounding it. Usually the child is asked either to name the center letter or to visually match it to one of a number of possible letters. There is a change with age in the ability of children to ignore the irrelevant surrounding stimuli and selectively attend to the central item. To measure the extent of crowding, a comparison is made between the size or contrast needed for accurate visual matching of an isolated letter compared to the minimum size of a letter when it is surrounded by other letters or patterns. This ratio is called the "crowding ratio" and varies with the stimulus parameters of both the central letter and its surround. For letter displays the minimum crowding seen in adults is also shown by 6-year-olds with younger children showing much larger crowding effects. Interestingly, some dyslexics also show marked crowding effects under certain stimulus conditions (Atkinson, 1991, 1993).

Such effects can be thought of as selective attentional problems rather than as a simple loss of visual contrast sensitivity or acuity. Selective attention must also operate in tests of embedded figures, but as yet a united theoretical account of the processing necessary for success on these tests and those in overcoming crowding effects has not been put forward in detail. All such studies to date have a minimum age restraint of around 3 years, when a child first understands the concept of "a visual match." However, some of the same selection procedures must be undertaken by younger children and infants, and new paradigms and procedures are needed so that data on crowding, embededness, and visual distractability can be compared right across the infant and preschool age range.

MEASURES OF CHANGES IN FOCUSING ACCURACY OR ACCOMMODATION TO TARGETS ATTENDED

In general when adults attend to an object they not only foveate it, they also adjust their accommodation or focusing power to bring the image into sharp focus. This is brought about by adjusting the ciliary muscles to alter the curvature of the lens. In our laboratory we have developed a relatively novel indirect method for measuring shifts of attention by determining the accuracy of shifts of focus in infants of different ages. Again, a parallelism between attention and focusing accuracy is assumed in infants by analogy with adult data. In an early study of changes in accommodation with age (Braddick, Atkinson, French, & Howland, 1979) we found that even newborn infants will shift their focus in the appropriate direction for a target a short distance away from their eyes (up to around 75 centimeters), compared to a greater distance. However, only approximately 50% of newborns consistently accommodated out to 75 centimeters when tested on three to five separate occasions. By 3 months of age, nearly all infants accommodate consistently over near distances, and by 6 months of age infants accommodate over a greater range of target distances (out to around 150 centimeters). Calculations in which we have estimated whether their limited acuity and contrast sensitivity might account for their poor focusing ability, as well as measures of their accommodative range in the musculature, suggest that neither of these factors account for the improvements in accommodation with age. Similar results have been found by Banks (1980a, 1980b). By analogy to measures of the lateral visual field mentioned above, we can consider the idea of an "effective visual attentional field," measured on the midline in terms of target distance for accurate accommodation. From these measures of accommodation, it seems that this attentional field also increases with age and may be subject to the same attentional constraints as those affecting the extent of the lateral visual field.

In a number of studies of children with neurological deficits we have found that many show poor shifts of accommodation for targets at different distances (Atkinson & van Hof-van Duin, 1993). These children also show inability to make saccadic shifts to peripherally located targets and so show reduced lateral visual fields, particularly in competition conditions when both a foveal target and a peripheral target are presented together.

Once again, a parallel between changes in attentional control and changes in the accuracy of another system have been made, although our understanding of the underlying synergies between attention and accommodation are not complete even in the adult system (for reviews see Judge & Miles, 1981; Judge, 1990).

GENERAL CONCLUSIONS

Shifting visual attention can been conceptualized as a selection-for-action mechanism that enables the organism to select, prepare, and engage in a coherent motor activity, one taken from a range of potential actions. The role of this selective mechanism is to avoid interference between competing stimulus events so that perception, cognition, and action can be smooth and coordinated. This idea applies to both overt and covert shifts of visual attention. This selection-for-action principle has been demonstrated in this chapter in many paradigms concerning the saccadic eye movement system used to align an object or area of interest with the fovea for maximal visual processing. However, there are several constraints on such a system. First, when there are a number of potentially competing actions, there must be some form of priority assignment based on either internal states or relative salience of the competing stimuli. The salience of an event or stimulus in capturing attention depends on the stimulus parameters such as contrast, color, and size, whether it is dynamic or static and whether it is close in position or time to other stimulus events.

The main change in attentional control in infants would seem to be twofold. First, there are improvements in acuity and contrast sensitivity that change the relative salience of competing stimuli. Secondly, there is a development in the ability of the infant to shift its gaze between visual targets as well as to relinquish fixation from a central stimulus to refixate a peripheral target. This inability to disengage fixation may reflect the operations of the subcortical orienting system functioning without executive control from the cortex. Subcortical orienting has been demonstrated in both children with cortical damage and in children lacking an entire cerebral hemisphere. The role of the cortical orienting system is to inhibit the subcortical system so that saccades can be directed to other visual targets. The selection-for-action model is a perceptual motor theory holding that these different response patterns may be mediated by different mechanisms that have evolved to allow the organism to act appropriately under different circumstances. One question that arises is why in human development these interactions between cortical and subcortical mechanisms should start to develop so early in life, around 3 months of age, when all other motor control systems such as prehension and locomotion are so immature. It is possible that the head and saccadic eye movement control systems become functional early in development as a precursor of these more elaborate motor systems and that in some way these early systems set the learning rules for further coordination of motor systems.

Certainly, in terms of development of attention, the executive systems controlling shifts that start to function in the first few months of life continue to develop for a number of years. We still see changes in the ability to concentrate on and attend to certain parts of the visual array between 3 and 6 years of age, when the child is using the visual crowding paradigms discussed above. There are likely to be even later changes in attention after the age of 6 years to bring the child up to adult maturity.

Other paradigms discussed above—those looking at visual habituation and changing focus for different target distances—clearly have an attentional component to the changes that we see with age and between different infants of the same age. Remaining tasks for future research are to dissociate changes in sensitivity with age from changes in the various attentional control mechanisms and to link such changes to underlying neurophysiological modules in these diverse experimental paradigms. We are starting to answer these questions, combining information from multiple neuroscientific approaches. Hopefully, with the advent of new techniques and with new studies using older, well-tested methods, we will be able to link together the various paradigms to give a full account of the development of attention.

ACKNOWLEDGMENT

This research was supported by the Medical Research Council, UK.

REFERENCES

Allport, A. (1989). Visual attention. In M. I. Posner (Ed.), *Foundations of cognitive science*. Cambridge, MA: MIT Press.

Anker, S., Atkinson, J., & MacIntyre, A. M. (1989). The use of the Cambridge Crowding Cards in preschool vision screening programmes, ophthalmic clinics and assessment of children with multiple disabilities. *Ophthalmic and Physiological Optics, 9*(4), 470.

Atkinson, J. (1984). Human visual development over the first six months of life: A review and a hypothesis. *Human Neurobiology, 3,* 61–74.

Atkinson, J. (1991). Review of human visual development: Crowding and dyslexia. In J. F. Stein (Ed.), *Vision and visual dysfunction: Vol. 13. Vision and visual dyslexia*. New York: Macmillan.

Atkinson, J. (1992). Early visual development: Differential functioning of parvocellular and magnocellular pathways. *Eye, 6,* 129–135.

Atkinson, J. (1993). Vision in dyslexics: Letter recognition acuity, visual crowding, contrast sensitivity, accommodation, convergence and sight reading music. In S. F. Wright & R. Groner (Eds.), *Facets of dyslexia and its remediation: Studies in visual information processing*. Amsterdam: Elsevier.

Atkinson, J., Anker, S., Evans, C., Hall, R., & Pimm-Smith, E. (1988). Visual acuity testing of young children with the Cambridge Crowding Cards at 3 and 6 metres. *Acta Ophthalmologica, 66,* 505–508.

Atkinson, J., Anker, S., Evans, C., & McIntyre, A. (1987). The Cambridge Crowding Cards for preschool visual acuity testing. In *Transactions of the 6th International Orthoptic Congress*, Harrogate, England.

Atkinson, J., & Braddick, O. J. (1985). Early development of the control of visual attention. *Perception, 14,* 25.

Atkinson, J., Braddick, O. J., Anker, S., Hood, B., Wattam-Bell, J., Weeks, F., Rennie, J., & Coughtrey, H. (1991). *Visual development in very low birth weight infants.* Paper presented at the 3rd meeting of the Child Vision Research Society, Rotterdam, The Netherlands.

Atkinson, J., Hood, B., Braddick, O. J., & Wattam-Bell, J. (1988). Infants' control of fixation shifts with single and competing targets: Mechanisms of shifting attention. *Perception, 17,* 367–368.

Atkinson, J., Hood, B., Wattam-Bell, J., & Braddick, O. J. (1992). Changes in infants' ability to switch attention in the first three months of life. *Perception, 21,* 643–653.

Atkinson, J., Pimm-Smith, E., Evans, C., Harding, G., & Braddick, O. J. (1986). Visual crowding in young children. *Documenta Ophthalmologica Proceedings Series, 45,* 201–213.

Atkinson, J., & van Hof-van Duin, J. (1993). Assessment of normal and abnormal vision during the first years of life. In A. Fielder & M. Bax (Eds.), *Management of visual handicaps in childhood.* New York: Cambridge University Press.

Banks, M. S. (1980a). Infant refraction and accommodation. *International Ophthalmology Clinics, 20,* 205–232.

Banks, M. S. (1980b). The development of visual accommodation during early infancy. *Child Development, 51,* 646–666

Becker, W., & Jürgens, R. (1979). An analysis of the saccadic system by means of double step stimuli. *Vision Research, 19,* 967–983.

Braddick, O. J., & Atkinson, J. (1988). Sensory selectivity, attentional control, and cross-channel integration in early visual development. In A. Yonas (Ed.), *Minnesota Symposia on Child Development: Vol. 20. Perceptual development in infancy.* Hillsdale, NJ: Erlbaum.

Braddick, O. J., Atkinson, J., French, J., & Howland, H. C. (1979). A photorefractive study of infant accommodation. *Vision Research, 19,* 319–330.

Braddick, O. J., Atkinson, J., Hood, B., Harkness, W., Jackson, G., & Vargha-Khadem, F. (1992). Possible blindsight in infants lacking one cerebral hemisphere. *Nature (London), 360,* 461–463.

Bronson, G. W. (1974). The postnatal growth of visual capacity. *Child Development, 45,* 873–890.

Bronson, G. W. (1990). Changes in infants visual scanning across the 2- to 14-week period. *Journal of Experimental Child Psychology, 49,* 101–125.

Bushnell, I. W. R. (1979). Modification of the externality effect in young infants. *Journal of Experimental Child Psychology, 28,* 211–229.

Cascy, B. J., & Richards, J. E. (1988). Sustained visual attention in young infants measured with an adapted version of the visual preference paradigm. *Child Development, 59,* 1514–1521.

Clohessy, A. B., Posner, M. I., Rothbart, M. K., & Vecera, S. P. (1991). The development of inhibition of return. *Journal of Cognitive Neuroscience, 3,* 345–356.

Damasio, A. R., & Benton, A. L. (1979). Impairments of hand movements under visual guidance. *Neurology, 29,* 170–178.

De Renzi, E. (1982). *Disorders of space exploration and cognition.* New York: Wiley.

Finlay, D. C., & Ivinski, A. (1984). Cardiac and visual responses to moving stimuli presented either successively or simultaneously to the central and peripheral visual fields in four-month-old infants. *Developmental Psychology, 20,* 29–36.

Fischer, B. (1986). The role of attention in the preparation of visually guided eye movements in monkey and man. *Psychological Research, 48,* 251–257.

Foreman, N., Flelder, A., Price, D., & Bowler, W. (1991). Tonic and phasic orientation in full-term and preterm infants. *Journal of Experimental Child Psychology, 51*(3), 407–422.

Girton, M. R. (1979). Infants' attention to intrastimulus motion. *Journal of Experimental Child Psychology, 28,* 416–423.

Hainline, L. (1993). Conjugate eye movements in infants. In K. Simons (Ed.), *Early visual development, normal and abnormal.* Oxford: Oxford University Press.

Haith, M. M., Bergman, T., & Moore, M. J. (1977). Eye contact and early scanning in early infancy. *Science, 198,* 853–855.

Harris, P. L., & MacFarlane, A. (1974). The growth of the effective visual field from birth to seven weeks. *Journal of Experimental Child Psychology, 18,* 340–384.

Hikosaka, O., & Wurtz, R. H. (1983a–1983d). Visual and oculomotor functions of monkey substantia nigra pars reticulata—I–IV. *Journal of Neurophysiology, 49,* 1230–1301.

Hood, B. (1991). *Development of visual selective attention in the human infant.* PhD thesis, University of Cambridge, England.

Hood, B., & Atkinson, J. (1990a). Sensory visual loss and cognitive deficits in theselective attentional system of normal infants and neurologically impaired children. *Developmental Medicine and Child Neurology, 32,* 1067–1077.

Hood, B., & Atkinson, J. (1990b). Inhibition of return in infants. *Perception, 19,* 369.

Hood, B., & Atkinson, J. (1991a, April). *Shifts of covert visual attention in infancy.* Paper presented at the meeting of the Society for Research in Child Development, Seattle, WA.

Hood, B., & Atkinson, J. (1991). Shifting covert attention in infancy. *Transactions of the Annual Meeting of the Association for Research into Vision and Ophthalmology (ARVO), 965.*

Hood, B. M., & Atkinson, J. (1991, April). *Inhibition of return in 3-, 6-month-olds and adults.* Paper presented at the meeting of the Society for Research in Child Development, Seattle, WA.

Hood, B. M., & Atkinson, J. (1993). Disengaging visual attention in the infant and the adult. *Infant Behavior and Development, 16,* 405–422.

Horowitz, F. D., Paden, L., Bhana, K., & Self, P. (1972). An infant–control procedure for studying infant visual fixations. *Developmental Psychology, 7,* 90.

Hubel, D. H., LeVay, S., & Wiesel, T. N. (1975). Mode of termination of retinotectal fibres in macaque monkey: An autoradiographic study. *Brain Research, 96,* 25–40.

Johnson, M. H. (1990). Cortical maturation and the development of visual attention in early infancy. *Journal of Cognitive Neuroscience, 2,* 81–95.

Johnson, M. H., Posner, M. I., & Rothbart, M. K. (1991). Components of visual orienting in early infancy: Contingency learning, anticipatory looking, and disengaging. *Journal of Cognitive Neuroscience, 3,* 336–344.

Johnson, M. H., & Tucker, L. A. (1993). *The ontogeny of covert visual atten-*

tion: facilitatory and inhibitory effects. Paper presented at the meeting of the Society for Research in Child Development, New Orleans, LA.

Judge, S. J. (1990). Neurophysiology of vergence and accommodation. In Obrecht & Stark (Eds.), *Presbyopia research: From molecular biology to visual adaption.*New York: Plenum Press.

Judge, S. J., & Miles, F. A. (1981). Gain changes in accommodative vergence induced by alteration of the effective interocular separation. In Fuchs & Becker (Eds.), *Progress in oculomotor tesearch.* New York: Elsevier/North Holland.

Lewis, T. L., & Maurer, D. (1992). The development of the temporal and nasal visual fields during infancy. *Vision Research, 32,* 903–911.

Lewis, T. L., Maurer, D., & Blackburn, K. (1985). The development of the young infants' ability to detect stimuli in the nasal visual field. *Vision Research, 25,* 943–950.

Livingstone, M. S., & Hubel, D. H. (1988). Segregation of form, color, movement, and depth: Anatomy, physiology, and perception. *Science, 240,* 740–749.

Maunsell, J. H. R., & Newsome. W. T. (1987). Visual processing in monkey extrastriate cortex. *Annual Review of Neuroscience, 10,* 3416–3468.

Maurer, D., & Salapatek, P. (1976). Developmental changes in the scanning of faces by young infants. *Child Development, 47,* 523–527.

Maylor, E. A. (1985). Facilitatory and inhibitory components of orienting in visual space. *Attention and Performance, 11,* 189–204.

Milewski, A. (1976). Infants' discrimination of internal and external pattern elements. *Journal of Experimental Child Psychology, 22,* 229–246.

Mountcastle, V. B. (1978). Brain mechanisms for directed attention. *Journal of the Royal Society of Medicine, 71,* 14–28.

Perenin, M. T. (1978). Visual function within the hemianopic field following earlycerebral hemidecortication in man—II: Pattern discrimination. *Neuropsychologica, 16,* 697–708.

Perenin, M. T., & Jeannerod, M. (1978). Visual function within the hemianopic field following early cerebral hemidecortication in man—I: Spatial localization. *Neuropsychologica, 16,* 1–13.

Pollack, J. G., & Hickey, T. L. (1979). The distribution of retino-collicular axon terminals in rhesus monkey. *Journal of Comparative Neurology, 185,* 587–602.

Pöppel, E., Held, R., & Frost, D. (1973). Residual visual function after brain wounds involving the central visual pathways in man. *Nature (London), 243,* 295–296.

Posner, M. I. (1978). *Chronometric explorations of the mind.* Hillsdale, NJ: Erlbaum.

Posner, M. I., & Cohen, Y. (1980). Orienting of attention. *Quarterly Journal of Experimental Psychology, 32,* 3–25.

Posner, M. I., Inhoff, A. W., Friedrich, F. J., & Cohen, A. (1987). Isolating attentional systems: A cognitive-anatomical analysis. *Psychobiology, 15,* 107–121.

Posner, M. I., & Petersen, S. E. (1990). The attention system of the human brain. *Annual Revue of Neuroscience, 13,* 25–42.

Posner, M. I., Rafal, R. D., Choate, L. S., & Vaughan, J. (1985). Inhibition of return: Neural basis and function. *Cognitive Neuropsychology, 2,* 211–228.

Ptito, A., Lassonde, M., Leporé, & Ptito, M. (1987). Visual discrimination in hemispherectomised patients. *Neuropsychologica, 25,* 869–879.

Rafal, R., Calabresi, P., Brennan, C., & Sciolto, T. (1989). Saccade preparation inhibits reorienting to recently attended locations. *Journal of Experimental Psychology: Human Perception and Performance, 15,* 673–685.

Rafal, R., Henik, A., & Smith, J. (1991). Extrageniculate contribution to reflex visual orienting in normal humans: A temporal hemifield advantage. *Journal of Cognitive Neuroscience, 3,*

Richards, J. E. (1985). The development of sustained visual attention in infants from 14 to 26 weeks of of age. *Psychophysiology, 22,* 409–416.

Richards, J. E. (1987). Infant visual sustained attention and respiratory sinus arrhythmia. *Child Development, 58,* 488–496.

Richards, J. E. (1989). Development and stability in visual sustained attention in 14, 20 and 26-week-old infants. *Psychophysiology, 26,* 422–430.

Salapatek, P. (1975). Pattern perception in early infancy. In L. B. Cohen & P. Salapatek (Eds.), *Sensation to cognition* (Vol. I). New York: Academic Press.

Saslow, M. G. (1967). Effects of components of displacement-step stimuli upon latency of saccadic eye movements. *Journal of the Optical Society of America, 57,* 1024–1029.

Schiller. P. H. (1985). A model for the generation of visually guided saccadic eye movements. In D. Rose & V. G. Dobson (Eds.), *Models of the visual cortex.* Chichester: Wiley.

Schiller P. H., Malpeli, J. G., & Schein, S. J. (1979). Composition of geniculostriateinput to superior colliculus of the rhesus monkey. *Journal of Neurophysiology, 42,* 1124–1133.

Schwartz, T. I., Dobson, V., Sandstrom, D. J., & van Hof-van Duin, J. (1987). Kinetic perimetry assessment of binocular visual field shape and size in young infants. *Vision Research, 12,* 2163–2175.

Shallice, T. (1972). Dual functions of consciousness. *Psychological Review, 79,* 383–393.

Tronick, E. (1972). Stimulus control and the growth of the infant's effective visual field. *Perception and Psychophysics, 11,* 373–376.

Ungerleider L. G., & Mishkin, M. (1982). Two cortical visual systems. In D. G. Ingle, M. A. Goodale, & R, J, Q, Mansfield (Eds,), *Analysis of visual behavior.* Cambidge, MA: MIT Press.

Valenza, E., Simion, F., & Umilta, C. (in press). Inhibition of return in newborns. *Infant Behavior and Development.*

Van Essen, D. C., & Maunsell, J. H. R. (1983). Hierarchical organization and functional streams in the visual cortex. *Trends in Neuroscience, 6,* 370–375.

Van Hof-van Duin, J., & Mohn, G. (1986). Visual field measurements, optokinetic nystagmus, and the threatening response: Normal and abnormal development. *Documenta Ophthalmologica Proceedings Series, 45,* 305–315.

Weiskrantz, L. (1986). *Blindsight: A case study and implications.* Oxford: Clarendon Press.

Zeki, S. M. (1973). Colour coding in rhesus monkey prestriate cortex. *Brain Research, 53,* 422–427.

Zeki, S. M. (1977). Colour coding in the superior temporal sulcus of rhesus monkey visual cortex. *Proceedings of the Royal Society of London Series B197*, 195–223.

Zeki, S. M., & Shipp, S. (1988). The functional logic of cortical connections. *Nature, 335*, 311–317.

Zihl, J., & von Cramon, D., & Mai, N. (1983). Selective disturbance of movement vision after bilateral brain damage. *Brain, 106*, 313–340.

THREE

Selective Attention to Novelty as a Measure of Information Processing across the Lifespan

Joseph F. Fagan III
Jodi Haiken-Vasen

The thesis of the present chapter is that the observation of selective attention to novelty can provide a common measure of information processing from birth to senescence and across various cognitively disordered populations. Empirical tests of variables influencing cognitive functioning from one age to another during development usually involve different tasks or metrics. Hence, conclusions about cognition and age must be advanced with the caution that task differences or measurement differences are also present and may in part be responsible for the obtained results. The problem of varying tasks or metrics to study individual differences in cognition becomes particularly acute when one tests special groups who may not be able to comply with the requirements of the tests for reasons unrelated to cognitive functioning per se. Difficulty in compliance could result from anxiety, from a limitation in comprehension due to cultural circumstances, or from motoric inabilities to make responses. The point is that extraneous influences, which may vary with the requirements for particular cognitive tasks, may limit the conclusions with regard to the nature of cognitive development or individual differences in cognitive functioning.

There is a solution to the problem of different tasks and metrics for measuring cognitive functioning at various ages and with special populations. We show in the present chapter that processing of nonverbal, new information can be studied across age and in various cognitively disordered populations using a paradigm that involves the same materials and the same measure of performance. The paradigm is based on a test of selective attention to visual novelty that has been used extensively over the past 30 years to measure the encoding and retention of information during infancy. In such a selective attention test, an individual studies a picture for a specific period of time, after which that picture is paired with a new picture. Typically, more visual fixation is paid to the novel target when the two targets are paired.

In the present studies, we tested information processing by simply instructing participants who viewed novel and previously seen targets to "look at the pictures." Their level of naturally occurring differential fixation to novelty served as a measure of information processing. Within subjects, tests of selective attention to novelty were made under immediate and delayed pairings of previously seen and new targets to obtain estimates of encoding and retention of information.

As the chapter proceeds, we will show that infants, normal children of various ages, neurologically impaired children, normal young adults, young adults with acquired neurological impairment, and the normal elderly, depressed elderly, and demented elderly all devote more fixation to novel targets. Moreover, we will find that selective attention during infancy predicts later mental retardation on standard IQ tests, shows some improvement during early development and some decrement with old age, and is compromised by early neurological impairment, dementia, and acquired neurological deficit. We will also point out that, aside from being applicable from birth to senescence, testing of selective attention to novelty has the additional practical advantage of having been used with nonhuman primates. Thus, tests of theories of cognitive functioning employing a common method and metric can ultimately be made not only across age but across species.

PARADIGM

Our studies of selective attention to novelty as a measure of information processing throughout the lifespan are based on a specific paradigm developed by Fantz (1956) to study the visual interests of infants. Fantz assumed that if an infant looks more at one stimulus than another, the infant must be able to differentiate between them.

While differential fixation to one stimulus over the other indicates perception and discrimination, the further assumption may be made that an unequal distribution of attention paid to a novel and a previously exposed target indicates that some information about the previously exposed target has been encoded and retained. One way to test visual information processing is to expose the infant to a target for a certain period of time (the familiarization period) and then to present the infant with the previously exposed target and a novel stimulus simultaneously (Fagan, 1970). Such presentations may be immediate or delayed in order to study the retention of information over time (Fagan, 1973). Infants typically devote the greater part of their visual fixation to the novel target when tested with this paired-comparison approach. Complete details of paired-comparison testing with infants are provided by Fagan (1990).

The general method of testing, based on the Fagan Test of Infant Intelligence (Fagan & Detterman, 1992), was the same for all studies reviewed in the present chapter. An observer viewed the eyes of each participant through a peephole in the center of a stage while the participant viewed pairs of photographs of unfamiliar faces, as illustrated in Figure 3.1. Participants were administered multiple pairs of novel and previously exposed targets. The session began with children or adults being allowed to study a picture until 5 seconds of actual looking were recorded (12–20 seconds of familiarization are usually given for infants). That picture was then quickly paired twice with the same novel picture for two 2-second pairings. Then, the next problem was administered. A total of 10 such immediate tests of selective attention to novel and previously exposed targets constituted the beginning of a test session. Following the 10 immediate visual selectivity tests, a series of 8–10 pairings of novel

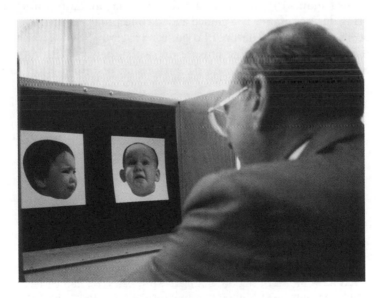

FIGURE 3.1. The testing situation.

with previously exposed targets took place. In each case, a picture which appeared during the earlier, immediate tests of selective attention was paired with a new picture. Either participants were not told what to do (e.g., infants) or, if able to talk and hear, were given very nondirected instructions such as, "Here are some pictures. You can look at them."

Visual novelty preference scores were defined as the percentage of total fixation paid to the novel target (i.e., fixation to the novel target divided by fixation to the novel plus fixation to the familiar target). The use of percentage scores rather than differences in raw looking times to express novelty preference scores has been the usual practice in studies of infants' information processing. For a more detailed discussion of scoring procedures the reader is referred to Fagan (1990).

INFANCY

Studies of the infant's preference for novelty have shown that the encoding and retention of information is a robust phenomenon during infancy. From birth, infants are capable of encoding and retaining some aspects of visual information. With age, increasingly subtle distinctions among visual stimuli are noticed and encoded. By the age of 5 months, infants are capable of recognizing previously seen targets after periods of hours, days, and even weeks, and such memory is not easily disrupted (see the review by Fagan, 1984b). The fact that we can measure information processing during infancy has gained added conceptual significance in light of a recent theory on the nature of cognition (Fagan, 1984a, 1991, 1992). Figure 3.2 presents a graphic illustration of the theory. Within this theory, cognition is assumed to be the processing of information to gain

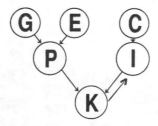

FIGURE 3.2. A model of cognition. Cognitive processes (P), influenced by genetics (G) and environment (E), interact with information (I) to produce knowledge (K). Information comes from the culture (C) and from previous relevant knowledge.

knowledge. The source of cognitive continuity lies in a small set of basic processes for acquiring information. The processes are innate, relatively automatic, dependent on neural integrity, and common to all ages. According to the model, new knowledge (K) is gained as a result of an interaction between the basic cognitive processes (P) and the information (I) made available for the individual to process. The neural integrity underlying the basic processes may be affected for good or ill by genetic endowment (G). Processing is also affected by specific environmental factors (E) that act directly on the central nervous system, such as trauma, drugs, or the presence of teratogens. The amount and quality of information provided to the learner will vary with cultural factors (C) that may be associated with demographic characteristics such as race, birth order, and socioeconomic status. Information is also made up of previous relevant knowledge.

According to the theory outlined in Figure 3.2, the origins of intelligence lie in the infant's ability to process information. An important prediction of the theory is that individual differences in measures of information processing during infancy should correlate with later individual differences in the amount of knowledge gained over time. Individual differences in attention to novelty during infancy, for example, should lead to later differences on conventional tests of intelligence. Intelligence tests usually include tests of knowledge retrieval (e.g., vocabulary tests). Infants who processed information faster or better than other infants should, as children, have gained more knowledge over time.

In fact, measures of visual novelty preference derived during infancy are related to later intellectual functioning. Various meta-analyses (Bornstein & Sigman, 1986; Fagan & Singer, 1983; McCall & Carriger, 1993) have found median correlations of about .45 between infant performance on tests of selective attention to novelty and later IQ. Those correlations are quite robust, occurring across sexes, races, levels of socioeconomic status, birth orders, ages at early test, ages at later test, various visual novelty tasks, different methods of assessing early performance, different outcome measures, and different laboratories. In short, there is a significant and well-established link between early preferences for visual novelty and later intelligence.

NORMAL DEVELOPMENT: FROM PRESCHOOL TO COLLEGE

Before we discuss the relationship between attention to novelty and cognitive ability in special populations of children and adults, it is important to consider the normal developmental trajectory observed in the measurement of preference for novelty. In the present section, data on the development of selective attention to novelty will be presented from preschool-aged children to college students.

Specifically, in a recent unpublished study, we observed selective attention to novelty in a sample of 115 subjects ranging in age from 3 years, 1 month to 23 years. The procedure used to map the development of preference for novelty through childhood and into young adulthood was the same as that previously described for infants with one exception. Instead of presenting the targets manually on a wooden stage, the pictures were digitized and presented on a laptop computer. The experimenter observed the child's or adult's eyes and recorded the eye movements by pressing the buttons on a computer mouse. Once again, visual novelty preference scores were defined as the percentage of total fixation paid to the novel targets (i.e., fixation to the novel target divided by the fixation to the novel plus fixation to the previously exposed target). Each participant received 20 visual novelty preference scores (10 immediate, 10 delayed). A preliminary analysis was performed to examine whether race or gender systematically influenced attention to novelty tasks. There was no effect of race or gender on mean fixation to novelty scores. Therefore, race and gender were not considered in subsequent analyses.

The first question we asked was whether normal children and adolescents would show a preference for novel targets as do infants. The ten immediate trials and the ten delayed trials were combined to produce two mean novelty preference scores: immediate and delayed. Based on the individual means for the 10 novelty preference scores included in the immediate and delayed portions of the tasks, the subjects' mean percentage of total fixation time to novel targets were 59.7% ($N = 115, SD = 6.7\%$, range = 46.8–80.7%) and 56.2% ($N = 115, SD = 6.5\%$, range = 40.7–73.6%). The means were tested against a chance level of 50%. The comparison yielded significant results for both the immediate ($t = 15.52$, $df = 114, p < .001$) and the delayed ($t = 10.23, df = 114, p < .001$) portions of the test as the children and adolescents in the sample showed a significant preference for the novel stimulus.

The main analysis of the data examined the developmental trends in performance across age for the immediate and delayed portions of the tasks. The subjects were combined into five groups based on their age (see Table 3.1 for mean ages and age ranges). The statistical analysis took the form of a between-subject (age group) and within-subject (immediate/delayed test trials) analysis of variance (ANOVA). The ANOVA was undertaken to examine whether the participants differed systematically in their mean preference for novelty as a function of age or retention interval. A significant effect for age group was demonstrated ($F(4,110) = 3.43, p < .011$). The five age group's mean preferences for novelty are

TABLE 3.1. Age Groups (Years, Months)

Age group	Mean age	SD	Range
1	4,8	0,8	3,1–4,11
2	6,0	0,7	5,0–6,11
3	8,2	0,10	7,0–9,4
4	12,5	1,4	10,6–14,11
5	19,8	1,4	18,0–23,0

listed in Table 3.2. Results show that there is an increase in the percentage of time the participants fixated on the novel stimulus, which is primarily due to the higher performance of the college students as compared to the children.

Results for retention interval indicated that there was a significant difference between the entire sample's performance when the test trial immediately followed the familiarization trial than when the test trial was presented after about a 4-minute delay ($F(1,110) = 31.34, p < .0001$). The subjects looked significantly less at the novel target after a delay between familiarization of the previously exposed stimulus and its paired comparison with the novel stimulus. Presumably, recognition of the old picture is more difficult as time elapses from its first presentation. The interaction between age group and the immediate and delayed portions of the test was not significant.

Empirically, the results demonstrate that children and college students look significantly longer at a new stimulus than at a previously exposed one, as do infants. Empirically, selective attention to novelty is behavior (selective fixation) influenced by a past event (having studied a picture earlier) in a situation in which there is no instruction to retrieve the past event. Such memory-based performance is usually labeled "implicit" mem-

TABLE 3.2. Selective Attention to Novelty over Age for Immediate and Delayed Testing

Age group	Immediate % to novel (± SD)	Delay % to novel (± SD)	Total % to novel (± SD)
1	58.5 (± 5.6)	54.3 (± 5.0)	56.4 (± 3.8)
2	59.1 (± 4.7)	55.2 (± 5.4)	57.1 (± 4.0)
3	58.0 (± 5.6)	54.1 (± 5.4)	56.1 (± 4.1)
4	61.4 (± 7.5)	55.4 (± 6.9)	58.4 (± 6.3)
5	61.3 (± 8.9)	60.5 (± 7.2)	60.9 (± 7.4)

ory. Conceptually, then, our data suggest that some components of implicit memory differ between children and college students, which is contrary to the conclusions of other researchers (Carroll, Byrne, & Kirsner, 1985; Parkin & Streete, 1988; Naito, 1990).

MENTAL RETARDATION

A number of implications for our understanding of mental retardation flow from viewing intelligence as processing. One implication has to do with the definition of mental retardation. According to the theory noted earlier and illustrated in Figure 3.2, mental retardation is assumed to be a deficit in processing (P). The deficit in P can be caused by a genetic defect (G) or by a toxic, traumatic, or infectious environmental event acting on the brain (E) or by some interaction of genetic and specific environmental factors. It is important to note here that mental retardation, in this theory, is not defined as a deficit in knowledge but as a deficit in processing. A low score on a conventional intelligence test is a sign of mental retardation only if the low score is a result of a deficiency in information processing. Theoretically, a low IQ score can also result from inadequate information provided by the child's culture. Thus, a low IQ score may mean mental retardation (poor processing) or ignorance (poor information) or both.

The theory would predict that processing early in life will lead to low intellectual achievement (i.e., a low IQ) later in life. Such a relationship has been demonstrated using the Fagan Test of Infant Intelligence, which has proved useful for the prediction of later IQ scores in individual cases. Fagan and Detterman (1992) summarized estimates of the predictive validity of the Fagan Test for later mental retardation from studies of 128 infants originally tested at 3, 4, 5, and 7 months (Fagan & Montie, 1988); 20 infants tested at 5 and 7 months (Fagan & Montie, 1988); and 241 infants tested at 6, 7, 9, and 12 months (Fagan & Detterman, 1992). The infants were followed to 3 years of age and then given the standard test of intelligence. For our present purposes, we can summarize the utility of the Fagan Test for the prediction of mental retardation in individual children, by combining these three samples and then dividing the 389 children in the total sample into two categories defined by IQ at age 3: IQ ≤ 70, a conventional estimate of mental retardation ($n = 26$), and IQ > 70 ($n = 363$).

In this combined analysis, the incidence of mental retardation at the age of 3 years was quite low at 6.6%. However, the Fagan Test, given at the age of 6–12 months, was highly sensitive to low IQ scores measured at 3 years. A mean novelty-preference score of ≤53% correctly identified 22 out of 26, or 85%, of the children who later obtained IQ scores

≤70. Thus, sensitivity (correctly identifying a child as mentally retarded) was 85%. Also, the test was as predictive for children with mild retardation (IQ = 50–70) as it was for children with severe retardation (IQ < 50). The test also had high specificity in identifying 336 out of 363, or 93%, of the normal children as normal. A false positive rate of 7% would not be unusual given the low incidence of mental retardation in the sample.

Rose, Feldman, and Wallace (1988) provide an independent replication of the clinical utility of tests of early visual information processing for the prediction of individual IQs. In their study, novelty-preference scores of ≤ 54% correctly predicted 23 out of 31 children with 3-year IQs ≤ 85 (a 74% sensitivity rate), and scores greater than 54% predicted 30 out of 36 children with IQs > 85 (an 83% specificity rate).

In summary, tests of information processing based on an infant's preference for visual novelty indicate that mental retardation, defined as poor processing, can be detected during the first year of life and that poor information processing early in life leads to low achievement on standard tests of intelligence later in life. Such results stand in contrast to repeated attempts over the past 50 years to predict later intelligence from tests of sensorimotor functioning during infancy, attempts that have resulted in no substantial prediction. The reader is referred to a review by Fagan and Singer (1983) of more than 100 such studies and Fagan, Singer, Montie, and Shepherd (1986, Table 2) for a direct comparison of the predictive value of information processing tests with sensorimotor tests within the same population of infants at risk for mental retardation.

The discovery that poor information processing can be identified during infancy should allow a more efficient approach to understanding the causes of mental retardation. Using information processing tests to detect infants at risk for later retardation could cut the lead time for longitudinal prospective studies of conditions leading to mild mental retardation from 6 or more years to 1 year or less (see Fitzhardinge, 1980, p. 1, on the gap in time in assessing mild intellectual impairment). Even very limited success in research in the etiology of mental retardation and in the prevention of some conditions leading to mental retardation would be of enormous social benefit. In fact, if conditions causing poor information processing could be prevented for only 1% of infants at risk for retardation, we would save more children from mental retardation than are now saved by screening and treatment for phenylketonuria, one of the known and treatable early causes of mental retardation (Fagan, 1991).

NEUROLOGICALLY IMPAIRED CHILDREN

After exploring the development of preference for novelty in normal children, our research team focused on selective attention to novelty on the part of neurologically impaired children (see Holland, Fagan, & Wiznitzer, 1994). We wanted to find out if such children would be able to be tested, would selectively attend to novelty, and would differ from normal controls.

The sample included 34 children. Of these 34 subjects, 18 were being treated by a pediatric neurologist for any one of a variety of disorders including seizures, metabolic disorders, autism, or autistic spectrum disorders. These latter two categories included 12 of the 18 impaired children. Rough estimates of mental age were available for 7 of the 12 autistic children. These mental ages ranged from 1.8 to 4.3 years with a mean of 2.5 (SD = 0.9). Mean chronological age for the same 7 children was 4.1 years (SD = 0.9). The estimated mean IQ was 59.3 (SD = 12.4, range = 50–85). The remaining 16 children constituted a normal comparison group of similar chronological age to the impaired group. The total sample of 34 ranged in age from 2.3 to 13.2 years. The mean age of the 18 impaired children was 6.01 years (SD = 3.04). The mean age of the 16 comparison children was 5.3 years (SD = 1.4).

Each child was given a number of preference for novelty tests on a laptop computer following the general procedure described earlier.

The mean novelty preference scores for each group of children at each retention interval are listed in Table 3.3. The comparison children showed a significant preference for novelty under both immediate and delayed testing (t = 10.2, df = 15, p < .001, and t = 3.8, df = 15 p < .01, respectively) the neurologically impaired children showed a significant preference for novelty only when tested immediately (t = 1.8, df = 17, p < .05). Lack of preference for novelty under delayed testing was probably due to a floor effect for the impaired children, given their low attention to novelty on immediate testing and some falloff over delay.

An ANOVA of groups (impaired, control) by retention interval (immediate, delayed) resulted in a significant group effect ($F(1,31)$ = 16.8, p < .001), with normals devoting more attention to novelty (58.4%) than

TABLE 3.2. Mean Novelty-Preference Scores for Neurologically Impaired and Normal Children under Immediate and Delayed Testing

		Immediate	Delayed
Normal	M	61.4	55.3
	SD	4.5	5.6
Impaired	M	54.0	49.1
	SD	9.3	5.8

TABLE 3.4. Estimates of Sensitivity to Neurological Impairment and Specificity for Normality for a Test of Selective Attention to Novelty

	Impaired	Normal	
≤ 55.7	16	4	Sensitivity 89%
> 55.7	2	12	Specificity 75%
			Validity 82%

did neurologically impaired children (51.8%). In general, children did better on immediate testing than after a delay ($F(1,31) = 10.8, p < .002$). There was no significant interaction of groups by retention interval, although this must be qualified by the fact that the impaired children were at a floor (50% is chance) under delayed testing.

For the purposes of prediction of abnormality or normality in individual cases, we found that a novelty preference score of 55.7% maximized the sensitivity of the test to neurological impairment while maintaining specificity to normality. The results are noted in Table 3.4. Specifically, of the 18 impaired children, 16 scored at or lower than 55.7% preference for novelty for a sensitivity of 89%. Of the 16 normals, 12 scored greater than 55.7% to the novel for a specificity of 75%. The overall validity of the test was 28 correct out of 34, or 82%. The 7 autistic children for whom some mental ages and IQs were available averaged 54.6% of fixation to the novel target ($SD = 2.4$) on tests of selective attention administered immediately after study. The correlation between their IQs and their attention to novelty on immediate tests was $r = .49$. The sample, of course, is too small to conclude that there is a relationship between selective attention to novelty and IQ within a group of autistic children, although the results are suggestive and encourage further study.

The present results, in which neurologically impaired children were compared with normals, agree with our previous work with infants showing selective attention to novelty to be indicative of level of cognitive functioning. In addition, we find that attention to novelty also provides a valid means for measuring cognitive functioning in individuals, such as autistic children, who may find it difficult or impossible to comply with the requirements of conventional tests of cognitive functioning.

NEUROLOGICALLY IMPAIRED ADULTS

A study by Fagan, Corrigan, and Layton (1992) sought to extend the construct validity of the assumption that selective visual attention to novelty reflects a basic process underlying cognitive functioning and is predictive of disordered cognitive functioning at any age. To do so we extended our testing to an adult sample chosen because they had experienced an injury during adulthood that produced neurological impairment. The specific hypothesis was that if selective attention to novelty reflects a basic process associated with potential for intellectual growth and which is subject to decline with early neurological damage (e.g., damage attendant on mental retardation or autism), it should also be associated with severity of brain damage and with concurrent cognitive functioning within a population of adults with acquired neurological impairment.

The sample included 41 adults with mean age of 31.6 years (SD = 9.1) and a mean educational level of 13 years (SD = 1.8). Of these 41 adults, 27 had a history of closed head injury (usually from automobile accidents), 2 had neurological damage resulting from anoxic encephalopathy, 7 had damage as a result of an aneurysm, 4 had a history of open head injury (gunshot wounds), and 1 subject had damage resulting from a seizure disorder. All were referred for neuropsychological evaluation from an outpatient brain injury rehabilitation program at a major university teaching hospital. The mean time since injury was 157.3 weeks (SD = 168.8, range = 8–692). Information on length of coma, one estimate of severity of brain damage, was available for 23 of the 27 closed head injury patients (mean length of coma was 31.3 days; SD = 35.9, range = 0–120).

Participants obtained 26 visual novelty preference scores (10 immediate, 16 delayed). The mean of the 26 scores was taken as the estimate of selective attention to novelty for each individual. Based on these individual means, the total group of 41 participants averaged 58.1% of total fixation to novel targets (SD = 5.4, range = 47.6–69.8). When tested against a chance value of 50%, the group mean of 58.1 proved to be significantly greater than a chance value of 50% (t = 9.1, df = 40, p < .001), indicating that, for the group, selective visual fixation to novelty did occur.

Of the 41 adults, 31 had received an extensive battery of conventional cognitive tests including tests of memory, attention, visual–spatial functioning, and executive functioning. One neuropsychologist and two neuropsychology trainees who were blind to the identity of the person rated the conventional test protocols of the 28 patients on a 5-point scale for overall level of cognitive functioning: a rating of 1 indicated a severe problem in function, and a rating of 5 indicated no problem. We used the mean of the ratings over the three experts as a general estimate of the client's cognitive functioning.

The 28 people rated for cognitive functioning by the three neuropsychologists on the 5-point scale averaged 3.2 points (SD = 1.0, range = 1.4–4.4). The three judges were highly agreed as to ratings for the 28 individuals with an average interjudge correlation of .79. Scores on the selective attention test proved to have concurrent validity for the prediction of cognitive functioning and/or severity of brain damage. Specifically, selective attention to novelty was significantly correlated with mean ratings of cognitive functioning ($r = .54$, $df = 27$, $p < .001$) and with length of coma ($r = -.62$, $df = 24$, $p < .0001$).

The conventional cognitive battery could also be divided into five different types of tests measuring primary memory, secondary memory, frontal lobe functions, visual–spatial abilities, or language fluency. Selective attention to novelty was most associated with secondary memory and frontal lobe functioning and moderately with primary memory. No relationship appeared to exist with visual–spatial abilities and language fluency. In effect, the results indicate that selective attention to novelty seems to be most related to what is usually called secondary memory.

In summary, our results indicate that adults with acquired neurological impairment are responsive to visual novelty and that selective attention to novelty is highly associated with severity of brain damage and/or level of cognitive functioning within such a neurologically impaired population.

DEMENTED/DEPRESSED ELDERLY

Our final study in the series (Fagan & Kennedy, 1994) took us to the end of the age scale as we tested selective attention to novelty on the part of normal elderly, depressed elderly, and depressed, demented elderly. The sample included 35 elderly with a mean age of 74.9 years ($SD = 7.9$) and a mean educational level of 11.7 years ($SD = 3.7$). Of the 35 subjects, 12 were normal elderly who lived at home. The remaining 23 of the 35 elderly had been living at home but were now inpatients in a psychiatric geriatric unit, because all 23 had been diagnosed as clinically depressed according to DSM-III-R criteria. In addition, 14 of the 23 had been diagnosed as demented according to DSM-III-R criteria. For ease of exposition, we will refer to the normal elderly as the *normal group,* the nondemented, depressed patients as the *depressed group,* and the depressed patients with dementia as the *dementia group.* Analyses indicated no significant age or educational differences among the groups.

Each subject received 20 novelty preference scores, 10 on immediate testing of selective attention and 10 on delayed testing. For the purposes of analyses the mean of the 10 immediate scores and the mean of the 10 delayed scores were computed for each subject and formed the basis for all subsequent analyses.

**TABLE 3.5. Mean Selective Attention
to Novelty in Elderly**

Group	n	Immediate	Delay
Normal	12	65.7%	61.9%
Depressed	9	63.1%	58.9%
Demented	14	57.9%	53.9%

Mean preference for novelty scores for each group (normal, depressed, demented) at each point of testing (immediate, delayed) are listed in Table 3.5 along with the number of subjects in each condition. One feature to note from Table 3.5 is that each mean score listed for subjects indicates more attention to novel than to familiar targets. In fact, the lowest score listed (53.9%, for the group with dementia under delayed testing) is itself significantly greater than a chance value of 50% ($t(13) = 2.1, p < .05$). Thus, the tendency for the elderly in the present study was to devote more attention to novelty, as has been the case with various other samples.

The main analysis was conducted by entering the mean novelty preference scores for each person into an ANOVA of groups (normal, depressed, dementia) by time of testing (immediate, delayed). Both main effects emerged as significant: the group effect ($F(2,32) = 9.0, p < .001$) and the effect of time of testing ($F(1,32) = 8.6, p < .005$). The interaction between groups and time of testing was not significant. Within the general group effect, it was also the case that selective attention to novelty was lessened in dementia. Separate analyses comparing each nondemented group to the group with dementia indicated that the normals were superior in attention to novelty to the patients with dementia ($F(1,24) = 19.1, p < .0001$) and that depressed patients were also superior to the patients with dementia ($F(1,21) = 6.6, p < .01$). Thus, what emerges from the analyses is evidence for a deficiency in selective attention to novelty due to dementia.

NONHUMAN PRIMATES

Thus far we have presented data showing that differential responsiveness to a novel target relative to a previously exposed target is a correlate of cognitive functioning for humans of various ages. Ultimately, we wish to know the neural basis of cognition. One way to explore the neural basis of cognition is to pick a measure of cognition such as responsiveness to novelty and to show that similar behavior is elicited by the same paradigm for other species, particularly those for whom we have specific knowledge of the neural bases of information processing. Fortunately, there are parallels between humans and macaque or rhesus monkeys in responsiveness to visual novelty.

Gunderson and her associates have demonstrated a number of similarities for visual responsiveness to novelty on paired-comparison tests between human and pigtailed macaque infants. For example, Gunderson and Sackett (1984) showed that pigtailed monkeys differentiate among abstract stimuli on tests of novelty preference in the same order of task difficulty over age as do humans. One week of development of visual recognition in the pigtailed monkey corresponds approximately to 1 month of development in the human. Pigtailed monkeys can also recognize novel abstract patterns after 24 hours (Gunderson & Swartz, 1985). At 6 weeks of age (like 5- to 6-month-old humans), pigtailed monkeys need only 5 seconds of study time to differentiate between two widely different abstract patterns on pairings of a novel and a familiar target (Gunderson & Swartz, 1986). Bachevalier and her associates have also noted such similarities between human and monkey infants on paired-comparison tests in infant rhesus macaques (e.g., Bachevalier, 1990; Brickson & Bachevalier, 1984). Brickson and Bachevalier (1984) demonstrated that rhesus monkeys look reliably more often at a novel stimulus even at 5 days of age.

Moreover, as Fagan and his associates have demonstrated with human infants (as discussed earlier), Gunderson, Grant-Webster, and Fagan (1987) have shown that pigtailed macaque infants with developmental problems such as hypoxia or failure to thrive do not do as well on tests of visual novelty preference as do pigtailed infants with no history of developmental problems. In a study of some possible environmental determinants of mental retardation, Gunderson, Grant, Burbacher, Fagan, and Mottet (1986) found that crab-eating macaques exposed *in utero* to maternal subclinical levels of methylmercury were less responsive as infants to visual novelty. In both of the latter two studies of Gunderson et al., normal and at-risk monkeys were tested on stimuli adapted from the Fagan Test of Infant Intelligence.

The significance of the parallels between humans and monkeys in visual preferences for novelty for understanding the neural bases of cognition is discussed more fully in Fagan (1990). At this point, we wish to point out that we may be at the threshold of asking whether particular drugs impede or facilitate the monkey's visual responsiveness to novelty during infancy. Ultimately we may be asking such questions as: Can the neural pathways subserving preferences for novelty be safely scanned in the human infant, and can chemical intervention ultimately be found to facilitate intellectual development in the human infant? These and many other such questions represent a new and vital area for further interdisciplinary research.

SUMMARY

In the present chapter we have shown that information processing can be studied across age and in various cognitively disordered populations using a paradigm that involves the same materials and the same measure of performance. The paradigm is based on selective attention to visual novelty. The extent of naturally occurring differential fixation to novelty serves as a measure of information processing. Tests of selective attention to novelty made under immediate and delayed pairings of previously seen and new targets allow estimates of encoding and retention of information.

The study of information processing in the infant via the observation of preferences for novelty has led to the view that intelligence is continuous from infancy. The study of selective attention to novelty in the infant has also led to the development of a standard test of information processing that is valid for the prediction of later intellectual achievement. Normal children of various ages, autistic children, normal young adults, young adults with acquired neurological impairment, the normal elderly, the depressed elderly, and the demented elderly, like infants, also devote more fixation to new targets on tests of selective visual attention. Selective attention to novelty shows some improvement in comparison of children with college students and some decrement with old age, and it is compromised by autism, dementia, and acquired neurological deficit. With further empirical study of the parameters determining selective attention to novelty (e.g., study time, delay, type of stimuli to be distinguished), it may be possible to compare groups with one cognitive disorder to those with another cognitive disorder (e.g., the autistic with the demented with the head injured). Such comparisons may allow us to gain a better understanding of the underlying nature of the various disorders in terms of their communalities and differences. For the moment, they remain interesting empirical questions. Aside from being applicable from birth to senescence with humans, selective attention to novelty, as a measure of information processing, has the additional practical advantage of having been demonstrated by nonhuman primates. Thus, tests of theories of information processing employing a common method and metric can ultimately be made across species by employing tests of selective attention. Further studies will allow us to discover how selective attention to novelty correlates with other, more well-established information processing tasks and ultimately to gain some understanding of the neuroanatomy and neural processing underlying selective attention to novelty.

Our hope is to facilitate the study of information processing across and among the disciplines of cognition, neuropsychology, comparative psychology, and developmental psychology by employing selective attention to novelty as a common operational definition of information process-ing. The theory guiding our work sees intelligence as information process-ing. Thus, the prospect that intelligence can be studied from birth to senescence and across species using a common paradigm and a common metric should facilitate an interdisciplinary approach to the study of in-telligence.

ACKNOWLEDGMENT

The preparation of this chapter was supported in part by a Mental Retardation Training Grant from the National Institute on Child Health and Human Develop-ment (HD 07176) and by Grant P50 AGE 08012-07 from the National Institute on Aging.

REFERENCES

Bachevalier, J. (1990). Ontogenetic development of habit and memory formation in primates. In A. Diamond (Ed.), *The development and neural basis of higher cognitive function*. New York: New York Academy of Sciences.

Bornstein, M. H., & Sigman, M. D. (1986). Continuity in mental development from infancy. *Child Development, 57,* 251–274.

Brickson, M., & Bachevalier, J. (1984). Visual recognition in infant monkeys: Evidence for a primitive memory process. *Society for Neuroscience Abstracts, 10,* 137.

Carroll, M., Byrne, B., & Kirsner, K. (1985). Autobiographical memory and per-ceptual learning: A developmental study using picture recognition, naming latency, and perceptual identification. *Memory and Cognition, 13,* 273–279.

Fagan, J. F. (1970). Memory in the infant. *Journal of Experimental Child Psy-chology, 9,* 217–226.

Fagan, J. F. (1973). Infants' delayed recognition memory and forgetting. *Journal of Experimental Child Psychology, 16,* 424–450.

Fagan, J. F. (1984a). The intelligent infant: Theoretical implications. *Intelligence, 8,* 1–9.

Fagan, J. F. (1984b). Infant memory: History, current trends, relation to cogni-tive psychology. In M. Moscovitch (Ed.), *Infant memory*. New York: Ple-num Press.

Fagan, J. F. (1990). The paired-comparison paradigm and infant intelligence. In A. Diamond (Ed.), *The development and neural basis of higher cognitive func-tion*. New York: New York Academy of Sciences.

Fagan, J. F. (1991). Early development of higher cognitive functioning. In F. H. Morris, Jr. & M. A. Simmons (Eds.), *The term newborn*. Columbus, OH: Ross Laboratories.

Fagan, J. F. (1992). Intelligence: A theoretical viewpoint. *Current Directions in Psychological Science, 1,* 82–86.

Fagan, J. F., Corrigan, P. G., & Layton, B. S. (1992). Selective visual attention to novel targets predicts severity of brain damage and level of cognitive functioning in neurologically impaired adults. *Journal of Clinical and Experimental Neuropsychology, 14,* 36.

Fagan, J. F., & Detterman, D. K. (1992). The Fagan Test of Infant Intelligence: A technical summary. *Journal of Applied Developmental Psychology, 13,* 173–193.

Fagan, J. F., & Kennedy, J. S. (1994). *Selective attention as a measure of implicit and explicit memory in the demented or depressed elderly.* Paper presented at the Fifth Cognitive Aging Conference, Atlanta, GA.

Fagan, J. F., & Montie, J. E. (1988). Behavioral assessment of cognitive well-being in the infant. In J. F. Kavanagh (Ed.), *Understanding mental retardation: Research accomplishments and new frontiers.* Baltimore: Brookes.

Fagan, J. F., & Singer, L. T. (1983). Infant recognition memory as a measure of intelligence. In L. P. Lipsitt (Ed.), *Advances in infancy tesearch* (Vol. 2). Norwood, NJ: Ablex.

Fagan, J. F., Singer, L. T., Montie, J. E., & Shepherd, P. A. (1986). Selective screening device for the early detection of normal or delayed cognitive development in infants at risk for later mental retardation. *Pediatrics, 78,* 1021–1026.

Fantz, R. L. (1956). A method for studying early visual development. *Perceptual and Motor Skills, 6,* 13–15.

Fitzhardinge, P. (1980). Current outcome: ICU populations. In A. W. Brann & J. J. Volpe (Eds.), *Neonatal neurological assessment and outcome: Report of the 77th Ross Conference on Pediatric Research.* Columbus, OH: Ross Laboratories.

Gunderson, V. M., Grant, K. S, Burbacher, T. M., Fagan, J. F., & Mottet, N. K. (1986). The effect of low level prenatal methylmercury exposure on visual recognition memory in infant crab-eating macaques. *Child Development, 57,* 1076–1083.

Gunderson, V. M., Grant-Webster, K. S., & Fagan, J. F. (1987). Visual recognition memory in high- and low-risk infant pigtailed macaques. *Developmental Psychology, 23,* 671–675.

Gunderson, V. M., & Sackett, G. P. (1984). Development of pattern recognition in infant pigtailed macaques. *Developmental Psychology, 20,* 418–426.

Gunderson, V. M., & Swartz, K. B. (1985). Visual recognition in infant pigtailed macaques after a 24-hour delay. *American Journal of Primatology, 8,* 259–264.

Gunderson, V. M., & Swartz, K. B. (1986). The effects of familiarization time on visual recognition memory in infant pigtailed macaques. *Developmental Psychology, 22,* 477–480.

Holland, C., Fagan, J. F., & Wiznitzer, M. (1994). *Attention to novelty in neurologically impaired children.* Paper presented at the Gatlinburg Conference on Mental Retardation and Developmental Disabilities, Gatlinburg, TN.

McCall, R. B., & Carriger, M. S. (1993). A meta-analysis of infant habituation and recognition memory performance as predictors of later IQ. *Child Development, 64,* 57–59.

Naito, M. (1990). Repetition priming in children and adults: Age-related dissociation between implicit and explicit memory. *Journal of Experimental Child Psychology, 50,* 462–484.

Parkin, A., & Streete, S. (1988). Implicit and explicit memory in young children and adults. *British Journal of Psychology, 79,* 361–369.

Rose, S. A., Feldman, J. F., & Wallace, I. F. (1988). Individual differences in infant information processing: Reliability, stability and prediction. *Child Development, 59,* 1177–1197.

Selective Attention over the Lifespan

Darlene A. Brodeur
Lana M. Trick
James T. Enns

I n this chapter we attempt to highlight some of the emerging patterns we see in our research on the development of visual attention over the lifespan. We began our studies of visual attention in children over 10 years ago (e.g., Enns & Girgus, 1985; Enns & Brodeur, 1989), but it is only within the past few years that we have begun to compare the trends observed at the beginning of life with those at the other end of life (Brodeur & Enns, in press; Plude, Enns & Brodeur, 1994; Trick & Enns, in press; Trick, Enns & Brodeur, 1996). These studies have led us to be alternatingly optimistic and cautious about the possibility of linking behavioral changes over the lifespan to theories of development and attention.

Our motivation in this work has been threefold. First, there is a need to collect normative data on comparable tasks that measure attention over the lifespan. It is fair to say that far more is known about lifespan changes in basic visual and auditory function than is known about changes in attention (see Coren, Ward, & Enns, 1994, for typical textbook coverage). Yet, one observation that keeps driving us to collect more data is that the apparently limiting factor on performance in many developmental studies (even those putatively studying low-level sensory function) is something that can go by no other name than "attention."

A second motivation for these studies concerns theories of perceptual and cognitive development. Some theories propose that development primarily reflects the changing effects of experience and knowledge on task performance (Chi, 1977; Roth, 1983). In childhood, performance improves with age because of the associated changes occurring in various skill domains. The young child as "novice" eventually becomes the older child and young adult as "expert." Other theories account for lifespan change with general biological mechanisms that are believed to wax and wane in a large inverted-U shape (Kail & Salthouse, 1994; Salthouse, 1985, 1991). They begin with the premise that the speed of any performance is limited by the maximum rate at which elementary cognitive operations can be executed. This limit is set by factors that would have very general consequences, such as the number of transient cortical connections and the degree of neural myelinization; candidates in adulthood include increased neural noise through weakened inhibitory connections and decreased levels of key neurotransmitters. These two classes of developmental theory thus propose very different views on the issue of task-specific lifespan changes.

A third, and too often overlooked, motivation is that developmental studies provide a unique opportunity to test the validity of general theories of attention. Developmental studies do this in the same way as neuropsychological, cross-cultural, and species-comparative studies (Enns, 1993). First, important differences among participant groups are noted. Second, a mapping is established between theoretical constructs and these group differences. Finally, data are collected to determine whether performance on theory-relevant tasks is systematically related to the group differences. One of the unique strengths of developmental studies in this regard is the inherent continuity that can be studied, as the observer moves from childhood, to adulthood, and eventually to old age.

In this chapter we first summarize our views on what constitutes attention by focusing on three separable aspects of attention that are known to vary in childhood as well as in old age. We will then summarize several different views on "What develops?" as an account of age changes in these aspects of attention. Finally, we will present lifespan data from our labs on these attentional components, considering these data in light of the various theoretical viewpoints.

WHAT IS ATTENTION?

In order to investigate lifespan changes in attention, it is necessary to first come to some understanding about the concept of attention. At this point, we believe there is considerable consensus on the central concepts. That is, attention is seen by almost everyone to involve issues of *processing selectivity,* whether that selectivity concerns locations of the visual field for further inspection, shapes and objects that constitute "figure" amid other shapes and objects that constitute "ground," attributes of objects that are relevant to the performance of some task, or even actions that must be inhibited while other actions are performed. However, we acknowledge at the same time that there is considerably less consensus about the boundaries of the concept. Does attention always involve conscious awareness? How do biologically determined biases in selection (e.g., the orienting reflex to abrupt visual and auditory stimuli) interact with knowledge-based biases (e.g., the voluntary effort to keep fixation straight ahead while driving)? Our strategy has been to steer clear of the contentious border issues while trying to stay firmly rooted on the islands of agreement. This will be seen in the following subsections, as we describe the tasks we have studied and the dominant theoretical perspectives associated with each.

Covert Orienting

One aspect of attention is the ability to detect change in the environment, whether that change results from the sudden appearance of a new object or an attribute change in an existing object. The ability to shift visual attention toward the location of such a change without accompanying physical movements of the eye, head, and body has been called "covert orienting" by Posner (1980). In a typical covert orienting task, participants make a speeded response to the onset of a target, or to discriminate one of two possible targets. Response time (RT) and accuracy are measured. Cues are presented prior to the onset of the target, indicating possible target locations. Comparisons are made between trials in which the cue correctly indicates the subsequent target location (so-called *valid* trials), trials in which the cue incorrectly indicates one of the possible locations (so-called *invalid* trials), and trials in which no specific location is indicated by the cue stimulus (so-called *neutral* trials).

In studies of this kind, responses are typically fastest and most accurate when cues are valid, even if eye movements are prevented. According to Posner's (1980) theory of visual orienting (VO), this is because there is an attentional focus or spotlight that can be moved independently of eye movements. This spotlight is responsible for detailed analysis; objects falling within its focus receive enhanced perceptual processing. However, the spotlight cannot process every object in the image at once because the cognitive resources it demands are limited. Disengaging the focus from one location, moving the position of the focus in the visual field, and engaging the focus on a new location each require time and effort. Consequently, performance is expected to be best on valid cue trials, because the spotlight has been given a head start to move to the target location before the target actually appears. When there is no information about where to put the attentional focus (neutral trials)—or worse, incorrect information (invalid trials)—performance suffers because the attentional focus has to be disengaged from its location of current activity, moved to the location of the source of change, and reengaged on the new object.

Visual Search

Another aspect of attention is the ability to search for certain objects or attributes that are presented among other task-irrelevant objects or attributes. Visual search involves discriminating the presence versus the absence of a particular target item among a varying number of nontarget items (often called "distractors"). This task requires the ability to distinguish between targets and distractors, as well as the ability to deal with spatial uncertainty, multiple items, and displays that occupy large areas of visual space. Participants make a speeded response to indicate the presence or absence of the target on each trail. Again, response time and/or accuracy can be measured. The most important measure, however, is RT slope, which is a summary measure of the increase in task difficulty as a function of the total number of items in the display.

Previous research has revealed two broad patterns of performance (e.g., Treisman & Gelade, 1980). When targets and distractors differ by an easily discriminable feature such as brightness, color, size, or orientation, RT slopes are small or even zero. When targets and distractors are not easily discriminable or differ by a conjunction of features (e.g., a particular combination of brightness and orientation), RT slope is relatively large.

A popular interpretation of these results comes from feature integration theory (FIT; Treisman & Gelade, 1980). This theory proposes that visual features such as brightness and orientation are initially registered in separate topographically organized regions of the brain. Consequently, information from remote brain regions must be brought together (integrated) to determine that a particular conjunction of features all share the same location or belong to the same object. FIT proposes the existence of a master map of spatial locations to which all feature maps have access. However, the binding together of different features at one location is a serial operation that can only be performed in relatively small regions at a time (perhaps as small as that occupied by one object).

Thus, according to FIT, RT slopes in conjunction search are high because the effortful feature integration operation must be performed for each item in the display until the target is found. RT slopes in feature search, on the other hand, are low because targets can be identified on the basis of unique activity in a single feature map. No linkage between different feature maps is required and so display size is unimportant. Although FIT has undergone several modifications since its origin (Treisman, 1988; Treisman & Gormican, 1988; Treisman & Sato, 1990), it is now widely accepted that targets defined by conjunctions demand more attentional processing than those defined by features (see Bundesun, 1990; Duncan & Humphreys, 1989; Wolfe, 1994).

Visual Enumeration

A third component of attention is the ability to register the presence of two or more distinct items in a display. Visual enumeration is the term given to the ability to specify the number of target items in a spatial array. Like visual search, enumeration involves the ability to deal with multiple-item displays that cover extended areas. However, unlike visual search, participants must register the presence of every single target, not just the first they see. In order to avoid missing targets or enumerating them more than once, targets must be kept distinct from one another. This process is referred to as "individuation."

Typically, there are two patterns of response in tasks of this kind. When there are only a small number of targets (up to three to five for most adults), the error rate is minimal and the increase in RT with each additional item (the slope) is relatively shallow (40–100 milliseconds/item). When there are larger numbers (five or more) the error rate grows rapidly and the RT slope is much larger (250–300 milliseconds/item). "Subitizing" is the term given to the cognitive processes involved when the slope is shallow, and thus the "subitizing range" is the range over which this shallow slope remains linear. "Counting" is the term applied to the cognitive processes involved when the slopes are steeper, and the "counting range" refers to the numbers of items that are beyond the elbow in the RT function.

Interestingly, subitizing only occurs in some situations. Participants can subitize complex objects (i.e., with multiple contours) of varying sizes; they can subitize O targets in X distractors, and items of one color or orientation amid a variety of distractor items of other colors or orientations. However, when spatial attention is required to differentiate the target item as a whole from its background (e.g., the enumeration of nested concentric items) or to distinguish the target from distractors (e.g., the enumeration of O's in Q's, items connected by a line, or items with a particular conjunction of orientation and color), then subitizing does not occur (Trick & Pylyshyn, 1993). In these cases, the discontinuity in the RT function is absent; RT slopes are uniformly high throughout the number range, as if the more effortful counting process were used for both large and small numbers of items.

From this, Trick and Pylyshyn (1994a) inferred that subitizing is performed by a preattentive mechanism that individuates and selects a small number of distinctive items for further processing (Pylyshyn, 1989). This preattentive mechanism can be used for enumeration when the items to be enumerated are preattentively discriminable from distractors (Trick & Pylyshyn, 1994a), provided that the number of items does not exceed the limited number of internal reference tokens. When attention is required to discern individual items, either because they are spatially overlapping or not sufficiently distinct from distractors, or when the number of items exceeds the number of preattentive reference tokens, enumeration requires attention. The counting process therefore involves moving an attentional focus from location to location, using and reusing the same limited number of reference tokens at successive locations.

WHAT DEVELOPS?

Armed with this range of attentional measures, constructs, and theories, it makes sense to ask the question "What is developing?" when performance changes over the lifespan.

Developmental Theories

According to both the expertise and the speed of processing theories, RT in each of these tasks should vary in a U-shaped fashion over the lifespan. However, the reason for the U shape is very different for the two views. The speed of processing view makes this prediction because each task taps into a common set of cognitive operations—such as sensory registration, perceptual identification of shapes, response selection, and response execution—that are subject to slowing. The expertise view holds that increasing amounts of practice in childhood, together with the "use it or lose it" principle in old age, account for the U-shaped trend.

The two views differ in their predictions about the lifespan patterns for measures that are specifically attentional, for example, the RT difference between valid and invalid cues in covert orienting, the RT slope in visual search, or the subitizing and counting slopes in visual enumeration. The speed of processing view would contend that each of these measures should show a U-shaped function over the lifespan, since each involves neural processing of the sort that is speeded and slowed by developmental processes. The expertise view, on the other hand, permits more diversity: Some of the measures may not change at all over the lifespan (e.g., if they are tapping into operations that are not changed with practice and use); others may show improvement even into old age (e.g., if they reflect operations that are in consistent use throughout life); and others may show the familiar U shape (e.g., if the operations are exercised most vigorously in young adulthood).

Attention Theories

The three theories of attention we have summarized provide for a large number of theoretical constructs. These theories, however, are for the most part silent on the issue of development. This has given us opportunities to consider the possible lifespan course for each of them. In some cases, it is not too difficult to make a plausible conjecture based on other (non-developmental) characteristics that are claimed for the construct by the theory. For example, if a theory proposes that some operation is "low level" and therefore impervious to strategy and intention on the part of the observer, then it is tempting to hypothesize that this operation will show little developmental change. For the majority of the proposed attentional constructs, however, the question of developmental change is still open. Consequently, lifespan data can be used to evaluate the plausibility of the theories.

RESULTS OF LIFESPAN STUDIES

In the three studies described below we compared participants sampled from five different age groups with mean ages of 6, 8, 10, 22, and 72 years. For each task participants responded by pressing one of two keys. Their instructions were always to respond as quickly as they could, without sacrificing accuracy. These instructions were understood uniformly across the age groups, as shown by the levels of response accuracy. As a result, we will focus our discussion on the RT data, although it should be borne in mind that the patterns discussed were also always evident in the accuracy data.

Covert Orienting

Both theory and research point to an important distinction between orienting that is elicited by a *stimulus* cue (usually abrupt luminance transients at the location to be attended) and an *information* cue (typically arrows or digits at the center of gaze that refer to predesignated locations). Stimulus-induced shifts are often said to be reflexive because they are not easily influenced by higher level goals such as voluntary shifts in attention (Jonides, 1981; Jonides & Yantis, 1988; Muller & Rabbitt, 1989; Nakayama & Mackeben, 1989; Yantis & Jonides, 1984, 1990). Moreover, stimulus-driven shifts generally result in rapid effects of a short duration, whereas information cues produce effects that are slower to emerge and longer lasting (Jonides, 1981; Muller & Rabbitt, 1989; Nakayama & Mackeben, 1989; Posner & Cohen, 1984). These theoretical and empirical distinctions suggest that there should be greater change over the lifespan for stimulus-driven than for information-based orienting.

Consequently, Brodeur and Enns (in press) compared orienting to the two cues over a range of cue–target intervals from 133 to 800 milliseconds. Participants were instructed to press one key if the target was an O and another if the target was an X, and targets were centered in one of four locations: 2.0° left, 2.0° right, 6.0° left, or 6.0° right of fixation. Targets were preceded by 50-millisecond cues: stimulus cues in one condition and information cues in another. The stimulus cue was a small black disk that could appear at fixation (neutral cue) or at one of four target locations. The information cue was either an equal sign (neutral cue) or arrows pointing left or right. The cues were valid in 20% of the trials for stimulus cues (i.e., entirely nonpredictive), as compared to 80% of the trials for information cues (i.e., highly predictive).

Participants in both conditions were instructed to keep their eyes at fixation throughout the trial sequence and to blink, when necessary, between trials. Eye movements were monitored with a video camera. Participants in the stimulus-cue task were warned that there would be a flash of light before the target (the cue), but they were told to ignore it. In contrast, participants in the information cue condition were told to use the arrow cues as a very helpful indicator of the target's likely location.

The results indicated that stimulus-driven covert orienting undergoes relatively minor developmental change over the lifespan, as shown in Figure 4.1. All age groups showed an orienting effect, which diminished at longer intervals. This is consistent with previous reports made separately for children (Akhtar & Enns, 1989; Enns & Brodeur, 1989) and senior adults

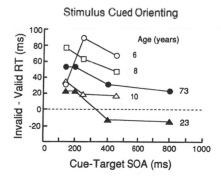

FIGURE 4.1. Orienting effects (invalid RT minus valid RT) in the stimulus-cuing condition of the covert orienting study. Children were tested at the three cue–target intervals of 133, 250, and 450 milliseconds; the adults were tested at the four cue–target intervals of 133, 200, 400, and 800 milliseconds (SOA = stimulus onset asynchrony). Adapted from Brodeur and Enns (in press).

(Hartley, Kieley, & Slabach, 1990; Hoyer & Familant, 1987; Madden, 1990). The young adults showed less orienting than the other groups did, perhaps because they were best able to follow the instructions to ignore the stimulus cues.

There were larger age-related changes for information cues. The young adult group demonstrated the most consistent orienting effects across the temporal intervals, as shown in Figure 4.2. By comparison, all three groups of children showed strong effects at short intervals with marked decreases in the effects after 200 milliseconds. Senior adults were different again, showing an information cue orienting effect only at the longest interval.

These results concur with those from previous studies on information cues. Children have often been reported to have difficulty sustaining strategic aspects of attention over time (e.g., Kupietz & Richardson, 1978), and senior adults have previously been shown to be slower in the use of information cues for spatial orienting (e.g., Hartley et al., 1990; Hoyer & Familant, 1987). However, contrary to theories that appeal to similar mechanisms for the reduced levels of performance at the beginning and end of life (e.g., cognitive slowing; see Kail, 1990, and Salthouse, 1985), these results suggest different underlying mechanisms. Children were able to make use of the information cue very rapidly (i.e., at least by 150 milliseconds), but they clearly had difficulty sustaining their attention voluntarily in the cued location. In contrast, older adults were simply unable to respond very quickly to the cue. A theory premised on a common mechanism for U-shaped age changes in information-based orienting would have difficulty accounting for the differences observed here.

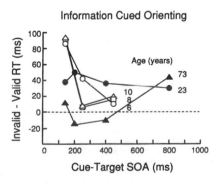

FIGURE 4.2. Orienting effects (invalid RT minus valid RT) in the information-cueing condition of the covert orienting study. Children were tested at the three cue–target intervals of 133, 250, and 450 milliseconds; the adults were tested at the four cue–target intervals of 133, 200, 400, and 800 milliseconds. Adapted from Brodeur and Enns (in press).

A second experiment looked more closely at the interaction between the two types of orienting. Stimulus and information cues were presented together in the same trial in the following sequence. An information cue was presented for 50 milliseconds upon the offset of the fixation marker. After a variable interval (140, 400 or 800 milliseconds), a stimulus cue was presented. The stimulus cue-to-target interval was a constant 133 milliseconds. Participants were instructed to use the information cue, as in the first experiment, and told that there would also be a task-irrelevant flash (the stimulus cue) on each trial.

Although the design and associated data in this experiment were complex, there were three clear findings. First, the presence of a neutral stimulus cue at a nontarget location (fixation) eliminated any of the effects of an information cue arrow for all participants. This suggests that the location of an abrupt stimulus cue can alter voluntary orienting for subjects of all ages. This effect can be thought of as akin to the reflexive orienting produced by an unexpected event (e.g., a bird or projectile in the periphery) during the performance of a task that requires voluntary concentration (e.g., a cognitive task such as reading or having a conversation).

Second, although stimulus-cuing effects were similar to those in the first experiment, information-cuing effects were larger, to the extent that all the age-related differences in information cuing seen previously disappeared. This suggests that stimulus cues can serve to prime or tune voluntary attentional mechanisms in some way, which can help compensate for any age related deficits. We speculate that it is the arousal properties of the abrupt cue onset that contribute to this finding.

Third, only young adults seem capable of at least partially discounting the information cue when the stimulus cue was valid. This is consistent with research involving other attention paradigm, showing young adults to be most flexible and adaptive in their approach to a task (e.g., Enns & Girgus, 1985; Guttentag, 1989; McDowd & Craik, 1988). In everyday terms it might be related to the ability to "stay on task" in the face of disruptive and unexpected visual events.

Visual Search

Two findings are well established in regard to this aspect of attention. One is that there is a U-shaped pattern of performance over the lifespan: Visual search speed improves in childhood and declines again in old age. The second finding is that in conjunction search tasks this pattern is true of both baseline RT (intercepts of the search function over display size) and the increase in RT with display size (RT slope). When feature search has been tested it seems only to be true of baseline RT (Plude et al., 1994). RT slopes in feature search tasks are almost flat for children as young as

5–6 years of age and in seniors as old as 80 years. This suggests minimally that not all aspects of the search task are subject to the same developmental limitations.

We considered the possibility that these age-related changes in RT slope in conjunction search might originate from a number of sources, including changes in peripheral acuity, eye movement speed, feature integration ability, attentional filtering of distractors, movement of the attentional focus, or responses to spatial uncertainty. In order to determine which, if any, of these factors were important, observers were tested on three variations of a search task (Trick & Enns, in press). In the first condition (Fixed Location — No Distractors) all uncertainty about the location of the target was eliminated. A single item always appeared at the center of the display, and observers indicated as rapidly as possible whether it was the target or not. If conjunction search was relatively more difficult than feature search for some age groups, it would suggest a fundamental difficulty in feature integration for that age group.

In a second task we added location uncertainty (Random Location — No Distractors). The single item now appeared in random locations anywhere in the display area, and observers judged whether it was the target or not. Two questions were of interest. First, did the addition of spatial uncertainty and increased foveal eccentricity influence any age groups disproportionately? Such a result would point to a fundamental difficulty in either peripheral acuity and/or moving attention to a new location in the visual field. Second, was the relationship between conjunction and feature search any different across ages in this task than the previous one? If so, it would suggest that the difficulty of feature integration for that age group was only observed when spatial attention was not already focused on the target location.

In the third task we added varying numbers of distractor items to the displays (Random Location — Distractors). The task was identical to the previous one except there were now an additional 1, 9, or 17 distractor items randomly positioned in the display on target-present trials. If the mere presence of distractors hindered search selectively for some age groups, it would indicate difficulty in ignoring items that were competing for attention. Furthermore, as the number of distractors increased, if conjunction search became disproportionately more difficult than feature search for some age groups, it would suggest a problem specific to voluntary movements of attention from one search item to another.

For all search tasks, participants were given the task of indicating the presence or absence of the same target — a dark outline circle. In feature search the distractors were randomly divided between light-gray outline circles and squares, making the target distinctive on the basis of brightness alone. In conjunction search the distractors were randomly divided between light-gray outline circles and dark-gray outline squares, making the target distinctive on the basis of a particular combination of brightness and shape.

The results from the three tasks are presented in Figures 4.3, 4.4, and 4.5. We found no evidence that the efficiency of feature integration changed with age. When a single item was presented at a fixed location in the display (Figure 4.3), conjunction search was indeed more difficult than feature search but the age of the observer had no effect on the degree of difficulty. Similarly, when a single item was presented at a random location, conjunction search was slower than feature search by approximately the same amount, and there was no age-related change in this difference.

Moreover, there was no evidence that age affected the efficiency of moving the attentional focus to a single display item. Responding to a single item in a random location was slower than responding to an item at a fixed location for all observers, but age played no role in this difference. This is an important finding because it rules out age differences in peripheral acuity (Akhtar, 1990), simple eye movement speed (Miller, 1973), and reflexive orienting to new stimuli (Enns & Brodeur, 1989) as sources for the age effects in search. At least such age differences are not evident when the search task involved responding to a single item in an otherwise empty display field.

In fact, the age differences in performance only emerged when there was more than one item in the display. There were two aspects to this effect. The first was evident only in children. We compared baseline performance in the Random Location—Distractor task (i.e., display size = 2) with performance in the Random Location—No Distractor task, as shown in Figure 4.4. The presence of a single distractor interfered markedly

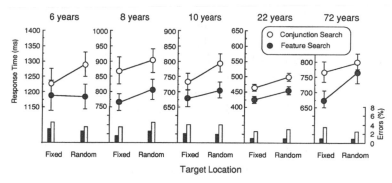

FIGURE 4.3. Mean correct RT and percentage errors in the two No Distractors search tasks. Bars represent standard errors of the mean. Adapted from Trick and Enns (in press).

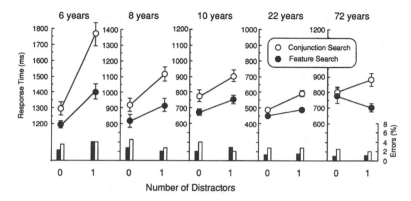

FIGURE 4.4. Mean correct RT and percentage errors in the Random Location–No Distractors task and the Random Location–One Distractor search task. Bars represent standard errors of the mean. Adapted from Trick and Enns (in press).

in the performance of the youngest children, particularly for conjunctions, and this type of interference decreased with age. This effect was not evident in senior adults.

This result thus reflects the difficulty children have in selecting a target from other candidate stimuli. Previous research suggests that children have trouble in this regard, even when targets appear at a predictable foveal location (see Enns, 1990, for a review). In contrast, senior adults are similar to young adults in their ability to ignore distractors in such tasks; this would explain why the size of the interference diminished with age (see Plude et al., 1994, for a review).

The second effect that emerged when distractor items were presented was apparent in both children and senior adults: the large RT slope in the conjunction search task shown in Figure 4.5. We attribute this slope effect to a difficulty in voluntary movements of attention from item to item. This conclusion is warranted because we were able to rule out differences in the processes of feature integration as well as in the processes involved in moving attention to a single item in a visual display. Both of these are ordinarily valid candidate mechanisms for explaining slope differences in conjunction search.

Visual Enumeration

How might subitizing and counting RT slopes be expected to change with age? Subitizing involves registering the targets preattentively as discrete items, individuating them, and selecting the appropriate number name response (Trick & Pylyshyn, 1994a). With the exception of response selec-

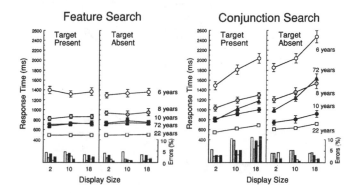

FIGURE 4.5. Mean correct RT and percentage errors in the Random Location–Distractor search task. The number of display items (Display Size) was varied randomly between 2, 10, and 18 in both features and conjunction search tasks. Bars represent standard errors of the mean. Adapted from Trick and Enns (in press).

tion, most of the current literature suggests that these processes change little with age. For example, visual search for simple features is comparable in children, senior adults, and young adults (see the previous study and Plude et al., 1994), and even very young infants can distinguish between two and three items (e.g., Starkey & Cooper, 1980; van Loosbroek & Smitsman, 1990). Therefore, the reported decline in the subitizing slope during childhood (Chi & Klahr, 1975; Svenson & Sjoberg, 1978) probably reflects improving efficiency in retrieving number names from memory and matching them to individuated items in order to select a response. Once the process of retrieving number names from memory is overlearned, however, there is no reason to expect it to deteriorate with normal aging and consequently no reason to expect the subitizing slope to increase again for senior adults. Thus, the subitizing slope should decline with age to adulthood and then stabilize.

In contrast, the counting process involves a number of operations in addition to those required for subitizing, including moving the attentional focus from item to item. The findings of the previous two studies would thus predict that counting slopes should be higher for both elderly subjects and children than they would be for young adults.

We investigated enumeration with a number discrimination task (Trick, Enns, & Brodeur, 1996). In each condition, random arrangements of one of two alternative numbers had to be discriminated by the observers: 1 versus 2; 3 versus 4; 6 versus 7; and 8 versus 9. The order of conditions was counterbalanced across observers.

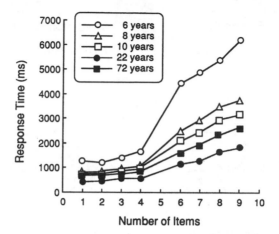

FIGURE 4.6. Mean correct RT in the number discrimination task as a function of the number of items and age of the subjects. Adapted from Trick, Enns, and Brodeur (1996). Copyright 1996 by the American Psychological Association. Adapted by permission.

RTs are shown in Figure 4.6 and RT slopes for the subitizing and counting ranges are presented in Table 4.1. The data revealed a different pattern over the lifespan for numbers in the subitizing range (one to four items) versus those in the counting range (six to nine items). The RT slope in the small number range decreased monotonically with age between 6 and 22 years and then did not decline significantly thereafter. In fact, the 72-year age group had the smallest slope estimates of all. This might be expected if the process that was changing with age involved matching individuated display items with number names retrieved from memory. Once this process becomes automatic, there would be no reason to expect it to deteriorate with age.

TABLE 4.1. Mean RT Slopes (Milliseconds per Additional Item) in the Number Discrimination Task

	Number of items	
Age (years)	1–4 range	6–9 range
6	159 (48)	547 (80)
8	106 (24)	438 (56)
10	85 (12)	399 (29)
22	62 (7)	260 (32)
72	51 (11)	354 (26)

Note. Standard error of the mean in parentheses.

In contrast, RT slopes in the large number range declined into young adulthood but then increased again in old age. Given that the position of the attentional focus has been shown to be important in the counting range (Trick & Pylyshyn, 1994b) and that other studies have shown children and elderly subjects to be less efficient at shifting attention (see the previous two subsections and Plude et al., 1994), it seems likely that attentional factors are responsible for this change. Though the counting process involves many other operations, such as storing and retrieving information from short-term memory and performing addition, attentional factors logically precede these operations. Therefore, it is parsimonious to conclude that voluntary control over spatial attention is a primary candidate for the U-shaped lifespan trend in counting slopes.

CONCLUSIONS

Implications for Theories of Development

It appears that the highly touted U-shaped pattern of performance over the lifespan accurately describes total response time and accuracy in our tasks but does not account for measures of performance that are specifically attentional.

Why is there a discrepancy between measures of overall task performance and finer grained measures of attention? We think the answer lies in the observation that a measure of overall task performance, in even the simplest of tasks, involves influential cognitive components that do indeed follow the U-shaped pattern predicted by both expertise-based and speed of processing theories. However, these components serve to obscure most of the theoretically interesting attentional effects.

For example, most of the response time measures reflect cognitive operations that are not of interest to the visual attention theorist. This would include the target identification stage, the response decision stage, and the response execution stage. In the case of visual search, these components are reflected in the baseline RT (intercept). The slope of the RT function over display size reflects the unique contribution of the increasing number of display items. If there is a measurable slope (and there is in virtually every search task we have ever seen) and this slope does not change with age despite large changes in baseline RT, then one is compelled to conclude that it reflects a cognitive operation that does not wax or wane over the lifespan. Exclusive reliance on overall response time would make it impossible to investigate the changes unique to attention. Instead, finer grained analysis is required.

The studies reported in this chapter employ measures useful for investigating age-related changes in the components of attention. We found that of our two measures of covert orienting, one of them changes very little with age (stimulus-cued orienting) whereas the other changes a great deal (information-based orienting). Furthermore, even the age changes in this latter case were not unidimensional over the lifespan. Children had more difficulty than young adults in sustaining their attention voluntarily to a cued location, whereas senior adults needed more time than did young adults to take advantage of the cue.

In visual search we found that targets defined by simple features showed no age-related change whereas search for conjunction-defined targets showed a U-shaped pattern. Closer examination of several possible reasons underlying this pattern pointed to a factor that appears to have much in common with information-based orienting. In visual search this manifested itself as a U-shaped trend in the ability to voluntarily shift attention among multiple items.

For visual enumeration we again found a dissociation for separate cognitive components. The enumeration of small numbers of items showed a monotonically improving trend even into old age, whereas the enumeration of larger numbers showed a U-shaped pattern. Once again, it appears that this pattern can be traced to difficulties directing the spatial focus of attention among multiple objects.

This diversity of lifespan patterns among components of visual attention can be understood from either an expertise or a speed of processing theory perspective, but it certainly complicates research in both areas. For example, for the expertise theory, it now becomes important to understand how factors of practice and knowledge preserve some aspects of attention while other aspects deteriorate. For the speed of processing view, it becomes important to understand why some cognitive operations are impervious to factors influencing neural conduction rates and conduction fidelity. Are different brain regions responsible for different attentional components? Do development and aging influence the neural speed and fidelity of these brain regions differentially? Though no data are available, it is tantalizing to hypothesize these kinds of connections, especially given the rapid growth in understanding of the neural bases of attention (e.g., Posner & Raichle, 1994; Zeki, 1994).

Implications for Theories of Attention

How do these lifespan data constrain theories of attention? Let us first consider feature integration theory (FIT; Treisman & Gelade, 1980), which proposes that RT slopes in conjunction search tasks reflect the incremental time associated with integrating visual features one item at a time. Furthermore, the initial location of the focus of attention should be critical for predicting performance, because features can only be integrated once attention is focused on the location of visual features in question. If this were true, then the difference between feature and conjunction search should have been larger in our Random Location task than in our Fixed Location task. The data did not support this prediction. This result, taken together with the failure to find age differences in feature integration itself, suggests that the mechanisms emphasized by FIT do not play a large role in age related trends in visual search. This should also lead researchers to question the degree to which feature integration is a "high-level" cognitive operation.

The implications for Posner's (1980) visual orienting (VO) theory are less specific. According to VO theory, conjunction search is less efficient than feature search because the target item does not trigger reflexive orienting mechanisms. As a consequence, observers must intentionally guide the spotlight of attention from item to item. This involves repeated uses of the *disengage, move,* and *engage* operations proposed by Posner and colleagues (Posner & Raichle, 1994; Posner & Petersen, 1990). The present studies suggest that the youngest and oldest participants had difficulty moving their attentional focus systematically through other items though they are capable of moving the focus in response to stimulus and information cues.

This difficulty could stem from any or all of Posner's three operations, which in itself suggests promising avenues for future research. For example, the *disengage* operation could be studied directly by using search tasks in which there are variable temporal gaps between the offset of a currently attended stimulus and the onset of a stimulus to be attended (Fisher & Breitmeyer, 1987; Kingstone & Klein, 1993). Similarly, the *move* operation could be studied by manipulating the spacing and configuration of items in the display. Finally, the *engage* operation could be tested by comparing psychometric functions of visual acuity in regions of the display that were either attended or not attended. Some researchers have already begun to speculate on which subset of the three attention-orienting components are at issue when age differences are found, but at this point the directly relevant research has yet to be done.

REFERENCES

Akhtar, N. (1990). Peripheral vision in young children: Implications for the study of visual attention. In J. T. Enns (Ed.), *The development of attention: Research and theory* (pp. 139–158). Amsterdam: Elsevier.

Akhtar, N., & Enns, J. T. (1989). Relations between covert orienting and filtering in the development of visual attention. *Journal of Experimental Child Psychology, 48,* 315–334.

Brodeur, D., & Enns, J. T. (in press). Covert visual orienting across the lifespan. *Canadian Journal of Experimental Psychology.*

Bundesun, C. (1990). A theory of visual attention. *Psychological Review, 97,* 523–547.

Chi, M. (1977). Age differences in the speed of processing: A critique. *Developmental Psychology, 13,* 543–544.

Chi, M., & Klahr, D. (1975). Span and rate of apprehension in children and adults. *Journal of Experimental Child Psychology, 19,* 434–439.

Coren, S., Ward, L., & Enns, J. (1994). *Sensation and perception* (4th ed.). New York: Harcourt Brace.

Duncan, J., & Humphreys, G. (1989). Visual search and stimulus similarity. *Psychological Review, 96,* 433–458.

Enns, J. T. (1990). Relations among components of visual attention. In J. T. Enns (Ed.), *The development of attention: Research and theory* (pp. 139–158). Amsterdam: Elsevier.

Enns, J. T. (1993). What can be learned about attention from studying its development? *Canadian Psychology, 34,* 271–281.

Enns, J. T., & Brodeur, D. A. (1989). A developmental study of covert orienting to peripheral visual cues. *Journal of Experimental Child Psychology, 48,* 171–189.

Enns, J., & Girgus, J. (1985). Developmental changes in selective and integrative visual attention. *Journal of Experimental Child Psychology, 40,* 319–337.

Fischer, B., & Breitmeyer, B. (1987). Mechanisms of visual attention revealed by saccadic eye movements. *Neuropsychologia, 25,* 73–83.

Guttentag, R. (1989). Age differences in dual task performance: Procedures, assumptions, and results. *Developmental Review, 9,* 146–170.

Hartley, A., Kieley, J., & Slabach, E. (1990). Age differences and similarities in the effects of cues and prompts. *Journal of Experimental Psychology: Human Perception and Performance, 16,* 523–537.

Hoyer, W., & Familant, M. (1987). Adult age differences in the rate of processing expectancy information. *Cognitive Development, 2,* 59–70.

Jonides, J. (1981). Voluntary versus automatic control over the mind's eye's movement. In J. Long & A. Baddeley (Eds.), *Attention and performance* (pp. 187–204). Hillsdale, NJ: Erlbaum.

Jonides, J., & Yantis, S. (1988). Uniqueness of abrupt visual onset in capturing attention. *Perception and Psychophysics, 43,* 346–354.

Kail, R. (1990). More evidence for a common, central constraint on speed of processing. In J. T. Enns (Ed.), *The development of attention: Research and theory* (pp. 159–173). Amsterdam: Elsevier.

Kail, R., & Salthouse, T. A. (1994). Processing speed as a mental capacity. *Acta Psychologica, 86,* 199–225.

Kingstone, A., & Klein, R. (1993). Visual offsets facilitate saccadic latency: Does predisengagement of visuospatial attention mediate this gap effect? *Journal of Experimental Psychology: Human Perception and Performance, 19,* 1251–1265.

Kupietz, S., & Richardson, E. (1978). Children's vigilance performance and inattentiveness in the classroom. *Journal of Child Psychology and Psychiatry, 19,* 145–154.

Madden, D. (1990). Adult age differences in the time course of visual attention. *Gerontology, 45,* 9–16.

McDowd, J., & Craik, F. (1988). Effects of aging and task difficulty on divided attention performance. *Journal of Experimental Psychology: Human Perception and Performance, 14,* 267–280.

Miller, L. K. (1973). Developmental differences in the field of view during covert and overt search. *Child Development, 44,* 247–252.

Muller, H., & Rabbitt, P. (1989). Reflexive and voluntary orienting of visual attention: Time course of activism and resistance to interruption. *Journal of Experimental Psychology: Human Perception and Performance, 15,* 315–330.

Nakayama, K., & Mackeben, M. (1989). Sustained and transient components of focal visual attention. *Vision Research, 29,* 1631–1647.

Plude, D., Enns, J. T., & Brodeur, D. A. (1994). The development of selective attention: A lifespan overview. *Acta Psychologica, 86,* 227–272.

Posner, M. I. (1980). Orienting of attention. *Quarterly Journal of Psychology, 32,* 3–25.

Posner, M. I., & Petersen, S. E. (1990). The attention system of the human brain. *Annual Review of Neuroscience, 13,* 25–42.

Posner, M. I., & Raichle M. E. (1994). *Images of mind.* New York: Freeman.

Posner, M. I., & Cohen, Y. (1984). Components of visual orienting. In H. Bouma & D. Bowhuis (Eds.), *Attention and performance* (pp. 531–556). Hillsdale, NJ: Erlbaum.

Pylyshyn, Z. (1989). The role of location indexes in spatial perception: A sketch of the FINST spatial-index model. *Cognition, 32,* 65–97.

Roth, C. (1983). Factors affecting developmental changes in the speed of processing. *Journal of Experimental Child Psychology, 35,* 509–528.

Salthouse, T. (1985). Speed of behavior and its implications for cognition. In J. E. Birren & K. W. Schaie (Eds.), *Handbook of the psychology of aging* (2nd ed., pp. 400–426). New York: Van Nostrand Reinhold.

Salthouse, T. (1991). *Theoretical perspectives on cognitive aging.* Hillsdale, NJ: Erlbaum.

Starkey, P., & Cooper, R. (1980). Perception of number by human infants. *Science, 210,* 1033–1035.

Svenson, O., & Sjoberg, K. (1978). Subitizing and counting processes in young children. *Scandinavian Journal of Psychology, 19,* 247–250.

Treisman, A. (1988). Features and objects: The fourteenth Bartlett memorial lecture. *Quarterly Journal of Experimental Psychology, 40A,* 201–327.

Treisman, A., & Gelade, G. (1980). A feature integration theory of attention. *Cognitive Psychology, 12,* 97–136.

Treisman, A., & Gormican, S. (1988). Feature analysis in early vision: Evidence from search asymmetries. *Psychological Review, 95,* 15–48.

Treisman, A., & Sato, S. (1990). Conjunction search revisited. *Journal of Experimental Psychology: Human Perception and Performance, 16,* 459–478.

Trick, L., & Enns, J. T. (in press). Lifespan changes in attention: The visual search task. *Cognitive Development.*

Trick, L., Enns, J. T., & Brodeur, D. A. (1996). Lifespan changes in visual enumeration: The number discrimination task. *Developmental Psychology, 32,* 925–932.

Trick, L., & Pylyshyn, Z. (1993). What enumeration studies can show us about spatial attention: Evidence for a limited capacity *preattentive* processing. *Journal of Experimental Psychology: Human Perception and Performance, 19,* 331–351.

Trick, L., & Pylyshyn, Z. (1994a). Why are small and large numbers enumerated differently? A limited capacity preattentive stage in vision. *Psychological Review, 101,* 80–102.

Trick, L., & Pylyshyn, Z. (1994b). Cueing and counting: Does the position of the attentional focus affect enumeration? *Visual Cognition, 1,* 67–100.

van Loosbroek, E., & Smitsman, A. (1990). Visual perception of numerosity in infancy. *Developmental Psychology, 26,* 911–922.

Wolfe, J. M. (1994). Guided search 2.0: A revised model of visual search. *Psychonomic Bulletin and Review, 1,* 202–238.

Yantis, S., & Jonides, J. (1984). Abrupt visual onsets and selective attention: Evidence from visual search. *Journal of Experimental Psychology: Human Perception and Performance, 10,* 601–620.

Yantis, S., & Jonides, J. (1990). Abrupt visual onsets and selective attention: Voluntary versus automatic allocation. *Journal of Experimental Psychology: Human Perception and Performance, 16,* 121–134.

Zeki, S. (1994). *A vision of the brain.* London: Blackwell.

SECTION III
INFANCY, ATTENTION, AND PSYCHOPATHOLOGY

FIVE

Attention Regulation in Infants Born at Risk

PREMATURITY AND PRENATAL COCAINE EXPOSURE

Linda C. Mayes
Marc H. Bornstein

The capacity to attend to the outside world is fundamental to infants' learning about the world, themselves, and those adults who care for them. When actively attending, infants are processing information, inviting social interactions, and observing and experiencing the effects of their own actions on the inanimate and animate environment. Prerequisite to every theory of learning and implicit in every theory of social development are states of arousal (or level of alertness) and attention. For infants and young children, concepts of arousal and attention regulation are closely related (Thoman & Ingersoll, 1989). An alert, optimally aroused state is necessary for infants' sustained attention to objects or people, and the capacity to attend in infancy has predictive validity for broader cognitive and social functions. Attention measured in infancy has been shown to relate to exploration, problem solving, and intelligence (Bornstein, 1985a, 1989a; Bornstein & Mayes, 1992; Fenson, Sapper, & Minner, 1974; Pêcheux & Lécuyer, 1983; Tamis-Lemonda & Bornstein, 1993); and the infants' capacity for sustaining an alert, attentional state supports ongoing and extended interactions with adults (Papoušek & Papoušek, 1995).

This chapter reviews studies of attentional regulatory mechanisms and relations among visual attention, information processing, and social interaction in two groups of infants at risk for central nervous system impairments: infants born prematurely and infants exposed to cocaine prenatally. These two groups were chosen because, for both, specific perinatal events make it plausible to hypothesize impairments in attentional regulation. For preterm infants, these perinatal events include the effects of respiratory distress, overall cardiovascular compromise, and complications such as intraventricular hemorrhage on those central nervous system functions serving arousal and attention regulation. In the case of prenatal cocaine exposure, the specific effects of cocaine on monoaminergic neurotransmitter systems and cocaine-related reduction in placental blood flow may both contribute to impairments in arousal and attention regulation. We first discuss the concept of attention in infancy. Next, for preterm and cocaine-exposed infants, separately, we review demographics, developmental biology, and arousal regulation and attention. Last, we consider remediation in these two at-risk conditions through environmental intervention including changes in parenting behaviors.

THE CONCEPT OF ATTENTION IN INFANTS

Attention is not a unitary process but encompasses many components including concentration or focused attention and sustained, selective, or divided attention; and attention is related to interest and varying degrees of volition. Attention involves multiple independent but interactive psychological processes (Posner & Boies, 1971) controlled by different neurological systems that are distinct but also interactive (Pribram & McGuinness, 1975). It is part reflex, part native preference, and part learned. Attention serves as a principal gauge of perceptual functioning in infancy and is a standard index of infants' state of arousal and affect. In this overview, we focus on two modes of attention: (1) selective and (2) intensive or sustained functions of attention, referring respectively to which aspects of stimuli infants direct their attention to versus how long they attend to different aspects (Bashinski, Werner, & Rudy, 1985; Berlyne, 1970; Haith, 1980). Sustained attention is presumed to involve active encoding of incoming information as is measured in habituation procedures, whereas selective attention involves orienting to stimuli and perhaps discriminating the novel from the familiar. From the neonatal period, babies both select and actively seek out certain information in their environment (Haith, 1980). Since it is not possible to attend to all stimuli at once, selectivity in attending protects the infant from being overwhelmed by multiple incoming stimuli. The balance between selective attention (as measured by latency to visual fixation) and sustained attention (as measured by duration of visual fixation toward a given stimulus) is mediated in part by stimulus properties such as complexity and in part by characteristics such as neurological maturity of the infant (Cohen, 1972, 1973). Selective and sustained attentional phases and shifts between them are also indexed by physiological measures such as heart rate (Casey & Richards, 1988; Richards, 1987; Ruff, 1988).

Much early work in studies of infancy was devoted to selective attention, that is, to what objects or aspects of objects infants preferred or found most engaging (e.g., Fantz, Fagan, & Miranda, 1975). Infants' visual preferences are in part determined by stimulus characteristics such as complexity (e.g., colors, patterns, number of perceptual modalities involved; Banks & Salapatek, 1981). Sustained attention depends on the frequency and duration of stimulus exposure and typically declines with increasing or ongoing exposure to the stimulus as incoming information is encoded. Such a decline in attention with continuous stimulus exposure in infancy defines the habituation response (Bornstein, 1985b; Cohen, 1976; Lewis, Goldberg, & Campbell, 1969; Mayes & Kessen, 1989). What mediates the habituation response is not well understood, although Sokolov (1969) proposed that the decrement in attention reflects an active, central-neurological process of constructing and comparing central representations of incoming information. Novel stimuli elicit central processes of constructing a central representation. As stimulus exposure continues and the representation increases in fidelity, the constructed representation is continuously compared to incoming information. Attention declines when the central representation sufficiently matches the external stimulus. As sustained attention declines, infants either stop attending altogether or reorient to a novel stimulus—the dual and complementary processes of habituation and novelty responsiveness. Individual differences in sustained attention, as indexed by differences in the initial length of time attending to an object, the peak length of the look, the accumulated amount of looking time toward an object, or the recovery of attention when a new object is presented (each obtained during a habituation paradigm), discriminate among populations of infants differing in risk status (Sigman, 1976; Sigman & Parmelee, 1974; Vietze, McCarthy, McQuiston, MacTurk, & Yarrow, 1983) and are moderately predictive of later childhood cognitive functioning (Bornstein & Sigman, 1986).

Arousal and arousal regulation have been incorporated in dual models of attention. The capacity to attend is directly linked to the development of control of states of sleep and wakefulness (Thoman & Ingersoll, 1989). The selective aspects of attention involve not only the physical orienting of receptors toward an object or event but also phasic alterations in central and autonomic nervous system activity (Ruff, 1988) or phasic alterations in states of arousal. Sustained attention also requires tonic maintenance of states or arousal. The relation between arousal regulation and selective and sustained attention is a ∩-shaped one, with both lower or higher states of arousal resulting in less visual fixation regardless of stimulus properties (Pribram & McGuiness, 1975; Ruff, 1988). Infants who are more easily overaroused in the face of novel stimuli will not be able either to select stimuli to attend to or to maintain a sustained attentional state. In these instances, the infant's capacity to modulate attention is impaired because of impaired arousal regulation, with the attendant implications for decreased information processing during diminished sustained attention.

In order to incorporate notions of arousal and activation into a unified model of attention, Posner and Petersen (1990) proposed three interactive attentional systems within the brain: an anterior system, a posterior system, and a vigilance network. The posterior system controls orienting to events in the external environment; the anterior system is involved in the detection of stimuli and processing of information; and the vigilance system optimizes arousal states. Each system depends on the other two for optimal functioning. For example, diminished or exaggerated arousal impairs both orienting to and selection of events necessary for the infant to attend to a novel stimulus. Similarly, the engagement or disengagement of attentional mechanisms as regulated by the posterior system gates the processing of novel stimuli by the anterior system, that is, the posterior system contributes to the ability of the anterior system to move on to another situation (Posner & Petersen, 1988). At birth, these three networks are not functionally mature, and rapid changes in function occur in the first postnatal months (Johnson, Posner, & Rothbart, 1991). For example, the latency to examine or explore an object decreases with age (Ruff, 1986a), a finding interpreted as suggesting a greater degree of arousal or ease of attaining an alert state, which in turn contributes to quicker organization of exploratory or examining responses.

Thus, attention in infants is indexed by temporal measures based on looking that include latency to explore, duration of individual looks and accumulated looking time, the rate of decrement in looking times, and the magnitude of recovery in looking time when new stimulus material is available for view. These measures are presumed to reflect interrelated processes of arousal regulation, orienting or selective attention, and sustained attention with the encoding of incoming information. Because individual differences in latencies to looking and exploration (selective attentional processes) and in duration of visual fixations (sustained attention) have their origins in part in perinatal factors, these indices are appropriate to study in preterm infants and in infants with complicated perinatal environments such as those exposed prenatally to drugs such as cocaine.

ATTENTION IN PRETERM INFANTS

Demographics of Prematurity

Approximately 10% of all newborn infants in the United States are born at a gestational age less than 37 weeks (Goldberg & Divitto, 1983, 1995). Estimates of morbidity and mortality among preterm infants are most often expressed in terms of the more readily measured birthweight and not gestational age. Between 80% and 85% of infants weighing 1,000-1,500 grams at birth survive the perinatal period, but only 50–60% of infants less than 1,000 grams do so. The accumulated evidence from several decades of study indicates that preterm infants are at higher risk than term infants for physical, emotional, social, and/or psychological impairments (Rose, 1983a; Friedman, Jacobs, & Wertmann, 1981). These risks include abnormalities in neurological development, poor physical growth, delayed or impaired intellectual development (particularly in very-low-birthweight infants), increased incidence of delayed language development, learning disabilities, and problems in conduct and socialization in later childhood and early adolescence (Caputo, Goldstein, & Taub, 1981; Goldson, 1992; Lubchenco, 1976). Among the very-low-birthweight group, the incidence of severe-to-moderate neurological sequelae is high. Approximately 11% of infants born weighing less than 1,000 grams have serious neurological problems including blindness, mental retardation, and cerebral palsy, and an additional 15% have less severe handicaps such as learning disabilities or medication-responsive seizure disorders (Goldberg & Divitto, 1983; Goldson, 1992).

The relation between prematurity and later developmental delays or physical and neurological impairments is an interactive one reflecting the degree of prematurity (e.g., gestational age, birthweight, adequacy of intrauterine growth for gestational age), related perinatal complications, changes in medical care, and quality of the postnatal environment (Goldberg & Divitto, 1995). A number of complications associated with prematurity greatly increase the risk for later physical and neurological impairments and developmental delays, and the risks for these complications further increase as infants are born at increasingly earlier gestational ages. For example, the very-low-birthweight infant is at greater risk for intraventricular hemorrhage, bronchopulmonary dysplasia, and apnea, which in turn increase the risk for a number of serious later impairments including blindness, seizures, chronic lung disease, intellectual deficits, and poor physical growth (Goldson, 1992).

Since the early 1960s, extensive changes in the medical management of the preterm infant during the neonatal period have eliminated or diminished conditions such as excessive use of oxygen, inadequate postnatal nutrition, hypothermia, and hyperbilirubinemia that were associated with severe disabilities including retrolental fibroplasia and blindness or choreoathetosis and severe neurological deficits (Bornstein & Lamb, 1992; Fitzhardinge et al., 1976). Because of these and other changes in medical management, preterm infants born in the last decade have demonstrated an overall improved outcome, including marked reductions in neonatal mortality and in the incidence of severe neurological and sensory deficits such as spastic diplegia or blindness (Horwood, Boyle, Torrence, & Sinclair, 1982). However, intellectual impairments, perceptual–motor difficulties, and specific delays in language and socialization skills remain a significant problem (Fuller, Guthrie, & Alvord, 1983; Klein, Hack, & Breslau, 1989; Largo et al., 1986), and as more very-low-birthweight infants survive, the incidence of attentional, perceptual, and cognitive dysfunctions has apparently increased (Goldson, 1992; Wallace, Escalona, McCarton-Daum, & Vaughan, 1982).

Developmental Biology of Prematurity

How the degree of prematurity, including associated perinatal complications and variations in medical management, specifically alters brain development and psychological function is not well understood. Until very recently, most studies of preterm infant outcome focused on measures such as developmental competency and cognitive performance that did not assess either specific areas of brain function or neuropsychological integrity such as arousal or attention. With these more global measures and limited understanding of how specific events and interventions affect brain development and function in prematurity, prediction of later neurodevelopmental outcome for the preterm infant has been limited. For example, even severe neurological insults that are more common in preterm infants, such as intraventricular hemorrhage, do not invariably have negative outcomes (Gardner & Karmel, 1983).

In addition to being based on a rather limited understanding of how the multiple variables influencing the preterm infant's extrauterine course interact, studies of preterm infant development are most often based on the assumption that these infants are functionally equivalent to term infants when their chronological age is corrected for degree of prematurity. In other words, an 8-week-old preterm infant born at 32 weeks of gestation is considered equivalent to a term neonate at 40 weeks of gestation in terms of neurobehavioral, motor, and perceptual development. This notion presumes that the preterm infant is simply an immature term infant who completes intrauterine development in an extrauterine environment on the same gestational timetable. Thus, scores on measures such as the Bayley Scales of Infant Development (1969, 1993) are corrected for gestational age with the assumption that such a correction in effect "normalizes" the score and allows comparison to term infants (DiPietro & Allen, 1991).

However, the preterm infant is born before many organ systems are physiologically coordinated and adapted for extrauterine life, and the preterm's extrauterine experiences and associated complications may actually alter the course and duration of subsequent developmental sequences (Gardner & Karmel, 1983; Goldberg & DiVitto, 1995), including those processes subserving the regulation of states of arousal and attention. The interventions necessary to ensure the survival of the preterm infant may act both to rearrange functional connections in brain maturation and to reorganize and redirect the development of neuropsychological capacities. This is likely true even if the preterm infant has a completely uncomplicated perinatal course. For example, early brain development is influenced by sensory stimulation (Greenough, Black, & Wallace, 1987). Preterm infants are often born as much as 10–12 weeks early and are therefore exposed to levels of environmental stimulation from which they would normally be shielded. If the sensory systems are fully functional, preterms are protected. If, however, the sensory systems are not fully functional, preterm infants may be adversely affected simply by the level of environmental stimulation, as, for example, in the neonatal intensive care unit (Thoman, 1993)

Arousal Regulation and Attention in Preterm Infants

The possibility of altered neuropsychological functions reflecting different patterns of brain organization are suggested in studies of arousal and attention regulation in preterm infants (Thoman, 1981). On measures of attentional regulation and reaction to stimuli, preterm infants show delays and deficits when compared to term infants who are seen at the same postconceptional age. Compared to term infants, preterm infants show differences in selective attention: They are overall less reactive to stimuli; they are less likely to orient to, or select, aspects of stimuli (Gardner & Karmel, 1983); and they are less likely to notice or respond to novel stimuli and spend less time exploring novel objects (Sigman & Parmelee, 1974; Rose, 1983a; Ruff, 1986a, 1988). Preterm infants frequently express visual preferences that differ from term infants seen at equivalent postconceptional ages. Preterm infants show a longer latency before visually exploring an object or stimulus as indexed by behavioral measures of visual fixation and cortical evoked potentials, and they take longer to organize and activate an exploratory response toward a novel object (Ruff, 1986b). The latency of the visually evoked cortical potential correlates with conceptional age (Umezaki & Morell, 1970). Differences in selective attention or in latencies to attend to a test stimulus also vary according to the severity of complications for preterm infants (Ruff, 1988). For example, preterm infants with intraventricular hemorrhage or respiratory distress require significantly more time to shift attention to test stimuli than do either term infants or preterm infants with no perinatal complications (Landry, Leslie, Fletcher, & Francis, 1985).

During sustained attentional states, apparent differences in visual fixations obtain between term and preterm infants. When compared to term infants at birth, 3- to 4-week-old preterm infants show longer visual fixations for both an initial look at a novel stimulus and for subsequent fixations toward the stimulus (Sigman, Kopp, Littman, & Parmelee, 1977). By the age of 4 months, no differences in visual fixation lengths are apparent between term and preterm infants, but preterm infants fail to show a novelty preference for more complex stimuli after familiarization with simple stimuli (Sigman & Parmelee, 1974). Similarly, Caron and Caron (1981) found that term infants seen four times between 12 and 15 months of age recognized the invariant feature of a previous stimulus whereas preterm infants tested at equivalent conceptional ages did not. Preterm infants also habituate less efficiently (Bornstein, 1985b; Friedman, Jacobs, & Wertmann, 1981; Kopp, Sigman, Parmelee, & Jeffrey, 1975; Sigman et al., 1977) and show apparent deficits in immediate recognition memory when compared to term infants (Rose, Gottfried, & Bridger, 1979; Rose, 1980).

The potential implications of these deficits in habituation, visual recognition memory, and novelty responsiveness is the suggestion that preterm infants are slower than conceptional age-equivalent term infants at encoding information. That is, in similar periods of sustained, intensive attention to a stimulus, preterms encode information less efficiently (Sigman, 1983). With an increased amount of time to become familiar with the object, however, preterm infants show similar novelty preferences and recovery of attention to novel information to twin infants. Preterm infants are also able to attend selectively to novel information and to encode and retrieve it, but they do so more slowly than conceptional age-equivalent term infants and require significantly more familiarization time, a difference that persists throughout the first year of life (Rose, 1983b; Rose, Feldman, McCarton, & Wolfson, 1988; Rose & Feldman, 1990).

Additional explanations for differences between preterm and conceptional age-equivalent term infants in selective attention and information encoding during sustained attention involve differences in the regulation of states of arousal. Impairments or delays in the regulation of arousal states may impede selective attention to novelty and information encoding during any sustained attentional phase and appear as an apparent delay in information processing (Sigman, 1983). There is a similar relation between visual fixation and states of arousal for preterm and term infants. However, for the preterm infant, there are differences in the range and threshold for optimal states of arousal which facilitate selective and sustained attention and information encoding (Gardner & Karmel, 1983). The preterm infant achieves an optimal arousal state less frequently than term infants do and has a more narrow range of optimal arousal for selectively attending to a stimulus and for sustaining attention.

ATTENTION AND PRENATAL COCAINE EXPOSURE

Demographics of Prenatal Cocaine Exposure

In many inner-city populations, nearly 50% of women giving birth report or test positive for cocaine use at the time of delivery (Amaro, Fried, Cabral, & Zuckerman, 1990; Osterloh & Lee, 1989). In a study of consecutively recruited women in routine prenatal care, 17% reported use of cocaine during pregnancy (Frank et al., 1988). National estimates across all socioeconomic groups suggest that 10–20% of infants are exposed to cocaine prenatally (Chasnoff, Landress, & Barrett, 1990). Most often, infants exposed prenatally to cocaine are also exposed to a number of other risk factors that may also contribute to impaired development (Mayes, 1992; Mayes, Granger, Bornstein, & Zuckerman, 1992). These include exposure to other substances of abuse including alcohol and tobacco as well as opiates, marijuana, and amphetamines. Mothers who abuse cocaine often have associated health problems including a higher incidence of HIV-positive serology with or without AIDS-related illnesses, and they have pregnancies more often complicated by preterm delivery and intrauterine growth retardation. Postnatally, infants exposed to cocaine continue to be exposed to ongoing parental substance abuse, are more often neglected and abused, and have parents with more frequent depression and higher overall stress and anxiety (Mayes, 1995). Any one of these factors may also influence the development of early arousal and attentional regulatory functions in these infants.

Developmental Biology of Prenatal Cocaine Exposure

An increasing number of studies in both human and animal models has reported potential cocaine-related teratological effects on the developing fetal brain (Dow-Edwards, 1991; Mayes, 1992; Zuckerman & Frank, 1992). Although the reports to date have been essentially inconclusive as to the presence of one or more cocaine-specific effects or to critical issues such as the timing or dose of exposure, findings from four domains suggest arousal and attentional regulation as a function particularly vulnerable to the teratological effects of prenatal cocaine exposure.

The first line of evidence comes from findings about the effects of cocaine or crack on developing neurotransmitter systems in fetal brain. Cocaine and crack are central nervous system stimulants that act through the monoaminergic neurotransmitter systems including dopamine, norepinephrine, and serotonin (5-hydroxytryptamine, or 5-HT) (Gawin & Ellinwood, 1988; Wise, 1984). The primary central nervous system action of cocaine occurs at the level of neurotransmitter release, reuptake, and recognition at the synaptic junction. Cocaine blocks the reuptake of dopamine, norepinephrine, and 5-HT by the presynaptic neuron (Swann, 1990), a process that is primarily responsible for the inactivation of neurotransmitters. Blocking reuptake leaves more dopamine, norepinephrine, and 5-HT available within the synaptic space (and thus in the peripheral blood as well) and results in enhanced activity of these agents in the central nervous system (Goeders & Smith, 1983) with associated physiological reactions (e.g., tachycar dia and vasoconstriction with hypertension; see Richie & Greene, 1985) and behaviors (e.g., euphoria and increased motor activity). Within the various dopamine-rich areas of the brain, certain areas of the prefrontal cortex (mesocortical system) are somewhat insensitive to the effects of cocaine on dopamine reuptake whereas other areas such as the nigrostriatal system are 100% sensitive to the effect (Hadfield & Nugent, 1983). The dopamine-rich nigrostriatal system projects from cell bodies in the substantia nigra to the corpus striatum and innervates the prefrontal cortex, nucleus accumbens, amygdala, and septum (Goeders & Smith, 1983; Shepherd, 1988). Each of these midbrain areas is involved in a number of basic neuropsychological functions including arousal and attentional modulation as well as the reinforcing properties basic to stimulant addiction in adults.

In fetal brain development, the maturation of those areas of the brain subserving arousal and attention regulation is controlled in part by dopamine, 5-HT, and norepinephrine. Each of these neurotransmitters plays a critical role in defining brain structure and neuronal formation by influencing cell proliferation, neural outgrowth, and synaptogenesis (Lauder, 1988, 1991; Mattson, 1988). Cocaine readily crosses the placenta as well as the blood–brain barrier, and brain concentrations of cocaine have been reported as high as four times that of peak plasma levels (Farrar & Kearns, 1989). Thus, cocaine may affect the formation and remodeling of brain structures through this effect on the release and metabolism of monoamines. Additionally, cocaine may influence the actual ontogeny of the neurotransmitter systems and thus again modify those areas of the brain most

involved in arousal and attention regulation. Prenatal treatment of the pregnant rat with cocaine results in an increase in serotonergic and cate-
cholaminergic fiber densities in selected brain areas involved in arousal and
attention regulation including the parietal cortex, the hippocampus, and
the cingulate cortex (Akbari & Azmitia, 1992; Akbari, Kramer, Whitaker-
Azmitia, Spear, & Azmitia, 1992. Similarly, cocaine administration to
the rat pup during the early postnatal period of synaptogenesis in the forebrain, a period roughly equivalent to the third trimester for the human
fetus, shows greatest change in brain activity in those dopamine-rich areas
of the brain (Dow-Edwards, Freed, & Milhorat, 1988; Dow-Edwards,
1989). By altering monoaminergic neurotransmitter control of brain mor-
phogenesis, chronic exposure to cocaine *in utero* may adversely affect the
regulation of arousal and attention in the developing nervous system.

The second line of evidence potentially linking prenatal cocaine exposure and arousal/attentional regulatory mechanisms derives from studies
of behavioral responses of pre- and postnatally treated animals. Several
measures of arousal, activity, and attention/learning have been examined
in prenatally and immediately postnatally cocaine-treated animals. Adult
animals exposed to cocaine prenatally show depressed hippocampal function that is involved in the consolidation of memories (Dow-Edwards,
Freed, & Fico, 1990) and is an area rich in monoaminergic neurotransmitter activity. Behaviorally, those animals exposed to cocaine in infancy
show abnormal adult behavioral responses in a number of situations including decreased activity level (Dow-Edwards, 1989), impaired associative or conditioned learning (Spear, Kirstein, & Frambes, 1989), and
diminished behavioral response to other stimulants such as amphetamines
(Dow-Edwards, 1988; Hutchings & Dow-Edwards, 1991).

The third line of evidence for an effect of cocaine on central mechanisms subserving arousal and attention regulation comes from neuropsychological studies of adults who are chronic cocaine abusers. Such
long-term cocaine abuse is reportedly associated with impairments in
memory and attention. Twenty cocaine abusers selected for absence of
previous learning difficulties, major Axis I disorders, or dependence on
other drugs displayed more problems in attention, concentration, and
memory retrieval when compared to age and education matched non-drug-
using controls (O'Malley, Adamse, Heaton, & Gawin, 1992). Similar findings have been reported for amphetamine abusers (Rylander, 1969), a drug
with central nervous system effects comparable to those of cocaine.

Finally, the effect of cocaine on fetal development may be expressed
through the norepinephrine-related effects of cocaine on vascular tone.
These consist of decreased uteroplacental blood flow, severe uteroplacental
insufficiency (acute and chronic), maternal hypertension, and fetal
vasoconstriction (Moore, Sorg, Miller, Key, & Resnik, 1986; Woods,

Plessinger, & Clark, 1987), in turn resulting in a relative state of fetal hypoxia. The effect of cocaine use on placental blood flow probably contributes to the adverse relation between cocaine and fetal growth (low birthweight, microcephaly, and intrauterine growth retardation) reported now by several investigators (Fulroth, Phillips, & Durand, 1989; Hadeed & Siegel, 1989; MacGregor, Keith, Bachicha, J. A., & Chasnoff, 1987; Mayes, Granger, Frank, Bornstein, & Schottenfeld, 1993; Oro & Dixon, 1987; Ryan, Ehrlich, & Finnegan, 1987). Infants whose intrauterine growth was retarded from multiple causes show persistent problems with irritability and distractibility well into the first year of life (Watt & Strongman, 1985; Watt, 1987). Also, because of the effect of cocaine on overall adult nutrition, compliance with prenatal care, and the usual association between cocaine use and use of other drugs such as alcohol, tobacco, and opiates (Frank et al., 1988; Amaro, Zuckerman, & Cabral, 1989), women using cocaine while pregnant are in an overall poorer state of health, which in turn increases the risk of impaired fetal outcome and intrauterine growth retardation.

Attention and Arousal Regulation in Prenatally Cocaine-Exposed Infants

Behavioral and cognitive outcome measures beyond the neonatal period in studies of children exposed to cocaine prenatally have for the most part utilized general measures of developmental competency (Mayes, 1996), and few have examined arousal regulation or selective and sustained attention per se. On general measures of developmental competency, such as the Bayley Scales of Infant Development (1969) that index information processing and indirectly attention, few differences are apparent between cocaine and non-cocaine exposed infants (Chasnoff, Griffith, Freier, & Murray, 1992). In older babies, however, it has been reported that, despite no apparent differences on either motor or mental indices on the Bayley Scales (1969), cocaine-exposed 24-month-olds appear to have more difficulty attending to several objects at the same time and in structuring an approach to a nonfamiliar task on their own in the context of the developmental assessment (Hawley & Disney, 1992).

In the few studies examining functional components of attention in prenatally cocaine-exposed infants, impairments have been reported in startle responsivity and reactivity to novelty as indices of arousal regulation and in habituation and recognition memory as processes that involve both selective and sustained attention. Anday, Cohen, Kelley, and Leitner (1989) reported that cocaine-exposed newborns were more reactive to reflex-eliciting stimuli as well as to specific auditory stimuli. In the neonatal period, findings of neurobehavioral impairments as measured by the Brazelton Neonatal Behavioral Assessment Scales (NBAS) have been inconsistent. Chasnoff, Griffith, MacGregor, Dirkes, and Burns (1989) found impairments of orientation, motor, and state regulatory behaviors on the NBAS. In contrast, Coles, Platzman, Smith, James, and Falek (1992) reported that NBAS scores fell within a clinically normal range regardless of cocaine or alcohol exposure, but she did not examine the habituation cluster for all infants. Eisen et al. (1990), studying neonates who were urine screen positive only for cocaine at birth and whose mothers denied opiate use, found significant deficits in cocaine-exposed infants in habituation performance as assessed by the NBAS. Similar findings were reported by Mayes and colleagues (1993). Impairments in habituation in the neonatal period likely reflect a combination of impaired regulation of arousal states and of selective and sustained attentional processes.

Links between the dopaminergic system and attentional mechanisms that are likely to involve the habituation process (Coles & Robbins, 1989) make it plausible to hypothesize that prenatal cocaine exposure could affect the infant's early habituation performance. The habituation response in infants, in turn, provides information about aspects of sustained and selective attention (Bornstein & Mayes, 1992). Only three studies have examined habituation and attentional processes in cocaine-exposed infants after the neonatal period. Struthers and Hansen (1992) reported impaired recognition memory among cocaine- or amphetamine-exposed infants compared to a non-drug-exposed group between 7 and 8 months of age. Similarly, Alessandri, Sullivan, Imaizumi, and Lewis (1993) reported delays in novelty responsiveness and recognition memory well into the second half of the first year of life. Recognition memory tasks rely in part on habituation processes and, while measuring infant responsiveness to novel versus familiar stimuli rather than decrement of attention over time, nevertheless require an integrated capacity to attend selectively to novel information. Mayes, Bornstein, Chawarska, and Granger (1995) found that, compared to the non-drug-exposed group, infants exposed prenatally to cocaine are significantly more likely to fail to begin a habituation procedure and significantly more likely to react with irritability early in the procedure. However, the majority of infants reached the habituation criterion, and among those who did no significant differences emerged between cocaine and non-cocaine-exposed infants in habituation or in recovery to a novel stimulus. Thus, for at least a subgroup of cocaine-exposed infants, initial reactivity and selectivity toward novel stimuli appear impaired.

Findings from different perspectives point to a possible relation between prenatal cocaine exposure and impaired arousal and attentional regulation in infants in the first year. However, as a caveat, it is important to note that establishing cause–effect relations between prenatal cocaine exposure and attentional deficits is problematic given the number of additional variables that might affect vulnerability in such neurodevelopmental outcomes. In addition to a direct effect on developing monoaminergic neurotransmitter systems in fetal brain, prenatal cocaine exposure may potentially affect attentional regulation indirectly because of the general effects of cocaine on placental blood flow, fetal nutrition, and thus fetal brain growth.

Continued maternal postnatal use of cocaine affects the child's caregiving environment at two levels that may contribute to attentional regulation. Adults who are under the influence of cocaine are less able to respond adequately to their children at any given time (Bauman & Dougherty, 1983; Burns, Chethik, Burns, & Clark, 1991), and a few studies are now available detailing the specific ways in which cocaine influences parenting behaviors (Mayes, 1995). Second, the effects of cocaine on memory and attention in adults (O'Malley et al., 1992) impair the adult's ability to care for a child. More generally, because of the lifestyle adjustments necessary with cocaine use — including, for example, prostitution, crime, exposure to violence, and the overwhelming power of the addiction — the overall environment for these children is often chaotic, violent, and neglectful (Black & Mayer, 1980; Regan, Leifer, & Finnegan, 1984). Specific outcomes in children such as attentional regulation are influenced by maternal interactive style (Bornstein, 1985a; Bornstein & Tamis-LeMonda, 1990; Tamis-LeMonda & Bornstein, 1989). Similarly, the psychological/personality factors that lead an adult to substance abuse may have genetic as well as experiential implications for the fetus. For example, attention deficits or chronic affective disorders in the adult, both of which may be partially mediated by cocaine (Khantzian, 1983; Khantzian & Khantzian, 1984; Rounsaville, Weissman, Kleber, & Wilbur, 1982), are associated with genetic risks for similar disorders in the child, and these disorders, particularly depression, also impinge on the adult's capacity to care adequately for the child (Fendrick, Warner, & Weissman, 1990; Field, 1995). Because of the effects of substance abuse on maternal behavior as well as on more general environmental factors, sorting out the biological effects of prenatal cocaine exposure on development in children from effects mediated by the influence of cocaine on the caregiving environment requires detailed studies of maternal style in conjunction with infant attentional regulation and information processing.

EFFECTS OF PARENTING ENVIRONMENT ON INFANT AROUSAL AND ATTENTION

The rapid postnatal maturation of attentional systems affords a productive source of study for examining interactions between genetic and/or prenatal factors and the postnatal caregiving environment. Different amounts and types of adult intervention may have negative effects on infants' regulation of arousal and selective and sustained attention to social and nonsocial stimuli and situations. Parental activities such as pointing, demonstrating, holding an object for the child, or physically restraining the child all affect an infant's ability to sustain attention to objects (Bornstein & Tamis-LeMonda, 1990; Landry, Chapieski, & Schmidt, 1986; Tamis-LeMonda & Bornstein, 1989). Such parental behaviors appear also to contribute to the relation between attention and later cognitive performance. Bornstein (1985a; also Bornstein & Ruddy,1984; Bornstein & Tamis-LeMonda, 1989, 1990, 1994; Tamis-LeMonda & Bornstein, 1989) assessed maternal "didactics"—how mothers engage their infants' attention to properties, objects, and events in the environment. Mothers who are active in this role significantly, and independently of the contribution of attention measures, can influence their infants' cognitive development across the early years of life. More attentive and responsive parents tend to support and encourage more attentive responses from their infants. Transactionally, more attentive infants have parents who are more attentive to them and more positive in their responses: that is, infants' own attentional organization may influence parents' efforts (Bornstein, 1989a, 1989b).

For infants at risk for attentional impairments because of perinatal risks—prematurity or prenatal cocaine exposure—the parenting environment may be crucial for mitigating (or exacerbating) biological vulnerabilities. More data are available about biological–environmental interactions for preterm infants than for those exposed prenatally to cocaine. In the absence of a clear organic basis for abnormal development, such as blindness or severe motor impairments, the degree to which preterm infants develop well or poorly is in part a function of the parenting environment the baby encounters after leaving the intensive care nursery. The postnatal development of preterm infants provides extensive support for interactive or transactional processes (Goldberg & Divitto, 1995; Infant Health and Development Program, 1990; Sameroff & Chandler, 1975). Preterm babies placed in enriching supportive homes tend to do well, whereas those placed in depriving environments tend to develop more poorly (Kopp, 1983; Sameroff, 1983; Sigman & Parmelee, 1979). The preterm infant's postnatal outcome is only indirectly related to pre- and perinatal complications and is mediated by parent—child interactions, which are in turn influenced by many factors including the status of the infant at birth and the severity of the nursery course (Goldberg & Divitto, 1995; Minde, Whitelaw, Brown, & Fitzhardinge, 1983).

The attentional impairments found in preterm infants in nonsocial situations also influence parent–infant interactions. Preterm infants are generally less alert and less responsive than their term peers (Goldberg

& Divitto, 1995), and these differences are accentuated when the preterm infant has experienced a medically compromised perinatal course (Minde et al., 1983). Thus, the preterm infant is generally available for social interaction less frequently and for briefer periods of time. Limits in the perceptual and cognitive skills of preterm infants may also modify the impact of parent behaviors on the preterm infant. Field (1982) conceptualized the preterm infant as having a relatively high threshold to adult social stimulation coupled with a low tolerance for stimulation. In response to the differences in stimulation tolerance and perceptual and cognitive skills, mothers of preterm infants appear to take a more active role with their infants than do mothers of term infants; the former direct attention more (Barnard, Bee, & Hammond, 1984; Field, 1979), hold and touch more, and provide more tactile and kinesthetic stimulation (Crnic, Greenberg, Ragozin, Robinson, & Basham, 1983). These strategies in parental activity increase the amount of mutual gaze between mother and infant, and in effect structure the infants' attention (Goldberg & Divitto, 1995). In one study, by 8 months of age preterm infants engaged in mutual gaze with their parents more than did a comparison term group (Mann & Plunkett, 1992, cited in Goldberg & Divitto, 1995). Differences in parental activity also influence preterm infants' performance on novelty preference and exploration tasks (Landry,1986; Landry, Chapieski, & Schmidt, 1986; Landry, Garner, Denson, Swank, & Balwin, 1993; Rose, 1980; Sigman, 1983); more parental encouragement improves the infant's performance on exploratory tasks.

To date, no published studies have examined how prenatal cocaine exposure influences infants' capacities to respond in social interactions or whether or how possible impairments in attention-related functions, such as reactivity, affect infant behavior in social situations (Mayes, 1995). The few studies of social interactions between prenatally cocaine-exposed infants and their parents focus primarily on maternal behavior and the lack of contingent responsiveness (Burns & Burns, 1988; Burns et al., 1991). In most cases, mothers of these infants are by definition active cocaine abusers, which may influence their own ability to attend to the infant.

CONCLUSIONS

Prematurity and prenatal exposure to cocaine provide models for studies of relations among arousal regulation and attention in situations of biological risk. Even if the accumulated evidence is still scant, it seems that infants in both conditions express at least early attentional impairments but with different components of attention and with potentially different implications for later development. Preterm infants show less efficient encoding during sustained attention and longer latencies to shifting attention. In contrast, based on the few data available to date, cocaine-exposed infants may exhibit arousal regulation problems, which in turn affect their attention. If a cocaine-exposed infant is able to attend to a stimulus, differences in behaviors reflective of information processing or encoding do not seem apparent when compared to non-drug-exposed infants.

Both groups also provide models for how parenting behaviors may influence infant arousal and attention regulation and how parents alter their behaviors in response to infants' attentional characteristics. These interactions are currently more widely studied in the parents of preterms, and findings suggest that parental activity with the preterm infant may ameliorate attentional deficits seen in nonsocial situations. Whether or not the same is true for the potential arousal regulation difficulties of cocaine-exposed infants has not been explored. Both groups present models for studying factors such as degrees of medical compromise and postnatal stress that in an ancillary way diminish or augment attentional problems.

Finally, attention is also an index of central arousal regulation. Apparent problems in visual attention or in encoding information in infants born at risk may be in part a reflection of impairments in the regulation of arousal. Impairments at the level of arousal regulation will in turn influence infant capacities for both sustained and selective attention. It is possibly through this type of pathway that the detrimental effects of high-risk status on learning and social interaction may be mediated. Influencing attentional regulation through better modulation of arousal is an outcome that may be achieved in some part through shaping parenting interactions with infants. Impairments in the regulation of arousal states may have implications for later development, not necessarily in terms of overall cognitive competency, but rather in terms of attention regulation and learning difficulties.

REFERENCES

Akbari, H. M., & Azmitia, E. C. (1992). Increased tyrosine hydroxylase immunoreactivity in the rat cortex following prenatal cocaine exposure. *Developmental Brain Research, 66,* 277–281.

Akbari, H. M., Kramer, H. K., Whitaker-Azmitia, P. M., Spear, L. P., & Azmitia, E. C. (1992). Prenatal cocaine exposure disrupts the development of the serotonergic system. *Brain Research, 572,* 57–63.

Alessandri, S. M., Sullivan, M. W., Imaizumi, S., & Lewis, M. (1993). Learning and emotional responsivity in cocaine-exposed infants. *Developmental Psychology, 29,* 989–997.

Amaro H., Fried, L. E., Cabral H., & Zuckerman B. (1990). Violence during pregnancy and substance use. *American Journal of Public Health, 80,* 575–579.

Amaro, H., Zuckerman B., & Cabral H. (1989). Drug use among adolescent mothers: Profile of risk. *Pediatrics, 84,* 144–151.

Anday, E. K., Cohen, M. E., Kelley, N. E., & Leitner, D. S. (1989). Effect of in utero cocaine exposure on startle and its modification. *Developmental Pharmacology and Therapeutics, 12,* 137–145.

Banks, M. S., & Salapatek, P. (1981). Infant pattern vision: A new approach based on the contrast sensitivity function. *Journal of Experimental Child Psychology, 31,* 145.

Barnard, K. E., Bee, H. L., & Hammond, M. A. (1984). Development of changes in maternal interactions with term and preterm infants. *Infant Behavior and Development, 7,* 101–113.

Bashinski, H. S., Werner, J. S., & Rudy, J. W. (1985). Determinants of infant visual fixation: Evidence for a two-process theory. *Journal of Experimental Child Psychology, 39,* 580–598.

Bauman, P. S., & Dougherty, F. E. (1983). Drug-addicted mothers' parenting and their children's development. *International Journal of the Addictions, 18,* 291–302.

Bayley, N. (1969). *Bayley Scales of Infant Development.* New York: Psychological Corporation.

Bayley, N. (1993). *Bayley Scales of Infant Development* (2nd ed.). San Antonio: Psychological Corporation (Harcourt, Brace).

Berlyne, D. B. (1970). Attention as a problem in behavior therapy. In D. I. Mostofsky (Ed.), *Attention: Contemporary theory and analysis* (pp. 25–29). New York: Appleton-Century-Crofts.

Black, R., & Mayer, J. (1980). Parents with special problems: Alcoholism and opiate addiction. *Child Abuse and Neglect, 4,* 45–54.

Bornstein, M. H. (1985a). How infant and mother jointly contribute to developing cognitive competence in the child. *Proceedings of the National Academy of Sciences (U.S.A.), 85,* 7470–7473.

Bornstein, M. H. (1985b). Habituation as a measure of visual information processing in human infants: Summary, systemization, and synthesis. In G. Gottlieb & N. Krasnegor (Eds.), *Development of audition and vision during the first year of postnatal life: A methodological overview* (pp. 253–295). Norwood, NJ: Ablex.

Bornstein, M. H. (1989a). Stability in early mental development: From attention and information processing in infancy to language and cognition in childhood. In M. H. Bornstein & N. A. Krasnegor (Eds.), *Stability and continuity in mental development: Behavioral and biological perspectives* (pp. 147–170). Hillsdale, NJ: Erlbaum.

Bornstein, M. H. (1989b). Attention and memory. *Pediatric Annals, 18,* 317–314.

Bornstein, M. H., & Lamb, M. E. (1992). *Development in infancy: An introduction* (3rd ed.). New York: McGraw-Hill.

Bornstein, M. H., & Mayes, L. C. (1992). Taking a measure of the infant mind. In F. Kessell, M. H. Bornstein, & A. Sameroff (Eds.), *Contemporary constructions of the child: Essays in honor of William Kessen* (pp. 45–56). Hillsdale, NJ: Erlbaum.

Bornstein, M. H., & Ruddy, M. (1984). Infant attention and maternal stimulation: Prediction of cognitive and linguistic development in singletons and twins. In H. Bouma & D. Bouwhuis (Eds.), *Attention and performance* (pp. 433–445). London: Erlbaum.

Bornstein, M. H., & Sigman, M. D. (1986). Continuity of mental development from infancy. *Child Development, 57,* 251–274.

Bornstein, M. H., & Tamis-LeMonda, C. S. (1989). Maternal responsiveness and cognitive development in children. In M. H. Bornstein (Ed.), *Maternal responsiveness: Characteristics and consequences* (pp. 49–61). San Francisco: Jossey-Bass.

Bornstein, M. H., & Tamis-LeMonda, C. S. (1990). Activities and interactions of mothers and their firstborn infants in the first six months of life: Covariation, stability, continuity, correspondence, and prediction. *Child Development, 61,* 1206–1217.

Bornstein, M. H., & Tamis-LeMonda, C. S. (1994). Antecedents of information-processing skills in infants: Habituation, novelty responsiveness, and cross-modal transfer. *Infant Behavior and Development, 17,* 371–380.

Burns, W. J., & Burns, K. A. (1988). Parenting dysfunction in chemically dependent women. In I. Chasnoff (Ed.), *Drugs, alcohol, pregnancy, and parenting* (pp. 159–171). London: Kluwer.

Burns, K., Chethik, L., Burns, W. J., & Clark, R. (1991). Dyadic disturbances in cocaine-abusing mothers and their infants. *Journal of Clinical Psychology, 47,* 316–319.

Caputo, D. V., Goldstein, K. M., & Taub, H. B. (1981). The development of prematurely born children through middle childhood. In S. Friedman & M. Sigman (Eds.), *Preterm birth and psychological development* (pp. 353–368). New York: Academic Press.

Caron, A. J., & Caron, R. F. (1981). Processing of relational information as an index of infant risk. In S. L. Friedman & M. Sigman (Eds.), *Preterm birth and psychological development.* New York: Academic Press.

Caney, B. J., & Richards, J. E. (1988). Sustained visual attention in young infants measured with an adapted version of the visual preference paradigm. *Child Development, 59,* 1514–1521.

Chasnoff, I. J., Griffith, D. R., Freier, C., & Murray, J. (1992). Cocaine/poly-drug use in pregnancy: Two-year follow-up. *Pediatrics, 89,* 284–289.

Chasnoff, I, Griffith, D. R., MacGregor, S., Dirkes, K., & Burns, K. (1989). Temporal patterns of cocaine use in pregnancy. *Journal of the American Medical Association, 261,* 1741–1744.

Chasnoff, I. J., Landress, H. J., & Barrett, M. E. (1990). The prevalence of illicit drug or alcohol abuse during pregnancy and discrepancies in mandatory reporting in Pinellas County, Florida. *New England Journal of Medicine, 322,* 102–106.

Cohen, L. B. (1972). Attention-getting and attention-holding processes of infant visual preferences. *Child Development, 43,* 868–879.

Cohen, L. B. (1973). A two process model of infant visual attention. *Merrill–Palmer Quarterly, 19,* 157–180.

Cohen, L. B. (1976). Habituation of infant visual attention. In R. J. Tighe & R. N. Leaton (Eds.), *Habituation: Perspectives from child development, animal behavior, and neurophysiology* (pp. 207–238). Hillsdale, NJ: Erlbaum.

Coles, B. J., & Robbins, T. W. (1989). Effects of 6-hydroxydopamine lesions of the nucleus accumbens septi on performance of a 5-choice serial reaction time task in rats: Implications for theories of selective attention and arousal. *Behavioral Brain Research, 33,* 165–179.

Coles, C. D., Platzman, K. A., Smith, I., James, M. E., & Falek, A. (1992). Effects of cocaine and alcohol use in pregnancy on neonatal growth and neurobehavioral status. *Neurotoxicology and Teratology, 14,* 23–33.

Crnic, K. A., Greenberg, M. T., Ragozin, A. S., Robinson, N. M., & Basham, R. B. (1983). Effects of stress and social support on mothers of premature and fullterm infants. *Child Development, 54,* 209–217.

DiPietro, J. A., & Allen, M. C. (1991). Estimation of gestational age: Implications for developmental research. *Child Development, 62,* 1184–1199.

Dow-Edwards, D. (1988). Developmental effects of cocaine. *National Institute on Drug Abuse Research Monograph, 88,* 290–303.

Dow-Edwards, D. (1989). Long-term neurochemical and neurobehavioral consequences of cocaine use during pregnancy. *Annals of the New York Academy of Sciences, 562,* 280–289.

Dow-Edwards, D. (1991). Cocaine effects on fetal development: A comparison of clinical and animal research findings. *Neurotoxicology and Teratology, 13,* 347–352.

Dow-Edwards, D. L., Freed, L. A., & Fico, T. A. (1990). Structural and functional effects of prenatal cocaine exposure in adult rat brain. *Developmental Brain Research, 57,* 263–268.

Dow-Edwards, D., Freed, L. A., & Milhorat, T. H. (1988). Stimulation of brain metabolism by perinatal cocaine exposure. *Brain Research, 470,* 137–141.

Eisen, L. N., Field, T. M., Bandstra, E. S., Roberts, J. P., Morrow, C., Larson, S. K., & Steele, B. M. (1990). Perinatal cocaine effects on neonatal stress behavior and performance on the Brazelton Scale. *Pediatrics, 88,* 477–480.

Fantz, R. L., Fagan, J. F., & Miranda, S. B. (1975). Early visual selectivity. In L. B. Cohen & P. Salapatek (Eds.), *Infant perception: From sensation to cognition* (pp. 249–345). New York: Academic Press.

Farrar, H. C., & Kearns, G. L. (1989). Cocaine: Clinical pharmacology and toxicology. *Journal of Pediatrics, 115,* 665–675.

Fendrick M., Warner V., & Weissman M. (1990). Family risk factors, parental depression, and psychopathology in offspring. *Developmental Psychology, 26,* 40–50.

Fenson, L., Sapper, V., & Minner, D. G. (1974). Attention and manipulative play in the 1-year-old child. *Child Development, 45,* 757–764.

Field, T. M. (1979). Interaction patterns of preterm and fullterm infants. In T. M. Field, A. M. Sostek, S. Goldberg, & H. H. Shuman (Eds.), *Infants born at risk.* Jamaica, NY: Spectrum.

Field, T. M. (1982). Affective displays of high risk infants during early interactions. In T. M. Field & A. Fogel (Eds.), *Emotion and early interaction.* Hillsdale, NJ: Erlbaum.

Field, T. M. (1995). Psychologically depressed parents. In M. H. Bornstein (Ed.), *Handbook of parenting: Vol. 4. Applied and practical parenting* (pp. 85–100). Hillsdale, NJ: Erlbaum.

Fitzhardinge, P. M., Pape, K., Arstikaitis, M., Boyle, M., Ashby, B., Rowley, A., Netley, C., & Sawyer, P. R. (1976). Mechanical ventilation of infants less than 1501 gm birthweight: Health, growth, and neurologic sequelae. *Journal of Pediatrics, 88,* 531–541.

Frank, D. A., Zuckerman B. S., Amaro H., Aboagye K., Bauchner, H., Cabral, H., Fried, L., Hingson, R., Kayne, H., & Levenson, S. M. (1988). Cocaine use during pregnancy: Prevalence and correlates. *Pediatrics, 82,* 888–895.

Friedman, S. L., Jacobs, B. S., & Werthmann, M. W. (1981). Sensory processing in pre- and full-term infants in the neonatal period. In S. L. Friedman & M. Sigman (Eds.), *Preterm birth and psychological development* (pp. 159–178). New York: Academic Press.

Fuller, P. W., Guthrie, R. D., & Alvord, E. C. (1983). A proposed neurological basis for learning disabilities in children born prematurely. *Developmental Medicine and Child Neurology, 25,* 214–231.

Fulroth R., Phillips B., & Durand, D. J. (1989). Perinatal outcome of infants exposed to cocaine and/or heroin in utero. *American Journal of Diseases of Children, 143,* 905–910.

Gardner, J. M., & Karmel, B. Z. (1983). Attention and arousal in preterm and full-term neonates. In T. Field & A. Sostek (Eds.), *Infants born at risk: Physiological, perceptual, and cognitive processes* (pp. 69–98). New York: Grune & Stratton.

Gawin, F. H., & Ellinwood, F. H. (1988). Cocaine and other stimulants. *New England Journal of Medicine, 318,* 1173–1182.

Goeders, N. E., & Smith, J. E. (1983). Cortical dopaminergic involvement in cocaine reinforcement. *Science, 221,* 773–775.

Goldberg, S., & Divitto, B. (1983). *Born too soon: Preterm birth and early development.* San Francisco: Freeman & Cooper.

Goldberg, S., & Divitto, B. (1995). Parenting children born preterm. In M. H. Bornstein (Ed.), *Handbook of parenting: Vol. 1. Children and parenting* (pp. 209–232). Hillsdale, NJ: Erlbaum.

Goldson, E. (1992). Follow-up of low birthweight infants: A contemporary review. In M. L. Wolraich & D. Routh (Eds.), *Advances in developmental and behavioral pediatrics* (Vol. 10, pp. 159–179). London: Jessica Kingsley.

Greenough, W. T., Black, J. E., & Wallace, C. S. (1987). Experience and brain development. *Child Development, 58,* 539–559.

Hadeed, A. J., & Siegel, S. R. (1989). Maternal cocaine use during pregnancy: Effect on the newborn infant. *Pediatrics, 84,* 205–210.

Hadfield, M. G., & Nugent, E. A. (1983). Cocaine: Comparative effect on dopamine uptake in extrapyramidal and limbic systems. *Biochemical Pharmacology, 32,* 744–746.

Haith, M. M. (1980). *Rules that babies look by.* Hillsdale, NJ: Erlbaum.

Hawley, T. L., & Disney, E. R. (1992). Crack's children: The consequences of maternal cocaine abuse. *Social Policy Report: Society for Research in Child Development, 6,* 1–21.

Horwood, S. P., Boyle, M. H., Torrence, G. W., & Sinclair, J. C. (1982). Mortality and morbidity of 500–1499 gram birth weight infants live-born to residents of a defined geographic region before and after neonatal intensive care. *Pediatrics, 69,* 613–620.

Hutchings, D. E., & Dow-Edwards, D. (1991). Animal models of opiate, cocaine, and cannabis use. *Clinics in Perinatology, 18,* 1–22.

Infant Health and Development Program. (1990). Enhancing the outcomes of low-birth-weight, premature infants: A multisite, randomized trial. *Journal of the American Medical Association, 263,* 3035–3042.

Johnson, M. H., Posner, M. I., & Rothbart, M. K. (1991). Components of visual orienting in early infancy: Contingency learning, anticipatory looking and disengaging. *Journal of Cognitive Neuroscience, 3,* 335–344.

Khantzian, E. J. (1983). An extreme case of cocaine dependence and marked improvement with methylphenidate treatment. *American Journal of Psychiatry, 140,* 784–785.

Khantzian, E. J., & Khantzian, N. J. (1984). Cocaine addiction: Is there a psychological predisposition? *Psychiatric Annals, 14,* 753–759.

Klein, N., Hack, M., & Breslau, N. (1989). Children who are very low birthweight: Development and academic achievement at nine years of age. *Journal of Developmental and Behavioral Pediatrics, 10,* 32–37.

Kopp, C. B. (1983). Risk factors in development. In P. H. Mussen (Gen. Ed.), M. M. Haith & J. J. Campos (Eds.), *Handbook of child psychology: Vol. 2. Infancy and developmental psychobiology* (pp. 1081–1088). New York: Wiley.

Kopp, C. B., Sigman, M., Parmelee, A. H., & Jeffrey, W. E. (1975). Neurological organization and visual fixation in infants at 40 weeks conceptional age. *Developmental Psychobiology, 8,* 165–170.

Landry, S. H. (1986). Preterm infants' responses in early joint attention interactions. *Infant Behavior and Development, 9,* 1–14.

Landry, S. H., Chapieski, M. L., & Schmidt, M. (1986). Effects of maternal attention directing strategies on preterms' responses to toys. *Infant Behavior and Development, 9,* 257–269.

Landry, S. H., Garner, P. W., Denson, S., Swank, P. R., & Baldwin, C. (1993). Low birth weight infants' exploratory behavior at 12 and 24 months: Effects of intraventricular hemorrhage on mothers' attention directing behaviors. *Research in Developmental Disabilities, 14,* 237–249.

Landry, S. H., Leslie, N., Fletcher, J. M., & Francis, D. J. (1985). Effects of intraventricular hemorrhage on visual attention in very premature infants. *Infant Behavior and Development, 8,* 309–321.

Largo, R. H., Molinari, L., Pinto, L. C., et al. (1986). Language development of term and preterm children during the first five years of life. *Developmental Medicine and Child Neurology, 28,* 333–350.

Lauder, J. M. (1988). Neurotransmitters as morphogens. *Progress in Brain Research, 73,* 365–387.

Lauder, J. M. (1991). Neuroteratology of cocaine: Relationship to developing monamine systems. *National Institute on Drug Abuse Research Monographs, 114,* 233–247.

Lewis, M., Goldberg, S., & Campbell, H. (1969). A developmental study of information processing within the first three years of life: Response decrement to a redundant signal. *Monographs of the Society for Research in Child Development, 34*(9, Serial No. 133), 1–41.

Lubchenco, L. O. (1976). *The high risk infant*. Philadelphia: Saunders.

MacGregor, S. N., Keith, L. G., Bachicha, J. A. & Chasnoff, I. J. (1987). Cocaine use during pregnancy: Adverse perinatal outcome. *American Journal of Obstetrics and Gynecology, 157,* 686–690.

Mattson, M. P. (1988). Neurotransmitters in the regulation of neuronal cytoarchitecture. *Brain Research Reviews, 13,* 179–212.

Mayes, L. C. (1992). The effects of prenatal cocaine exposure on young children's development. *Annals of the American Academy of Political and Social Science, 521,* 11–27.

Mayes, L. C. (1995). Substance abuse and parenting. In M. H. Bornstein (Ed.)., *Handbook of parenting: Vol. 4. Applied and practical parenting* (pp. 101–126). Hillsdale, NJ: Erlbaum.

Mayes, L. C. (1996). Exposure to cocaine: Behavioral outcomes in preschool aged children. In L. Finnegan (Ed.), *Behavioral studies of drug-exposed offspring* (NIDA Technical Symposium No. 164, pp. 211–229). Washington, DC: U.S. Government Printing Office.

Mayes, L. C., Bornstein, M. H., Chawarska, K., & Granger, R. H. (1995) Habituation and developmental assessments in three month olds exposed prenatally to cocaine. *Pediatrics, 95,* 539–545.

Mayes, L. C., Granger, R. H., Bornstein, M. H., & Zuckerman, B. (1992). The problem of intrauterine cocaine exposure. *Journal of the American Medical Association, 267,* 406–408.

Mayes, L. C., Granger, R. H., Frank, M. A., Bornstein, M. & Schottenfeld, R. (1993). Neurobehavioral profiles of infants exposed to cocaine prenatally. *Pediatrics, 91,* 778–783.

Mayes, L. C., & Kessen, W. (1989). Maturational changes in measures of habituation. *Infant Behavior and Development, 12,* 437–450.

Minde, K. K., Whiltelaw, A., Brown, J., & Fitzhardinge, P. (1983). Effect of neonatal complications in premature infants on early parent–infant interactions. *Developmental Medicine and Child Neurology, 25,* 763–777.

Moore, T. R., Sorg, J., Miller, L., Key, T., & Resnik, R. (1986). Hemodynamic effects of intravenous cocaine on the pregnant ewe and fetus. *American Journal of Obstetrics and Gynecology, 155,* 883–888.

O'Malley, S., Adamse, M., Heaton, R., & Gawin, F. H. (1992). Neuropsychological impairment in chronic cocaine abuse. *American Journal of Drug and Alcohol Abuse, 18,* 131–144.

Oro, A. S., & Dixon, S. D. (1987). Perinatal cocaine and methamphetamine exposure: Maternal and neonatal correlates. *Journal of Pediatrics, 111,* 571–578.

Osterloh, J. D., & Lee, B. L. (1989). Urine drug screening in mothers and newborns. *American Journal of Diseases of Children, 143,* 791–793.

Papoušek, H., & Papoušek, M. (1995). Intuitive parenting. In M. H. Bornstein (Ed.), *Handbook of parenting: Vol. II. Biology and ecology of parenting* (pp. 117–136). Hillsdale, NJ: Erlbaum.

Pêcheux, M. G., & Lécuyer, R. (1983). Habituation rate and free exploration tempo in 4-month-old infants. *International Journal of Behavioral Development, 6,* 37–50.

Posner, M. I., & Boies, S. J. (1971). Components of attention. *Psychological Review, 78,* 391–408.

Posner, M. I., & Petersen, S. E. (1988). Structures and functions of selected attention. In T. Boll & B. Bryant (Eds.), *Master lectures of clinical neuropsychology* (pp. 173–202). Washington, DC: American Psychological Association.

Posner, M. I., & Petersen, S. E. (1990). The attention system of the human brain. *Annual Review of Neuroscience, 13,* 25–42.

Pribram, K. H., & McGuinness, D. (1975). Arousal, activation, and effort in the control of attention. *Psychological Review, 82,* 116–149.

Regan, D., Leifer, B., & Finnegan, L. (1984). The incidence of violence in the lives of pregnant drug abusing women. *National Institute on Drug Abuse Research Monograph, 49,* 330.

Richards, J. E. (1987). Infant visual sustained attention and respiratory sinus arrhythmia. *Child Development, 58,* 488–496.

Richie, J. M., & Greene, N. M. (1985). Local anesthetics. In A. G. Gilman, L. S. Goodman, T. N. Rall, & F. Murad (Eds.), *The pharmacologic basis of therapeutics* (7th ed. pp. 309–310). New York: Macmillan.

Rose, S. A. (1980). Enhancing visual recognition memory in preterm infants. *Developmental Psychology, 16,* 85–92.

Rose, S. A. (1983a). Behavioral and psychophysiological sequelae of preterm birth: The neonatal period. In T. Field & A. Sostek (Eds.), *Infants born at risk; Physiological, perceptual, and cognitive processes* (pp. 45–67). New York: Grune & Stratton.

Rose, S. A. (1983b). Differential rates of visual information processing in fullterm and preterm infants. *Child Development, 54,* 1189–1198.

Rose, S. A., & Feldman, J. F. (1990). Infant cognition: Individual differences and developmental continuities. In J. Colombo & J. Fagen (Eds.), *Individual differences in infancy: Reliability, stability, prediction* (pp. 229–246). Hillsdale, NJ: Erlbaum.

Rose, S. A., Feldman, J. F., McCarton, C. M., & Wolfson, J. (1988). Information processing in seven-month-old infants as a function of risk status. *Child Development, 59,* 589–603.

Rose, S. A., Feldman, J. F., Wallace, I. F., & McCarton, C. M. (1989). Infant visual attention: Relation to birth status and developmental outcome during the first five years. *Developmental Psychology, 25,* 560–576.

Rose, S. A., Gottfried, A. W., & Bridger, W. H. (1979). Effects of haptic cues on visual recognition memory in full-term and preterm infants. *Infant Behavior and Development, 2,* 55–67.

Rounsaville, B. J., Weissman, M. M., Kleber, H. D., & Wilbur, C. (1982). Heterogeneity of psychiatric diagnosis in treated opiate addicts. *Archives of General Psychiatry, 39,* 161–166.

Ruff, H. A. (1986a). Components of attention during infant's manipulative exploration. *Child Development, 57,* 105–114.

Ruff, H. A. (1986b). Attention and organization of behavior in high risk infants. *Journal of Developmental and Behavioral Pediatrics, 7,* 298–301.

Ruff, H. A. (1988). The measurement of attention in high risk infants. In P. M. Vietze & H. G. Vaughan (Eds.), *Early identification of infants with developmental disabilities* (pp. 282–296). New York: Grune & Stratton.

Ryan, L., Ehrlich, S., & Finnegan, L. (1987). Cocaine abuse in pregnancy: Effects on the fetus and newborn. *Neurotoxicology and Teratology, 9,* 295–299.

Rylander, G. (1969). Clinical and medico-criminological aspects of addiction to central stimulating drugs. In F. Sjoquist & M. Tottie (Eds.), *Abuse of central stimulants* (pp. 251–274). Stockholm: Almquist & Wiksell.

Sameroff, A. J. (1983). Developmental systems: Contexts and evolution. In P. H. Mussen (Gen. Ed.), W. Kessen (Ed.), *Handbook of child psychology: Vol. 1. History, theory, and methods* (pp. 237–294). New York: Wiley.

Sameroff, A. J., & Chandler, M. J. (1975). Reproductive risk and the continuum of caretaking casualty. In F. D. Horowitz, E. M. Hetherington, S. Scarr-Salapatek, & G. M. Siegel (Eds.), *Review of child development research* (Vol. 4, pp. 187–244). Chicago: University of Chicago Press.

Shepherd, G. M. (1988). *Neurobiology* (2nd ed.). New York: Oxford University Press.

Sigman, M. (1976). Early development of preterm and fullterm infants: Exploratory behavior in eight month-olds. *Child Development, 47,* 606–612.

Sigman, M. (1983). Individual differences in infant attention: Relation to birth status and intelligence at 5 years. In T. Field & A. Sostek (Eds.), *Infants born at risk: Physiological, perceptual, and cognitive processes* (pp. 271–293). New York: Grune & Stratton.

Sigman, M., Kopp, C. B., Littman, B., & Parmelee, A. H. (1977). Infant visual attentiveness in relation to birth condition. *Developmental Psychology, 13,* 431–437.

Sigman, M., & Parmelee, A. H. (1974). Visual preferences of four-month-old premature and full-term infants. *Child Development, 45,* 959–965.

Sigman, M., & Parmelee, A. H. (1979). Longitudinal evaluation of the preterm infant. In T. M. Field, A. M. Sostek, S. Goldberg, & H. H. Shuman (Eds.), *Infants born at risk.* New York: Spectrum.

Sokolov, Y. N. (1969). The modeling properties of the nervous system. In M. Cole & F. Maltzman (Eds.), *A handbook of contemporary Soviet psychology* (pp. 671–704). New York: Basic Books.

Spear, L. P., Kirstein, C. I., & Frambes, N. A. (1989). Cocaine effects on the developing central nervous system: Behavioral, psychopharmacological, and neurochemical studies. *Annals of the New York Academy of Sciences, 562,* 290–307.

Struthers, J. M., & Hansen, R. L. (1992). Visual recognition memory in drug-exposed infants. *Journal of Developmental and Behavioral Pediatrics, 13,* 108–111.

Swann, A. C. (1990). Cocaine: Synaptic effects and adaptations. In N. D. Volkow & A. C. Swann (Eds.), *Cocaine in the brain* (pp. 58–94). New Brunswick, NJ: Rutgers University Press.

Tamis-LeMonda, C. S., & Bornstein, M. H. (1989). Habituation and maternal encouragement of attention in infancy as predictors of toddler language, play, and representational competence. *Child Development, 60,* 738–751.

Tamis-LeMonda, C. S., & Bornstein, M. H. (1993). Antecedents of exploratory competence at one year. *Infant Behavior and Development, 16,* 423–439.

Thoman, E. B. (1982). A biological perspective and a behavioral model for assessment of premature infants. In L. A. Bond & J. M. Joffe (Eds.), *Facilitat-*

ing infant and early childhood development (pp. 159–179). Hanover, NH: University Press of New England.

Thoman, E. B. (1993). Obligation and option in the premature nursery. *Developmental Review, 13,* 1–30.

Thoman, E. B., & Ingersoll, E. W. (1989). The human nature of the youngest humans: Prematurely born babies. *Seminars in Perinatology, 13,* 482–494.

Umezaki, H., & Morell, F. (1970). Developmental study of photic evoked responses in premature infants. *Electroencephalography and Clinical Neurophysiology, 28,* 55–63.

Vietze, P. M., McCarthy, M., McQuiston, S., MacTurk, R., & Yarrow, L. J. (1983). Attention and exploratory behaviors in infants with Down syndrome. In T. Field & A. Sostek (Eds.), *Infants born at risk: Physiological, perceptual, and cognitive processes* (pp. 251–268). New York: Grune & Stratton.

Wallace, I. F., Escalona, S. K., McCarton-Daum, C., & Vaughan, H. G. (1982). Neonatal precursors of cognitive development in low birthweight children. *Seminars in Perinatology, 6,* 327–333.

Watt, J. E. (1987). Temperament in small-for-dates and preterm infants: A preliminary study. *Child Psychiatry and Human Development, 17,* 177–189.

Watt, J. E., & Strongman, K. T. (1985). The organization and stability of sleep states in fullterm, preterm, and small-for-gestational-age infants: A comparative study. *Developmental Psychobiology, 18,* 151–162.

Wise, R. A. (1984). Neural mechanisms of the reinforcing action of cocaine. *National Institute of Drug Abuse Research Monographs, 50,* 15–33.

Woods, J. R., Plessinger, M. A., & Clark, K. E. (1987). Effect of cocaine on uterine blood flow and fetal oxygenation. *Journal of the American Medical Association, 257,* 957–961.

Zuckerman, B., & Frank, D. A. (1992). Prenatal cocaine and marijuana exposure: Research and clinical implications. In I. S. Zagon & T. A. Slotkin (Eds.), *Maternal substance abuse and the developing nervous system* (pp. 125–154). San Diego, CA: Academic Press.

Attention and Information Processing in Infants with Down Syndrome

Philip R. Zelazo
Dale M. Stack

D own syndrome (DS) is a genetic disorder that represents about one-third of the moderately to severely retarded population (Rondal, 1988). Children born with DS have physical anomalies, peripheral pathological factors associated with defective speech (e.g., a protruding tongue, undersized mouth cavity), cardiac deficiencies, hypotonia, and sensory deficits. Hearing loss is common and impaired visual function also may occur. As development progresses, language delays and problems with learning are seen. Additional cognitive deficits commonly cited as related to DS include short attention span, slow reaction time, deficiencies in auditory–vocal processing, limitations in short-term memory, and reduced perceptual discrimination.

In this chapter we review research on attentional functioning in children with DS, underscoring the importance of attention and information processing for early cognitive development and its measurement. Moreover, we describe an alternative procedure to conventional tests of mental development that we use to assess information processing in normal and delayed infants and present our own data on attention in infants with DS that partially address limitations in the literature. The relation between the development of attention and atypical developmental processes is considered, and we suggest that assessment of information-processing abilities may provide a relatively unconfounded estimate of mental ability in infants with DS.

The study of "information processing," as the term is used here, is research that examines the mental activity that occurs during attention to events. Some studies have focused on age changes; others, on the determinants of both initial and sustained attention; and still others, on the information-processing characteristics operating during attention, processes such as detection, encoding, evaluation, storage, retrieval, and output (Kopp, 1987; Bornstein & Sigman, 1986; McCall & Carriger, 1993; Zelazo, 1988a, 1989). During the encoding phase infants create mental representations for the events that they attend to (Bornstein & Sigman, 1986; Zelazo, Kearsley, & Stack, 1995).

Three components are studied: (1) initial orientation, that is, the elicitation of attention toward a stimulus—a reflexive-like response; (2) sustained attention, when the bulk of information processing occurs and mental representations are formed; and (3) the termination of attention, which occurs when the information is redundant and the measures of attention (principally visual fixation and cardiac deceleration) decline from initial levels, that is, habituate. It is during the termination phase that novel events become compelling elicitors of attention.

DIFFICULTIES WITH THE STUDY OF ATTENTION AND INFORMATION PROCESSING IN CHILDREN WITH DOWN SYNDROME

A paucity of research on young children with DS and methodological problems with existing studies add to confusion about performance deficits associated with DS. The methodological issues involved in establishing the developmental course of attention among children with DS are formidable. It is not clear whether the appropriate comparison group should be matched on the basis of chronological age, mental age, or level of language development, for example. It may be that several comparison groups are needed to disentangle the areas of psychological deficits inherent in DS. Outcome measures are critical, and matching on the basis of processes related to the development of intelligence—attention, recognition memory, and information processing measures—are essential.

Most reviews and research on DS have been cross-sectional investigations; there have been few longitudinal studies allowing for examination of within-subject changes (Wagner, Ganiban, & Cicchetti, 1990). Longitudinal studies are rare for many reasons; perhaps the most important is the difficulty in obtaining large samples of DS children to follow over time. With an incidence of one DS child for every 1,500 births, it is necessary to have a very dense population center and generally to draw from multiple obstetric hospitals. A common census of 9,000 births would only yield about 6 children with DS—a minimal and statistically inadequate sample size for research.

Longitudinal studies offer the advantage of examining within-subject changes and individual differences, but they also have their drawbacks. Longitudinal research with DS children poses difficulties establishing appropriate comparison groups and ascertaining the most important variables for matching comparison subjects. Wagner et al. (1990) argue that over time normal subjects become inappropriate because of their relatively accelerated rate of development. In the past, studies have employed chronological-age-matched and mental-age-matched comparisons. However, matching is based on processes and behaviors that may not be related to later intelligence. We agree with Wagner et al. that matching on recognition memory and attention scores may circumvent possible confounded avenues of assessment. When mental abilities of children with DS are evaluated, there are several ways of confounding between measures used to infer their mental ability and characteristics of their disability that may lead to depressed estimates of their mental ability. For example, DS is associated with hypotonia leading to poor motor development, but motoric measures dominate virtually all conventional tests of both motor and mental development during the first year of life. It is methodologically inappropriate and intellectually unjustified to use motoric measures to infer mental ability among children with DS, yet there has been no alternative (cf. Zelazo, 1979, 1988a, 1989).

Overall group effects can establish that children with DS are different at one point in time. However, to establish that different cognitive processes are involved, it is necessary to show differential effects relative to matched comparison subjects over time on the same manipulated variable, yielding a statistical interaction (Wagner et al., 1990). In other words, to enable a true difference statement to be made, children with DS must perform better or worse than normally developing children on an independent variable, such as modality of presentation, that is tested at several points in time. To simply demonstrate overall lower levels of performance relative to comparison subjects on one occasion is not strong evidence for different processes in the two samples.

ATTENTION AND INFORMATION PROCESSING IN INFANTS WITH DOWN SYNDROME

Direct Evidence

Most research on attention and cognitive processes in people with DS has been conducted with the age range from middle childhood to adulthood (e.g., Boyd & Burack, 1993). The same experimental paradigms used to study attention and processing in normally developing infants have been used with DS infants, including the simultaneous paired comparison and sequential habituation–recovery procedures. Similarly, the study of attention and information processing among infants with DS involves the study of initial attention (the orientation phase), sustained attention (the familiarization phase), and the termination of attention (the habituation and recovery phase). One little-discussed problem with this research is that the use of static visual stimuli seriously limits the age range of infants studied. Static stimuli are habituated rapidly, often leading to boredom and protest among children older than 8–10 months. As a result, most of the research on infant attention, with both normally developing and infants with DS, is confined to children between 3 and 7 months of age (Zelazo, 1988a, 1988b, 1989).

Both age and stimulus limitations make the task of isolating differences between DS and normal infants complicated and often compound existing problems such as the inclusion of appropriate comparison groups. These problems render unrealistic the identification of specific cognitive processes to account for observed delays. As with normal infants, the mean duration of visual fixation is commonly used as a measure of attention and processing in infants with DS. According to Cicchetti and Ganiban (1990), infants with DS have long attention spans, as reflected in their durations of visual fixation (Cohen, 1981; Fantz, Fagan, & Miranda, 1975; Miranda & Fantz, 1973, 1974), implying that they are less distractible than matched samples of normal infants. However, the number of trials to habituation is also telling. For example, in a study by Cohen (1981), the number of trials to habituation were similar for normal infants and infants with DS but the fixation times were longer for DS infants, implying longer processing time. Similarly, in familiarization–novelty procedures, DS infants displayed longer fixation times but with less differential fixation (e.g., Miranda & Fantz, 1973).

In their now classic series of studies Miranda and Fantz (1973, 1974; Fantz et al., 1975) established that infants with DS had delayed recognition memory, implying delayed processing of visual stimuli relative to same-age normal infants. Using a visual preference method, they compared the relative lengths of visual fixation to 13 pairs of visual targets at 8 months and found differences in selective visual attention (Miranda & Fantz, 1973). On a familiarization–novelty procedure with repeated testings and immediate and delayed recall tests, Miranda and Fantz (1974) demonstrated that normal infants showed earlier novelty preferences than DS children at each of three age ranges (8–16, 17–29, and 30–40 weeks) and for three different levels of task difficulty. Whereas age and type of stimulus differentiated DS and normal infants, varying lengths of familiarization (30 and 60 seconds) and immediate versus delayed tests of recognition memory did not discriminate the groups. However, the interaction of age and stimulus meets the specifications for meaningful statistical interactions that Wagner et al. (1990) argue are essential for demonstrating that infants with DS have different information-processing capabilities.

Attention and information processing are informed by a comparison of children with DS with normally developing matched comparison subjects, but it is important also to compare children with DS to other handicapped populations—a strategy that Wagner et al. (1990) refer to as the "uniqueness question." Lewis and Brooks-Gunn (1984) studied children from 3 to 36 months of age in each of four groups: DS, cerebral palsy, developmentally delayed with unknown etiology, and multiply handicapped, using an habituation–recovery procedure. They argued that if habituation is a valid measure of CNS integrity, then different handicapped infants should show different attention patterns. They found differences in visual attention as a function of age. In particular, their data support the view that all handicapped infants, both DS and others, exhibit delays in information-processing skills at the ages tested. Interestingly, contrary to Cohen's (1981) findings in which DS infants looked longer relative to normally developing infants, Lewis and Brooks-Gunn found lower initial fixation times. Large age differences in response decrement and fixation were found in Lewis and Brooks-Gunn's study with no handicapped group differences reported. These results imply that the information-processing task they used was not sensitive to specific abilities or deficits although overall levels of general cognitive delay were detected. Nevertheless, consistent with more recent work, their results suggest that information processing can index mental age or general cognitive ability.

One avenue to evaluate individual differences in cognitive capacity is the examination of electrophysiological correlates of information processing. Schafer and Peeke (1982) showed that while nonretarded adults displayed rapid habituation of cortical evoked potentials, DS adults did not habituate. Based on these and other findings, Schafer and Peeke argued that DS is associated with deficient mechanisms of habituation.

To summarize, infants with DS display distinct visual preferences during the first year of life, with longer fixations and fewer shifts in gaze from a preferred visual pattern than normally developing infants, indicating clear differences in selective visual attention.

Several authors (e.g., Loveland, 1987; Cichetti & Sroufe, 1978) have suggested that the longer sustained levels of attention, slower habituation, and later ages of recovery to novelty displayed by infants with DS may be due to poorly developed forebrain inhibitory mechanisms that diminish their ability to control their states and actions. If these inhibitory mechanisms are impaired the ability to disengage from a task or to redirect attention may suffer. As a consequence, the DS infant may appear to be more attentive and less distractible than the normal infant (Cichetti &

Ganiban, 1990). Explanations based on inhibitory processes are consistent with Schafer and Peeke's (1982) argument that the absence of response decrement in adults with DS reflects deficient ability to adapt and inhibit neural responses to repetitive stimulation. Studies of infant information processing designed to examine predictions from this inhibition perspective are needed to identify and verify hypothesized deficits.

Indirect Evidence

Not only do infants with DS display longer fixation times to nonsocial stimuli (Fantz et al., 1975; Miranda & Fantz, 1974), implying slower information processing, they are more visually attentive in their social interactions (MacTurk, Vietze, McCarthy, McQuiston, & Yarrow, 1985; Vietze, McCarthy, McQuiston, MacTurk, & Yarrow, 1983). A number of studies that were initially designed with different objectives in mind and conducted in naturalistic settings have indirectly contributed to the data on the development of attention and processing in DS infants. For example, Landry and Chapieski (1989) examined mother–child joint attention interactions in toy-centered play. Using a sample of 12-month-old infants with DS and high-risk preterm infants matched for mental and motor ages, they found that infants with DS manipulated toys less, passively held toys, more, and looked longer at the toys in response to their mothers attention-directing behaviors than the matched-control infants. Moreover, infants with DS had difficulty engaging in joint attention when their mothers placed demands on them to shift attention between objects.

In a second study, Landry and Chapieski (1990) examined DS and high-risk preterms matched for mental age in two free-play conditions—one where the infant played alone with toys while the mother was present but did not interact, and another where she engaged her infant with the toys. They found that 6-month-old infants with DS played with toys less and looked at their mothers more whether their mothers were actively involved or not. Moreover, when mothers attempted to redirect their infants' attention, the DS infants showed fewer shifts of attention to a toy than did preterm infants, suggesting that DS infants have less mature attentional skills. Gunn, Berry, and Andrews (1982) found that 6- and 9-month-old DS infants in a 5-minute free-play situation spent almost half of the play session looking at their mothers, nearly twice the amount of the normally developing control children. Gunn et al. (1982) argue that these data indicate that the looking behavior of infants with DS in a naturalistic setting is more interpersonal than referential and thus limits exploration of their environment.

Vietze et al. (1983) examined the exploratory behavior of DS infants at 6, 8, and 12 months using problem-solving tasks that infants could interact with physically, each of which required different cognitive skills.

The tasks involved a 3-minute exploration of each of 12 toys (e.g., three men in a tub, peg board) taking place over two sessions. Social interactions, visual attention, exploratory, task, off-task, and social behaviors were measured. They found that looking was greatest at 6 months and declined with age. Exploratory and mastery behaviors tended to increase across age groups but only for some tasks. Vietze et al. (1983) compared their data to a normative data set of 6-month-old infants. The infants with DS looked at objects without manually exploring them for a third of the two 18-minute sessions, whereas normal infants looked for only a tenth of the time. Normal infants spent more time exploring the materials and engaging in mastery behavior. Possible explanations for these results include caregiver practices, hypotonia associated with DS, and greater effort required for infants with DS to contact and explore objects.

Because their previous findings might have been confounded by differences in developmental status, Vietze and his colleagues (see MacTurk et al., 1985) conducted a follow-up study with DS and normally developing infants matched on mental age. Infants with DS did not differ from the nonhandicapped infants in overall amount of behavior but varied considerably in the distribution of behavior. In particular, social behaviors were less frequent for infants with DS, although they looked at toys more frequently than did nondelayed infants. There were striking similarities in the way that DS and normal infants mastered the tasks; it was in the transitions to and from looking that differences were revealed. Children with DS "looked" before exploring or going off task; it appeared that "looking" was the hub of behavior organized for the children with DS, whereas "social behavior" was the hub for the nondelayed infants. These findings support the view that children with DS need more processing time to obtain the same information as that obtained by nondelayed children. In addition, MacTurk et al. highlight the potential importance that sequencing of exploratory activities may have in providing insight into cognitive competence and processing limitations.

Taken together, these findings indicate that processing differences in DS children are reflected in visual fixation and exploratory behavior. Lewis and Bryant (1982) extended these findings to the domain of tactual processing in a series of studies. They examined tactual–visual transfer in infants with DS of 13–35 months of age relative to normal infants matched on mental age. Such extensions inform the information-processing literature and provide support for the argument that deficits among DS children are central in origin.

Summary and Conclusions

Results from cross-sectional research indicate that children with DS show longer attention to visual stimuli in both paired-comparison and habituation–recovery paradigms. Moreover, they looked substantially longer at their mothers than did normal infants in naturalistic joint attention studies. Cichetti and Sroufe (1978) suggested that this phenomenon may be the result of delayed or deficient inhibitory capacities. More recently, Cichetti and Ganiban (1990) suggested that performance differences in children with DS are due to delayed development of higher level information-processing skills. However, a more parsimonious interpretation is that children with DS have slower processing speed. If they processed information more slowly because their neuronal impulses had greater difficulty crossing synapses or because myelination progressed more slowly, for example, they would take longer than normal infants to create mental representations for events. This slower processing speed would manifest itself by relatively longer durations of visual fixation during sustained attention phases of information-processing tasks, possibly more trials to criterion habituation, and less recovery to novelty in fixed trial procedures because they would have less complete mental representations for the standard stimuli. Longitudinal research on information processing in infants with DS may help to distinguish these interpretations.

LIMITATIONS OF PROCESSING MEASURES

Research on the determinants of attention holds promise as a direct probe of central processing ability and as a measure of mental facility because it can bypass the expressive confounding of traditional tests of intelligence. A likely candidate for the quantification of information-processing differences is speed of processing independent of whether inhibitory processes play a role. There is a long and extensive history of research on speed of information processing (Kail, 1991a, 1991b), but practically no research on processing speed during the second and third years of life (Zelazo et al., 1995). If developmental changes in speed of processing are measurable during the first 3 years of life, an alternative and psychometrically sound means to assess mental ability is possible. An information-processing measure, combined with conventional tests would afford greater diagnostic precision allowing a differential diagnosis of central processing delays from delayed expressive development (Zelazo & Kearsley, 1984; Zelazo, 1988a, 1989).

Despite the potential of information-processing measures as indices of central processing ability, a number of questions limit their validity and appropriateness (Clifton & Nelson, 1976; McCall, 1982; Reznick & Kagan, 1982; Sophian, 1980; Bornstein & Sigman, 1986). First, most studies used only one response system, visual fixation, thereby confounding the visual modality with a global central processing effect. One way to establish central processing is to demonstrate common responding across multiple response systems. However, those studies that used multiple systems such as visual fixation and heart rate deceleration produced different results for each response (e.g., Clifton & Nelson, 1976; McCall & Kagan, 1967). It is possible that visual fixation and heart rate follow different patterns and that either one may correlate with one or more other measures such as vocalization and / or smiling but not with themselves. There is ample evidence that multiple responses occur to the processing of visual and auditory events (Reznick & Kagan, 1982; Zelazo, Hopkins, Jacobson, & Kagan, 1974; Hopkins, Zelazo, Jacobson, & Kagan, 1976); it is less clear that they co-occur in simultaneous clusters, a demanding test of correlation. Thus, an unconfounded measure of central processing is needed.

A second limiting factor has been the use of two procedures — habituation and paired comparisons — to predict later intelligence. Bornstein and Sigman (1986) and McCall and Carriger (1993) performed syntheses and meta-analyses of infant studies predicting later intelligence and concluded that both the habituation and paired-comparison paradigms are equally predictive. Moreover, response to novelty is highly predictive of later mild, moderate, and severe mental retardation (Fagan & Detterman, 1992; Zelazo, Weiss, Papageorgiou, & Laplante, 1989).

We suggest, like Bornstein and Sigman (1986), that habituation to a repeated standard and recovery to a novel stimulus measure different aspects of a common process, namely, the creation of mental representations. Clusters of cognitive and affective responses including cardiac deceleration, smiling, positive vocalization, and often motoric gestures such as clapping or pointing occur during the peak of visual attention (Reznick & Kagan, 1982; Zelazo et al., 1974; Zelazo, 1988b) and can be used to infer mental representations. The use of expressive clusters to infer mental representations is contiguous and direct, in contrast to inferences from habituation (a marked decrement in responsiveness, and ultimately the absence of a response) and recovery (responsiveness to a different stimulus), which are removed in time and indirect logically.

A third limiting factor is the heavy reliance on static visual stimuli in most prior research of infant attention (e.g., Cohen, 1972; Fagan, 1984; Rose, Feldman, McCarton, & Wolfson, 1988; Rose, Feldman, Wallace, & McCarton, 1989). Indeed, children older than about 7 months do not attend as consistently as younger children to static visual stimuli, presumably because they get bored. Sequential stimuli are more compelling than static stimuli, reduce the speed with which the information can be processed, and permit a gradual unfolding of the mental representation process (Zelazo, 1979; 1988a). Laplante, Zelazo, and Gauthier (1989) showed 4-month-old infants both static stimuli used by Lewis and Brooks-

Gunn (1984) and sequential stimuli developed by Kagan, Kearsley, and Zelazo (1978). Infants looked proportionately longer, cried less, and were less likely to have the session terminated due to distress during the sequential events. These events remained interesting for children from about 3 through 36 months of age and produced greater affective responsiveness. Sequential stimuli have been used to evaluate rule transfer (McCarty & Haith, 1989) and predictability and its effects on infant visual expectations (Haith, Hazan, & Goodman, 1988; McCarty, 1989), as well as to determine whether event-related potentials can provide evidence for expectancy (Karrer et al., 1989).

A fourth limiting factor concerns the restricted age range during which current information-processing procedures are applicable. Most of the basic and applied information-processing research was conducted on children between the ages of about 3 to 7 months with a few exceptions (Lewis & Brooks-Gunn, 1984; Lewis, Goldberg, & Campbell, 1969; McDonough & Cohen, 1982; Kagan et al., 1978; Zelazo & Kearsley, 1984). It was established that processing speed increases from 22 to 32 months (Zelazo et al., 1995), but data are needed both before and after this age range to show not only that processing speed increases but that it can be measured. From a pragmatic perspective, there is a need for valid assessment of central processing ability among 18- to 36-month-olds when delays with walking and talking and behavior problems prompt both parents and pediatricians to question whether a child's mental development is delayed.

THE STANDARD–TRANSFORMATION–RETURN PROCEDURE

The limitations of the information-processing measures were addressed by developing sequential visual and auditory stimuli presented in a Standard–Transformation–Return (STR) paradigm and using clusters of behaviors to measure the speed with which mental representations are formed. The STR procedure elicits attention from children from the first through the third years of life (Kagan et al., 1978; Zelazo, 1979, 1988a), a prerequisite for the assessment of information-processing ability. A stimulus is repeated so that a child can build an expectancy (the S phase), assimilate changes to discrepant variations of the standard (the T phase), and recognize the reappearance of the standard following the discrepancy (the R phase). In order to both monitor this dynamic process and to strengthen the base on which inferences about central processing ability can be made, clusters of cognitive and affective behaviors, rather than single responses, are used. The STR procedure tests the integrity of the child's capacity to create mental representations for events and measures the speed at which these representations are formed and announced. Because mental representations for complex events are created during periods of sustained attention (cf. Cohen, 1972; Zelazo et al., 1974), the procedure was designed to maximize attention and responsiveness, thereby increasing its clinical usefulness.

We created a paradigm that was consistent with the assumption that infant attention is centrally mediated and that information-processing ability develops in a predictable pattern over the first 3 years of life. Another goal was to determine whether at-risk groups were different from normally developing children both in terms of sustained attention and speed of processing. If these goals could be achieved by identifying both age-appropriate and delayed processing using recognition clusters to visual and auditory sequences, the basis for an alternative test of infant–toddler mental development would be forged.

In the STR procedure, there are a series of five events, two visual and three auditory, that are alternated in a fixed order for all children. For each event there are six repetitions of the S phase, three repetitions of the T phase, and three reappearances of the standard stimulus during the R phase. The child observes the events in a room resembling a puppet theater while seated on the caregiver's lap. For example, in the light sequence (Figure 6.1) a rod is lifted through a 240° arc to make contact with and illuminate three colored bulbs (the S phase). During the T phase, the rod moves through the arc without the experimenter's hand and the bulbs light when the rod returns to the starting position. During the R phase, the original standard presentation reappears. In the car–doll event (Figure 6.2), a toy car rolls down the incline of a ramp and knocks over a Styrofoam figure on contact (the S phase). During the T phase, the car hits the doll but it does not fall. The three auditory events are tape-recorded

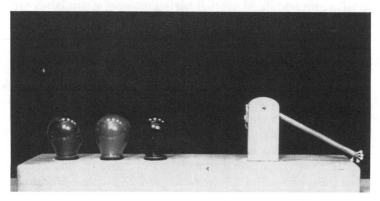

FIGURE 6.1. Sequential light stimulus.

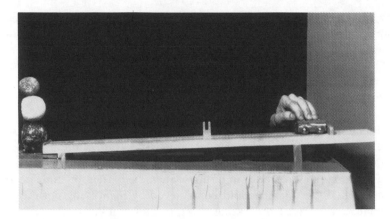

FIGURE 6.2. Sequential car–doll stimulus.

sequences of meaningful and nonmeaningful spoken phrases at different levels of developmental complexity.

The durations of multiple behavioral measures (e.g., visual fixation, smiling, vocalizing, pointing, clapping) are coded by observers behind the stage using button boxes, and beat-by-beat heart rate is measured throughout the procedure and timelocked with analogues of the stimulus events. Measures of attention—fixation to visual stimuli and "searching" to auditory stimuli equal to or greater than 80% of each trial—are used to ensure that an appropriate cardiac deceleration with one or more expressive behaviors announce a "true recognition cluster," that is, constitute a stimulus-related rather than artifactual response. The measures of attention and cardiac decelerations during specific segments of the sequences are common among all children, whereas a variety of expressive behaviors are used to accommodate individual variations among children's expressive patterns.

The validity of these procedures was established in several ways. In the first study, these procedures discriminated cross-sectional samples of normally developing children at 22, 27, and 32 months of age (Zelazo et al., 1995). Children were shown two sequential visual stimuli to assess whether their responses would reflect changes in processing speed. It was hypothesized that "first clusters" of recognition responses would be displayed earlier for older children and that this faster speed of processing would be reflected in both numbers of trials and latencies to the first recognition clusters. Both measures distinguished 22- from 27- and 32-month-olds during the S phase and 32- from 22- and 27-month-olds during the T phase.

In a second study, these normative data were used to distinguish intact from impaired information processors among a sample of 41 children with delays of unknown etiology on conventional developmental tests (Zelazo & Kearsley, 1984). No children had evidence of congenital or acquired disorders associated with mental or motor retardation. Children were enrolled at either 22 or 32 months of age. All children were evaluated using the STR procedure to determine whether their information-processing abilities were age appropriate or delayed. These children had delays on the Bayley Scale of Infant Mental Development (Bayley, 1969) of at least 4 or 5 months at 22 and 32 months of age, respectively. However, it was reasoned that children with intact-processing abilities had delays with the development of expressive behaviors rather than centrally mediated delays. All groups were given 10 months of parent-implemented treatment designed to stimulate productive language and age-appropriate object use and to eliminate maladaptive resistant and noncompliant behaviors (Zelazo, Kearsley, & Ungerer, 1984). The children were reevaluated at the end of active treatment, and follow-up evaluations were obtained 6 and 18 months after treatment.

Scores from the Bayley Mental (1969) and Stanford–Binet (Terman & Merrill, 1973) tests confirmed the predicted mental status (intact vs. impaired) × testing (entry, 10, 16, 28 months) interaction. Children whose information processing ability appeared age appropriate improved over testings, whereas children with impaired processing ability did not. Nine of ten children with impaired processing had delays that increased; only one child showed a temporary arresting of the delay. The mental status × testing interaction for delays on conventional tests ($F(3,111) = 20.96$, $p < .0001$) not only supported the validity of the test of central processing but demonstrated the effectiveness of the parent-implemented treatment procedures. Reductions from an initial mean delay of 8.0 to 0.4 months occurred for the intact group by the 18-month follow-up test, whereas the magnitude of the delays for the impaired group increased from a mean of 15.1 to 28.8 months. A mental status × testing interaction also occurred for rates of mental development ($F(3,111) = 9.22$, $p < .0001$). Rates increased for intact children from 0.70 (mental age divided by chronological age) at entry to 0.99 by the 18-month follow-up evaluation but remained low and stable for impaired processors.

Of the 41 children in the prospective sample, 31 (75.6%) displayed intact information-processing ability, indicating that conventional testing was misleading. Moreover, within the intact sample, 61% eliminated their delays and achieved intelligence test scores that equaled or exceeded their chronological ages by the 18-month follow-up. Follow-up evaluations 2 years later indicated that this pattern of results continued to hold as children entered school. The information-processing procedures identified children whose mental ability was intact despite significant expressive delays; the elimination of those delays with treatment in a substantial number of children demonstrates their validity experimentally.

THE STANDARD–TRANSFORMATION–RETURN PROCEDURE AS USED TO ASSESS INFANTS WITH DOWN SYNDROME

The study of attention and information processing provides the potential for a more precise assessment of the mental abilities of infants with DS. Conventional tests for assessing infant–toddler mental development are biased against children with developmental disabilities since they are confounded with the dominant disabilities displayed during the first 3 years of life (Zelazo, 1988a, 1989). Infants and toddlers in need of mental testing are children with delayed expressive language and/or motor development, and/or serious behavior problems, but conventional tests infer mental ability using these same domains of development: expressive language, motor facility, and compliance with an examiner. Tests such as the Bayley Scale of Mental Development measure motor facility during the first year, imitation and receptive language during the second year (requiring facility with object use and compliance with the examiner's requests), and expressive language during the third year (Zelazo, 1979, 1988a, 1989). Our research has shown that a child who is not talking may have intact mental ability; delayed expressive language may reflect an expressive problem that is experiential, even behavioral, in origin and need not imply delayed mental ability as assumed by conventional tests (Zelazo & Kearsley, 1984; Zelazo, 1979, 1989).

Down syndrome is characterized by hypotonia and expressive language delays. Our own research and clinical experience with developmentally delayed children indicates that these developmental delays are almost always associated with noncompliant/resistant behavior. Thus, children with DS almost uniformly have difficulties in at least two of these areas (motor and language), and often in all three (behavior). Unfortunately, these three areas are dominant avenues of measurement in conventional tests, including the second edition of the Bayley Scales of Infant Development (1993). One hope for breaking this impasse and circumventing these confounded avenues of assessment rests with measures of attention and central information processing. Information-processing procedures can allow a relatively unbiased assessment of mental ability independent of motor and expressive language delays and noncompliant behavior. Moreover, they may permit researchers to disentangle the precise cognitive deficiencies associated with DS.

Our own studies examining attention and information processing in infants with DS are preliminary but nonetheless reveal new findings. We examined whether information-processing ability discriminates infants with DS from a sample of normal infants matched on age, sex, socioeconomic status, and language of parents. In two studies with Trisomy 21 newborns

(Weiss, Laplante, & Eisen, 1989), habituation and recovery of localized headturning to laterally presented speech sounds and visual fixation to square-wave gratings were assessed and compared with full-term normal matched-control newborns. In the first study, an infant-controlled procedure was used to demonstrate orientation and habituation of headturning to spoken words ("tinder" or "beagle") across three phases: (1) repetition of a standard stimulus (orientation–habituation); (2) presentation of a novel stimulus (recovery); (3) return of the standard stimulus (dishabituation). Percentage of trial blocks with localized headturns served as the principal dependent measure. Comparable percentages of headturning occurred during initial familiarization trials; however, the degree of recovery to the novel word discriminated the two groups. Normal infants showed greater recovery to novelty than DS infants, and a similar tendency was shown during the dishabituation phase. The second study used the same procedure including infant controlled habituation with square-wave visual patterns presented in a viewing chamber. The percentage of visual fixation during each phase of the study was lower for the DS infants than for matched comparison infants, and there was poorer recovery to novelty and to the return of the standard stimulus. Together, these studies indicate that both normal and DS newborns displayed orientation and habituation of attention to auditory and visual stimuli. However, infants with DS displayed poorer recovery and dishabituation to both auditory and visual stimuli indicating poorer information processing as early as 48 hours after birth.

In a study with 4-month-olds (Weiss, Cohen, Eisen, & Swain, 1990), heart rate recordings of DS and matched infants were compared during three auditory events using the STR procedure. Infants with DS showed stable heart rates, little variability, and small cardiac decelerations relative to the comparison infants who displayed greater variability and large cardiac decelerations during initial orientation to the standard stimuli and to the introduction of stimulus changes. Four-month-olds with DS differ from normal infants in their cardiac responsiveness to auditory information, implying poorer processing and indicating that the poorer performances observed in newborns with DS continue to at least 4 months of age.

In a separate study, Stack, Laplante, and Zelazo (1991) examined 4-month-old infants with DS and normal infants' patterns of attention to sequential visual stimuli. Using the STR procedure, infants were presented with the car–doll and light stimuli described earlier. Duration and frequency of visual fixation and length of first gaze were examined. The patterns of attention across phases and events were similar for the two groups, but the overall level of attention was lower for infants with DS. The reduced level of attention to the sequential stimuli for DS infants implies that the poorer processing of visual stimuli observed with newborns continues to 4 months of age. Low levels of attention to the compelling sequential events for infants with DS appear inconsistent with prior studies that used static stimuli and reported higher levels of sustained attention. We believe that this result reflects poorer processing because the STR procedure is designed to maximize attention throughout all phases. Patterns of attention to sequential stimuli by normal children differ from those to static stimuli showing increases rather than decreases over age (Kagan et al., 1978). Moreover, the S phase of the STR procedure for children tested between 4 and 36 months is a familiarization—not a habituation— procedure. Attention, as measured by visual fixation greater than 80% of each trial, is used as a criterion to establish that other cognitive and affective behaviors such as cardiac decelerations, smiling, and vocalizing are stimulus related.

Finally, we attempted to partially address one of the major shortcomings in the existing research literature by examining the development of attention in children with DS longitudinally. We examined a sample of 11 children with DS and 11 normally developing comparison children matched for chronological age, sex, socioeconomic status (mother's educational level), and language at three ages: 13, 22, and 31 months (Zelazo, Stack, Rogers, & Reid, 1995). The lights and car–doll sequences were shown at all three ages. The mean percentages of fixation during the S, T, and R phases were analyzed for each stimulus over age.

Our preliminary data reveal that looking time to the sequential stimuli increases over age, unlike results reported for static visual stimuli. Moreover, levels of attention for the normally developing matched-comparison children are greater than for children with DS. Duration of visual fixation to the lights and car–doll stimuli are depicted in Figures 6.3 and 6.4 for each phase (S, T, and R) and age (13, 22, and 31 months). Children with DS display substantially lower levels of visual fixation at 13 and 22 months relative to comparison children. By 32 months, children with DS reach levels of attention comparable to those reached by normal 13-month-olds. The lower attention for infants with DS in the STR paradigm implies poorer information processing not only during the first year but at 13, 22, and 32 months. To pursue these data further, we will analyze latencies and trials to first cluster—our principal measures of central processing (Zelazo et al., 1995).

SUMMARY AND CONCLUSIONS

We have argued that conventional tests of mental development are inappropriate for children with delayed development (Zelazo, 1979, 1988a, 1989), but they are particularly biased against children with DS. Some

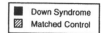

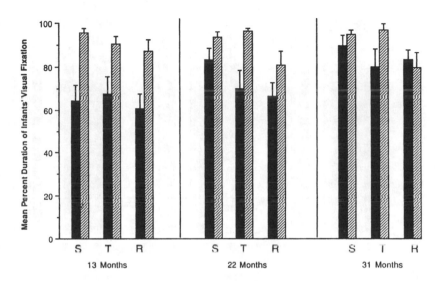

FIGURE 6.3. Mean percent duration of visual fixation to the light stimulus as a function of group (DS, matched control) for each phase (Standard, S; Transformation, T; Return, R) and age (13, 22, and 31 months).

of the generally poor performances of children with DS on conventional measures of motor and language development could be secondary to associated characteristics of the syndrome such as hypotonia, expressive language difficulties, and noncompliant behavior. For example, when children with DS were institutionalized, their scores on conventional tests were worse on average than when they were deinstitutionalized, revealing a role for experience, not just biology, in their poor intellectual performances (Stedman & Eichorn, 1964). An examination of information-processing abilities in a longitudinal sample of home-reared children with DS that used matched comparisons may help to disentangle these influences. We have done so using static visual stimuli at birth and two sequential visual stimuli at the ages of 4, 13, 22, and 31 months. The results consistently show shorter looking times for infants with DS. Preliminary results at 31 months for clusters of behaviors reflecting the formation of mental representations indicate that the relatively poor attention of DS infants reflects slow processing speed (cf. Zelazo et al., 1995). Thus, the STR procedure may help to clarify the nature of mental retardation in infants with DS.

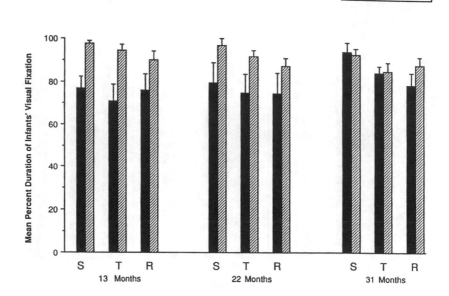

FIGURE 6.4. Mean percent duration of visual fixation to the car–doll stimulus as a function of group (DS, matched control) for each phase (S, T, R) and age (13, 22, and 31 months).

Measures of attention and information processing make at least two unique contributions to the understanding of cognitive development in children with DS; they represent the least confounded measure and are available from birth. The findings derived from the information-processing assessments are consistent with conventional wisdom; children with DS generally show less attention to sequential visual events than do normally developing children at the same age, and this deficit appears to be due to slower information-processing speed. Slower processing is a more parsimonious explanation than the inability to inhibit extraneous stimuli as postulated by Loveland (1987), Cichetti and Sroufe (1978), and McCall (1994). Inhibition as a solitary explanation is insufficient because it presumes a force that must be inhibited and constitutes a second mechanism in addition to an initial thrust to act. This initial force, we argue, is the tendency to process information. We do not exclude a role for inhibition; we only argue that it is a secondary factor (Zelazo et al., 1995).

The greater visual fixation to static stimuli for 3- to 10-month-old infants with DS relative to normal matched-comparison subjects is consistent with a slower information-processing interpretation. Static stimuli are redundant for the duration of exposure, reach a ceiling early, and require less time to process with age. The sequential stimuli used in the STR paradigm provide new information during the duration of initial exposure, are more complex, and take longer to reach a ceiling level. As a result, duration of attention among normal infants increases rather than decreases during the first year (Kagan et al., 1978; Zelazo, 1979). Therefore, the pattern of results reported in Figures 6.3 and 6.4 showing infants with DS achieving levels of attention at the age of 31 months that are comparable to those of normal infants reflects their longer period to achieve a ceiling level. Normally developing infants achieve peak levels of attention at 13 months that remain high and relatively stable through 31 months, whereas DS infants display an ascending pattern of attention from 13 to 22 to 31 months—a pattern not identified previously.

Several directions for future research can be highlighted. One is the longitudinal investigation of increased processing speed and the development of inhibition during cognitive transitions in large samples of children with DS. For example, Zelazo and Leonard (1983) note that the dramatic cognitive changes occurring between 9 and 13 months are preceded by inhibition of vocalization and quiet vigilance or wariness to both social (Roe, 1975) and nonsocial stimuli (Zelazo, 1982). Moreover, Zelazo et al. (1995) hypothesize that proactive inhibition from familiar to discrepant events is diminished around 30 months of age, allowing discrepant changes to be incorporated more rapidly into existing mental representations. Research is needed to document more precisely the interplay between processing speed and the onset of inhibition at these developmental transitions, particularly for children with DS. A second future direction is more interdisciplinary. The evidence that children with DS process information at a slower rate may offer a specific direction for researchers in the neurosciences to pursue. An investigation of the neurochemical mechanisms involved in facilitating processing speed may lead to direct benefit to children with DS and may inform us about the interplay between the development of processing speed and inhibition in normal children.

At least within the first few years of life, our data imply that for children with DS attention and information-processing ability—two central cognitive constructs—are delayed, not deficient. Whether this distinction holds throughout later development awaits further empirical study. The biases and confoundings addressed in this chapter with infants and toddlers apply to older children as well. When unconfounded measures of mental ability are developed, the negative expectations of DS suspended, and the debilitating consequences of hypotonia and expressive language difficulties on later cognitive development neutralized, we will be able to determine the developmental course of information-processing ability in children with DS. Does information-processing ability follow a slower but otherwise normal course of development or are there higher order information-processing abilities that are deficient? It is incumbent upon researchers to attempt answers in an unbiased way.

ACKNOWLEDGMENTS

We thank David Laplante and Michael Weiss for help with data collection, and Josée Brouillette, Peta Leclerc, Caroline Reid, Cheryl-Lynn Rogers, and Manon St. Germain for their aid with data reduction, analysis, graphics, and preparation of the manuscript. We also thank Yves Beaulieu for editorial comments and Mark Gross for computer programming. The support from the National Institute on Child Health and Human Development (Grant No. 1-R01-HD18029), Fonds de la Recherche en Santé du Québec (No. 881554), the Montreal Children's Hospital–McGill University Research Institute, and the Gustav Levinschi Foundation to Philip R. Zelazo is gratefully acknowledged. Finally, we express our thanks to Apostolos Papageorgiou and the staff at the Jewish General Hospital's maternity wards, and the parents and infants from the Montreal community who participated in our studies.

REFERENCES

Bayley, N. (1969). *Bayley Sales of Infant Development.* New York: Psychological Corporation.
Bayley, N. (1993). *Bayley Scales of Infant Development* (2nd ed.). San Antonio: Psychological Corporation (Harcourt, Brace).
Bornstein, M. H. (1990). Attention in infancy and the prediction of cognitive capacities in childhood. In J. T. Enns (Ed.), *The development of attention: Research and theory* (pp. 3–19). Amsterdam: Elsevier.
Bornstein, M. H., & Sigman, M. D. (1986). Continuity in mental development from infancy. *Child Development, 57,* 251–274.
Boyd, L. M., & Burack, J. A. (1993, March). *Selective attention and distractibility in children with Down syndrome.* Abstracts of the biennial meeting of the Society for Research in Child Development, New Orleans, LA.
Cicchetti, D., & Ganiban, J. (1990). The organization and coherence of developmental processes in infants and children with Down syndrome. In R. M. Hodap, J. A. Burack, & E. Zigler (Eds.), *Issues in the developmental approach to mental retardation* (pp. 169–225). New York: Cambridge University Press.
Cicchetti, D., & Sroufe, L. A. (1978). An organizational view of affect: Illustrations from the study of Down's syndrome infants. In M. Lewis & L. Rosenblum (Eds.), *The development of affect* (pp. 309–351). New York: Plenum Press.
Clifton, R., & Nelson, M. (1976). Developmental study of habituation in infants: The importance of paradigm, response system and state. In T. J. Tighe &

R. N. Leaton (Eds.), *Habituation: Perspectives from child development, animal behavior and neurophysiology* (pp. 159–205). Hillsdale, NJ: Erlbaum.

Cohen, L. B. (1972). Attention getting and attention-holding processes of infant visual preferences. *Child Development, 43,* 869–879.

Cohen, L. B. (1981). Examination of habituation as a measure of aberrant infant development. In S. L. Friedman & M. D. Sigman (Eds.), *Preterm birth and psychological development* (pp. 241–253). New York: Academic Press.

Fagan, J. F. (1984). Recognition memory and intelligence. *Intelligence, 8,* 31–36.

Fagan, J. F., & Detterman, D. K. (1992). The Fagan Test of Infant Intelligence: A technical summary. *Journal of Applied Developmental Psychology, 13,* 173–193.

Fantz, R. L., Fagan, J. F., & Miranda, S. B. (1975). Early visual selectivity as a function of pattern variables, previous exposure, age from birth conception and expected cognitive deficit. In L. B. Cohen & P. Salapatek (Eds.), *Infant perception: From sensation to cognition: Vol. 1. Basic visual processes* (pp. 249–345). New York: Academic Press.

Gunn, P., Berry, P., & Andrews, R. J. (1982). Looking behavior of Down syndrome infants. *American Journal of Mental Deficiency, 87*(3), 344–347.

Haith, H. M., Hazan, C., & Goodman, G. S. (1988). Expectation and anticipation of dynamic visual events by 3.5-month-old babies. *Child Development, 58,* 467–479.

Hopkins, J., Zelazo, P., Jacobson, S., & Kagan, J. (1976). Infant reactivity to stimulus-schema discrepancy. *Genetic Psychology Monographs, 93,* 27–62.

Kagan, J., Kearsley, R. B., & Zelazo, P. R. (1978). *Infancy: Its place in human development.* Cambridge, MA: Harvard University Press.

Kail, R. (1991a). Developmental change in speed of processing during childhood and adolescence. *Psychological Bulletin, 109,* 490–501.

Kail, R. (1991b). Development of processing speed in childhood and adolescence. In H. W. Reese (Ed.), *Advances in child development and behavior* (Vol. 23, pp. 151–185). New York: Academic Press.

Karrer, R., Ackles, P. K., Haughwout, P., Cook, K., Walker, M. A., & Barg, M. D. (1989). Event-related potential evidence for expectancy in six-month-old infants. *Society for Research in Child Development Abstracts, 281.*

Kopp, C. B. (1987). Developmental risk: Historical reflections. In J. D. Osofsky (Ed.), *Handbook of infant development* (2nd ed., pp. 881–912). New York: Wiley.

Landry, S. H., & Chapieski, M. L. (1989). Joint attention and infant toy exploration: Effects of Down syndrome and prematurity. *Child Development, 60,* 103–118.

Landry, S. H., & Chapieski, M. L. (1990). Joint attention of six-month-old Down syndrome and preterm infants: I. Attention to toys and mother. *American Journal on Mental Retardation, 94*(5), 488–498.

Laplante, D., Zelazo, P. R., & Gauthier, S. (1989). Normal, moderate and high-risk infant attention to sequential and static visual stimuli. *Society for Research in Child Development Abstracts, 291.*

Lewis, M., & Brooks-Gunn, J. (1984). Age and handicapped group differences in infants' visual attention. *Child Development, 55,* 858–868.

Lewis, M., Goldberg, S., & Campbell, H. (1969). A developmental study of learning within the first three years of life: Response decrement to a redundant signal. *Monographs of the Society for Research in Child Development,* *34*(Serial No. 133).

Lewis, V. A., & Bryant, P. E. (1982). Touch and vision in normal and Down's syndrome babies. *Perception, 11,* 691–701.

Loveland, K. A. (1987). Behavior of young children with Down syndrome before the mirror: Finding things reflected. *Child Development, 58,* 928–936.

McCall, R. B. (1982). Issues in the early development of intelligence and its assessment. In M. Lewis & L. Taft (Eds.), *Developmental disabilities: Theory, assessment and intervention* (pp. 177–184). New York: S.P. Medical and Scientific Books.

McCall, R. B. (1994). What process mediates predictions of childhood IQ from infant habituation and recognition memory? Speculations on the roles of inhibition and rate of information processing. *Intelligence, 18,* 107–125.

McCall, R. B., & Carriger, M. S. (1993). A meta-analysis of infant habituation and recognition memory performance as predictors of later IQ. *Child Development, 64,* 57–79.

McCall, R. B., & Kagan, J. (1967). Stimulus-schema discrepancy and attention in the infant. *Journal of Experimental Child Psychology, 5,* 381–390.

McCarty, M. E. (1989). Predictability and its effects on infant visual expectations. *Society for Research in Child Development Abstracts, 312.*

McCarty, M. E., & Haith, M. M. (1989). Rule transfer in the infant visual expectation paradigm. *Society for Research in Child Development Abstracts, 312.*

McDonough, S., & Cohen, L. (1982, March). *Use of habituation to investigate concept acquisition in cerebral palsied infants.* Paper presented at the Third International Conference on Infant Studies, Austin, TX.

MacTurk, R. H., Vietze, P. M., McCarthy, M. E., McQuiston, S., & Yarrow, L. J. (1985). The organization of exploratory behavior in Down syndrome and nondelayed infants. *Child Development, 56,* 573–581.

Miranda, S. B., & Fantz, R. L. (1973). Visual preferences of Down's syndrome and normal infants. *Child Development, 44,* 555–561.

Miranda, S. B., & Fantz, R. L. (1974). Recognition memory in Down's syndrome and normal infants. *Child Development, 45,* 651–660.

Reznick, J. S., & Kagan, J. (1982). Category detection in infancy. In L. Lipsitt (Ed.), *Advances in infancy research* (Vol. 2, pp. 79–111). Norwood, NJ: Ablex.

Roe, K. V. (1975). Amount of infant vocalization as a function of age: Some cognitive implications. *Child Development, 46,* 348–356.

Rondal, J. A. (1988). Down's syndrome. In D. K. M. Bishop and K. Mogford (Eds.), *Language development in exceptional circumstances* (pp. 165–176). Edinburgh: Churchill Livingstone.

Rose, S. A., Feldman, J. F., McCarton, C. M., & Wolfson, J. (1988). Information processing in seven-month-old infants as a function of risk status. *Child Development, 59,* 589–603.

Rose, S. A., Feldman, J. F., Wallace, I. F., & McCarton, C. (1989). Infant visual attention: Relation to birth status and developmental outcome during the first 5 years. *Developmental Psychology, 25,* 560–576.

Schafer, E. W. P., & Peeke, J. V. S. (1982). Down syndrome individuals fail to habituate cortical evoked potentials. *American Journal of Mental Deficiency, 87*(3), 332–337.

Sophian, C. (1980). Habituation is not enough: Novelty preferences, search and memory in infancy. *Merrill-Palmer Quarterly, 26,* 239–256.

Stack, D. M., Laplante, D., & Zelazo, P. R. (1991, August). *Four month Down syndrome infants attention to sequential visual stimuli.* Poster presented at the annual meeting of the American Psychological Association, San Francisco, CA.

Stedman, D. J., & Eichorn, D. H. (1964). A comparison of the growth and development of institutionalized and home-reared mongoloids during infancy and early childhood. *American Journal of Mental Deficiency Research, 69,* 391–401.

Terman, L. M., & Merrill, M. A. (1973). *Stanford–Binet Intelligence Scale: Manual for the Third Revision Form L-M.* Boston: Houghton, Mifflin Co.

Vietze, P. M., McCarthy, M., McQuiston, S., MacTurk, R., & Yarrow, L. J. (1983). Attention and exploratory behavior in infants with Down's syndrome. In T. Field & A. Sostek (Eds.), *Infants born at risk: Perceptual and physical processes* (pp. 251–268). New York: Grune & Stratton.

Wagner, S., Ganiban, J. M., & Cicchetti, D. (1990). Attention, memory, and perception in infants with Down syndrome: A review and commentary. In D. Cicchetti & M. Beeghly (Eds.), *Children with Down syndrome: A develop mental perspective* (pp. 147–177). New York: Cambridge University Press.

Weiss, M. J., Cohen, K. M., Eisen, L., & Swain, U. (1990, April). Heart rate variability discriminates 4-month Down syndrome and control infants. *Infant Behavior and Development, 13,* 666.

Weiss, M. J., Laplante, D., & Eisen, L. (1987). Habituation and recovery of Down's syndrome neonates' attention to auditory and visual stimuli. *Society for Research in Child Development Abstracts, 6,* 291.

Zelazo, P. R. (1979). Reactivity to perceptual-cognitive events: Application for infant assessment. In R. Kearsley & I. Sigel (Eds.), *Infants at risk: Assessment of cognitive functioning* (pp. 49–83). Hillsdale, NJ: Erlbaum.

Zelazo, P. R. (1982). The year old infant: A period of major cognitive change. In T. Bever (Ed.), *Regressions in development: Basic phenomena and theoretical alternatives* (pp. 47–79). Hillsdale, NJ: Erlbaum.

Zelazo, P. R. (1988a). An information processing paradigm for infant–toddler mental assessment. In P. M. Vietze & H. G. Vaughan, Jr. (Eds.), *Early identification of infants with developmental disabilities* (pp. 299–317). Philadelphia: Grune & Stratton.

Zelazo, P. R. (1988b). Infant habituation, cognitive activity and the development of mental representations. *European Bulletin of Cognitive Psychology, 8,* 649–654.

Zelazo, P. R. (1989). Infant–toddler information processing and the development of expressive ability. In P. R. Zelazo & R. G. Barr (Eds.), *Challenges to developmental paradigms: Implications for theory, assessment and treatment* (pp. 93–112). Hillsdale, NJ: Erlbaum.

Zelazo, P. R., Hopkins, J. R., Jacobson, S. N., & Kagan, J. (1974). Psychological reactivity to discrepant events: Support for the curvilinear hypothesis. *Cognition, 2,* 385–395.

Zelazo, P. R., & Kearsley, R. (1984). The identification of intact and delayed information processing: An experimental approach [Abstract]. *Infant Behavior and Development, 7,* 393.

Zelazo, P. R., Kearsley, R. B., & Stack, D. M. (1995). Mental representations for visual sequences: Increased speed of central processing from 22 to 32 months. *Intelligence, 20*(1), 41–63.

Zelazo, P. R., Kearsley, R. B., & Ungerer, J. A. (1984). *Learning to speak: A manual for parents.* Hillsdale, NJ: Erlbaum.

Zelazo, P. R., & Leonard, E. L. (1983). The dawn of active thought. In K. Fischer (Ed.), *Levels and transitions in children's development* (pp. 37–50). San Francisco: Jossey-Bass.

Zelazo, P. R., Stack, D. M., Rogers, C., & Reid, C. (1997). *A longitudinal investigation of Down syndrome infants' information processing.* Manuscript in preparation.

Zelazo, P. R., Weiss, M. J., Papageorgiou, A., & Laplante, D. (1989). Recovery and dishabituation of sound localization among normal, moderate and high risk newborns: Discriminant validity. *Infant Behavior and Development, 12,* 321–340.

Conceptual Relations between Attentional Processes in Infants and Children with Attention-Deficit/ Hyperactivity Disorder

A PROBLEM-SOLVING APPROACH

Jeffrey T. Coldren
Kris Corradetti

During the past 20 years, a phenomenal amount of research has been directed at the complex childhood disorder known as attention-deficit/hyperactivity disorder (ADHD). From this voluminous literature, researchers and clinicians have reported several consistent findings. First, ADHD affects a large number of children; approximately 3–5% of school-age children are estimated to have ADHD (Barkley, 1990, 1991), with one figure of its prevalence reaching as high as 20% (Ross & Ross, 1982). Second, there is also consensus that ADHD is highly disruptive and interferes with a child's functioning in intellectual, educational, family, and social domains. Children with ADHD show characteristics such as the inability to attend to certain portions of their environment, the inability to sustain attention over extended periods, impulsiveness, and excessively high levels of activity (Barkley, 1991). Third, most investigators generally agree that neurological, genetic, prenatal/perinatal, and environmental factors are likely to be involved as causative of ADHD (Barkley, 1990; Carlson, Jacobvitz, & Sroufe, 1995; Goodman & Stevenson, 1989; Hartsough & Lambert, 1985; Hynd, Hern, Voeller, & Marshall, 1991). And, fourth, once children have been identified as having ADHD, a variety of treatments including medication, school, and home-based programs may be implemented to reduce its deleterious consequences (Barkley, 1990). These programs have shown a wide range of effectiveness in treating children with the disorder (Rapport & Kelly, 1991; Whalen & Henker, 1980).

Despite the vast amount of understanding about ADHD, there is little regarding its age of onset. Detection of ADHD typically occurs around the time that the child enters formal schooling but may range between 3 to 9 years of age (Barkley, 1989, 1990; McGee, Williams, & Feehan, 1992). However, as detection of the disorder should not be confused with onset of the disorder, ADHD may exist during infancy prior to the point of detection. It appears to arise during infancy or very early childhood, but it is only detected in later childhood years because its symptoms or characteristics are not severe or problematic enough to warrant suspicion of ADHD (Barkley, 1989; Campbell, 1985; Jacobvitz & Sroufe, 1987; McGee et al., 1992).

Identifying the origins of ADHD during infancy prior to the development of severe symptoms later in life is important because a primary goal of developmental psychology is to optimize the outcome of children (Baltes, Reese, & Nesselroade, 1977). By the relatively late age when ADHD is usually identified, serious intellectual and scholastic problems or delays already may be well entrenched throughout a child's functioning. Studies of developmental psychopathology have convincingly shown that maladaptive behavior exhibited during a child's developmental history has the potential to affect future developmental tasks that must be faced by the child (Achenbach, 1992). Clearly, a more efficient strategy for preventing deleterious consequences associated with a childhood disorder is to understand how it may arise and find a way to predict its onset rather than waiting for its occurrence and associated problems (Carlson et al., 1995). Specifically, in the case of ADHD, this strategy would allow investigators to conceptualize how a child's inability to control attention at one age may relate to problems that prospectively can occur later in a child's developmental progress (Douglas, 1983). Once attentional difficulties have been identified, appropriate intervention can begin that may alleviate or prevent the developmental delay.

PURPOSE AND ORGANIZATION OF THE CHAPTER

The purpose of this chapter is to consider cognitive antecedents of ADHD in infancy. The goal is to identify attentional processes in infancy that may be related to attentional processes in ADHD later in childhood. In the next section, attentional processes thought to be deficient in children with ADHD will be identified. In the following major section, the attentional processes most likely to be deficient in children with ADHD will be related to comparable attentional processes in infancy. In particular, the discrimination problem-solving approach will be presented. Then, in the third major section below, communalities across the attentional processing of infants and ADHD will be discussed in order to identify the developmental processes involving attention from infancy to children with ADHD (Achenbach, 1992). In the final section, implications of the proposed approach will be considered and a research agenda toward predicting ADHD in childhood from infancy will be proposed.

IDENTIFYING DEFICIENT ATTENTIONAL FUNCTIONING IN CHILDREN WITH ADHD

Although investigators are able to agree upon the general characteristics associated with ADHD, there is little consensus about the precise nature of the cognitive processes that are at the core of the condition (Goodman & Poillion, 1992; Guevremont, DuPaul, & Barkley, 1990). Two areas of attention have been identified most often as being inappropriate or impaired in children with ADHD: sustained attention and selective attention.

Sustained Attention

Sustained attention or vigilance refers to an effort, resource, or capacity that is applied to tasks in varying degrees (Kahneman, 1973). There are numerous reports that children with ADHD are unable to adequately sustain attention to tasks for extended periods of time compared to children without ADHD (Douglas, 1983). They show less vigilance or persistence when engaged in a task, shift more frequently from one activity to another, and take an impulsive approach to tasks by using rapid, inaccurate responding. Sustained attention is usually measured in the laboratory by the continuous performance task (CPT). In this task, children are required to maintain their attention to a series of successively presented letters that are presented on a screen. Compared to children without ADHD, children with the condition have been found to more often fail to detect a series of letters that are the same (errors of omission) or mistakenly respond as if they were seen (errors of commission), and they show a faster rate of performance decrement over the course of the task (Douglas & Peters, 1979; Klee & Garfinkel, 1983; Seidel & Joschko, 1990; Sergeant & van der Meere, 1990). The presumed reason for these difficulties is the inability to appropriately maintain their attention for accurate detection of the stimuli over the entire presentation series.

Selective Attention

Attention also refers to selectivity: It functions to admit some limited amount of information to the information-processing system rather than all available stimulation (Enns, 1990). Under the rubric of selectivity, several finer distinctions may be made, including the concept of *filtering*—ignoring irrelevant information in order to process other more crucial information efficiently; *search*—looking for an object that may or may not be present; *integration*—responding to relations among individual stimulus features; and *priming*—which refers to the role that experience and response demands play in maintaining or switching attention over time (Enns, 1990; Enns & Cameron, 1987; Enns & Girgus, 1985).

Children with ADHD also have been reported to have difficulty in selective attention. Frequently, they have been found to be less able than children without ADHD children to attend to relevant portions of a stimulus display and to ignore irrelevant extraneous stimuli in the task environment. These types of attentional difficulties have been explored in the laboratory with sorting or classification tasks in which children are required to sort a series of stimuli into one of two groups based upon a specified dimension while distracting information is present. Compared to children without the condition, children with ADHD make more sorting errors due to the highly distracting effects of the dimensions of the interfering and irrelevant stimuli (Rosenthal & Allen, 1978, 1980; Strutt, Anderson, & Well, 1975). Moreover, in a dual-task paradigm, performace of children with ADHD on the primary task is more adversely affected by the secondary task than is that of children without ADHD. These results suggest that children with ADHD are deficient in the ability to selectively attend to some sources of stimulation over others (Schachar & Logan, 1990).

These findings regarding sustained or selective attention, however, are not clear cut; there is evidence to the contrary that did not support the existence of deficits in either sustained attention (Chee, Logan, Schachar, Lindsay, & Wachsmuth, 1989; van der Meere & Sergeant, 1988a) or selective attention (Douglas, 1983; Douglas & Peters, 1979; van der Meere & Sergeant, 1988b). For example, several investigators have reported that children with ADHD had slower response times (RTs) or made more errors in overall responding but otherwise showed no specific deficits involving selective attention in tasks such as letter identification or speeded classification (Hooks, Milich, & Lorch, 1994; Tarnowski, Prinz, & Nay, 1986; van der Meere & Sergeant, 1988b). Further, others studies have shown that children with ADHD detect fewer targets and have more omissions in CPT tasks but that their sustained attention does not decline at a faster rate than that of comparison children (van der Meere & Sergeant, 1988a). One consistent finding across studies of sustained or selective attention is that RTs of children with the condition are consistently either slower or more variable than children without it (Firestone & Douglas, 1975; Hynd et al., 1989; Mitchell, Chavez, Baker, Guzman, & Azen, 1990).

In evaluating the attentional difficulties of children with ADHD across these numerous studies, it may be concluded that they are more inefficient and variable in their expression of attentional skills, but it is apparent that neither sustained nor selective attentional components may be identified with certainty as a primary attentional problem (Goodman & Poillion, 1992; Halperin et al., 1990; Prior, Sanson, Freethy, & Geffen, 1985). The difficulty in understanding the impairments in attention in children with ADHD may be due to the fact that they show considerable variation in their performance under various situations or task demands (Douglas, 1983; Guevremont et al., 1990; Pearson & Lane, 1990; Rubenstein & Brown, 1984). For instance, in conditions that are self-paced, novel, contain high levels of repeated instructions, or involve a high rate of immediate reinforcement, the problems associated with ADHD are considerably reduced (Freibergs & Douglas, 1969); conversely, differences in performance involving sustained and selective attention are most readily observed in tasks that are dull, boring, or repetitive (Luk, 1985; Mitchell et al., 1990).

As a result of the ambiguity about the extent and exclusivity to which sustained and selective attention may be involved in the cognitive processing deficiencies associated with ADHD, a revised perspective on the cognitive difficulties of children with the condition has emerged. Investigators have argued that the search for the deficiency in ADHD should not focus directly upon either sustained or selective attention per se (Douglas & Peters, 1979). Instead, research should concentrate on the manner in which sustained or selective attentional processes may be used or deployed during the actual performance of tasks. This argument is based in the reasoning that attentional processes may be most validly understood as they are deployed under the demands of a particular task or to solve a particular problem. Within this view, a functional relationship exists among verbal or visual stimuli, a child's attention to the stimuli, and the consequences from the environment for the child's attention (Barkley, 1989, 1990, 1991). It is proposed that children with ADHD have difficulty involving the interaction of attentional factors with the demands of a particular task because they are unable to invest, organize, regulate, and maintain attention based upon its consequences (Burke, 1990; Douglas, 1983, 1988; Korkman & Peltomaa, 1991; Sergeant, 1988; Swanson et al., 1990). This problem in processing by children with ADHD could result in the failure to understand the consequences of attending to the most critical or relevant part of stimulation or failure to understand the consequences of attending to an inappropriate set of environmental stimuli.

Indeed, there is convincing evidence to support the view that children with ADHD have a great deal of difficulty on complex tasks that require the use of attentional skills (Douglas, 1980; Douglas & Benezra, 1990; Tant & Douglas, 1982). On tasks that require children to solve a problem involving multiple trials, such as identifying the correct picture from a stimulus array or matrix, the performance of children with ADHD was less efficient than that of comparison children (e.g., Douglas & Peters, 1979; Tant & Douglas, 1982). In these types of situations, the former made more errors, were less likely to correct errors, generated and employed less efficient problem-solving plans and strategies, and required more time to survey stimulus materials, formulate, and execute responses (Reardon & Naglieri, 1992; Swanson et al., 1991). Moreover, children with ADHD appear to have difficulty in organizing these individual components of cognitive processing into an overall problem-solving approach (Douglas & Peters, 1979). Whereas these difficulties may involve either sustained or selective attention, inaccurate conclusions may be reached if investigators seek to understand deficiencies in attentional components without also taking into account the task demands. A more fruitful approach, therefore, is to go beyond the search for deficient attentional components in children with ADHD to understand their functioning in a task.

THE NATURE AND PROCESSES
OF ATTENTION IN INFANCY

In order to identify conceptual relations in attentional processes between children with ADHD and infants, the purpose of this section is to discuss attentional processes in infancy that have analogues in the attentional functioning of children with ADHD. There is a great deal of information from the past 30 years that has documented several relatively sophisticated attentional abilities in infants. As in the literature on attention in ADHD in children, the functioning of sustained and selective attention in particular has dominated the investigation of attention in infancy. Infants are able to discriminate and selectively attend to stimuli containing both color and form features (see the reviews by Banks & Salapatek, 1983, Cohen & Salapatek, 1975, and Olson & Sherman, 1983). Infants are also able to adequately sustain their visual attention during task performance (Richards & Casey, 1992; Ruff, 1990; Weissberg, Ruff, & Lawson, 1990).

However, given that most of the studies of infant attention have involved either selective or sustained abilities, it is important to evaluate whether these components may be viable candidates to be conceptually linked to attention in ADHD. Indeed, several reasons may be offered that measures of sustained and selective attention from infancy may not be related to attention in ADHD. First, predictive relationships have been observed between attentional measures from infancy to childhood (Bornstein & Sigman, 1986; Colombo, 1993; McCall & Carriger, 1993; see also Fagan & Haiken-Vasen, Chapter 3, this volume); however, there is no comprehensive theory that specifies the development of either sustained or selective attentional processes across the ages (Thompson, Fagan, & Fulker, 1991). Second, there are considerable uncertainties about the role of sustained or selective attention in the functioning of children with ADHD. It makes little sense to attempt to relate selective or sustained attentional processes in infancy when their role in ADHD is indeed questionable. And, third, while the accumulation of data on the sustained and selective attentional capacities of infants was impressive and valuable, such studies gave only a partial portrait of cognitive functioning. Most studies of attention in infants emphasized what they *could do,* leading to the view that infants had competence in their attentional skills (Horowitz & Colombo, 1990). This emphasis, however, failed to consider how attentional processes may be actually used during the performance of tasks such as solving a problem. Therefore, to identify attentional processes in infancy that may be related to ADHD, it is necessary to know how infants' attentional skills may be used in the performance of tasks. In the next subsection, a recent series of studies on the attentional abilities of infants as they function toward the solution of problems will be reviewed. This approach is compatible with recent calls from investigators of ADHD to identify the function of attention under the demands of a particular task.

The Study of Discrimination Problem Solving in Infancy

In order to demonstrate that infants have impressive attentional skills and that they are able to use these skills in the service of solving problems, a discrimination problem-solving task was applied to infants. In brief, this task usually involves the presentation of two chromatic geometric stimuli; a response to one of these stimuli is rewarded, whereas a response to the other stimulus is not. The subject's task is to learn to respond on the basis of any one of the possible features irrespective of variation in the other irrelevant features. Specifically, the purpose was to test how infants would selectively attend to a particular stimulus feature that is relevant for solving a problem when other stimulus features are present and varied

(Neill, 1977; Well, Lorch, & Anderson, 1980; Wright & Vlietstra, 1975). The discrimination problem-solving task was used because this task has been central throughout the field of experimental child psychology since the 1930s and thus rests on a firm empirical and theoretical basis (Stevenson, 1983). Moreover, as the study of discrimination learning has remained so prominent throughout the years due to its empirical rigor, it offers investigators a specific methodology to determine the manner in which processes such as stimulus perception, selective attention, sustained attention, and representation operate together in order to solve a problem (Caron & Caron, 1978).

A set of experiments were performed in which 9-month-old infants were given two successive discrimination problems (Coldren & Colombo, 1994). The method was to simultaneously present infants with two visual stimuli, one to the left and one to the right of midline. The stimulus pairs consisted of colored geometric forms that may be described in terms of dimensions, such as form, color, or position. Each of these dimensions was composed of specific individual features, such as blue and green, triangle and circle, and left and right. Visual fixation to one of these stimuli was rewarded, whereas a response to the other stimulus in the pair was not. In order to solve these problems, infants must selectively direct their attention and respond on the basis of one of the possible features while simultaneously ignoring the variation in the other features. For example, if the correct feature was blue, the infants must respond to this feature by focusing on the color dimension while ignoring variation in the two other, irrelevant dimensions. Whenever infants visually fixated the stimulus containing the correct feature, auditory reinforcement (maternal speech) was presented synchronously with the onset and for the duration of the fixation (e.g., Colombo, Mitchell, Coldren, & Atwater, 1990).

Immediately following the completion of the first problem, a second followed in which contingencies for responding were shifted. In a reversal (R) or intradimensional (ID) shift, the experimenter trained the child to respond to a particular feature of a dimension (e.g., color — blue) and then switched reinforcement contingencies to another feature within the same dimension (e.g., color — green). In a nonreversal (NR) or extradimensional (ED) shift, the reinforcement was switched from a feature in one dimension (e.g., color — blue) to a feature on the opposite dimension (e.g., form — triangle).

From the use of the discrimination problem-solving task, three findings were noteworthy about infants' attentional processes as they function in the course of solving a problem (Coldren & Colombo, 1994):

1. Infants directed attention to the reinforced stimulus feature without being distracted by irrelevant features and dimensions on other dimen-

sions. From this finding, it was concluded that infants have the ability to selectively focus their attention on a feature in the presence of competing stimuli. This is an important ability that permits infants to focus on the most relevant portion of the available stimuli rather than being overwhelmed by stimulus input.

2. Infants showed better performance on R or ID shifts than on NR or ED shifts. This indicated that infants show an advantage in attending to features that appear on the same relevant dimension across training and test problems. That is, in addition to being able to parse individual stimulus features from the whole, infants are aware that particular features constitute separable dimensions and can direct their attention to those dimensions.

3. In attending to stimulus features and dimensions while solving the problem, infants' level of fixation hovered around chance levels (i.e., .50) prior to showing a precipitous rise at the point of problem solution. Theoretically, such a pattern of responding has been interpreted as evidence of the active selection and testing of responses until the one is found that is consistently reinforced (Zeaman & House, 1963; Gholson, 1980; Hayes, 1953). These data have led us to propose that preverbal infants use their attentional processes to solve discrimination problems in a manner that involves the selection and testing of stimulus features until they isolate the one relevant for solution (Coldren & Colombo, 1994).

COMMON GROUND:
A DYNAMIC PROBLEM-SOLVING
APPROACH TO ATTENTION

A common theme emerges from the preceding discussions of attention in children with ADHD and in infants. Investigators from both areas have independently arrived at the conclusion that assessments of attentional abilities are of limited value if they fail to take into account how attentional may actually be deployed under the demands of solving a particular problem or task. In children with ADHD, for example, the problems in attention associated are most clearly recognized and understood when they are viewed as they are actually deployed in the context of the demands of a task. In infants, for example, the study of attentional processes has revealed that they solve discrimination problems in a more sophisticated manner than previously thought possible. The findings from studies of discrimination learning suggest that infants have impressive attentional skills to select among the stimulus features and sustain their effort until the completion of the task. However, this finding is even more significant because it suggests that infants can use their selective attention actively, systematically, and flexibly in the face of changing stimuli over trials in order to find the one feature that is consistently reinforced and thereby is the solution to the problem.

Thus, investigators in both areas have gone beyond discovering the attentional capabilities by taking a dynamic approach to the assessment of cognition. Instead of simply observing the products of attentional functioning involving sustained or selective components in either children with ADHD or infants, a theme that has been common to both areas of research has been to explore the use and deployment of attention under the demands of solving a task. The point is not to measure static attentional products such as the observation of sustained or selective components of attention. Nor is the point to expect the subject to know how to perform the task at the outset of the experiment. The goal is to understand *how* attentional processes are used by either infants or children with ADHD during the solution to problems over trials (e.g., Brown, 1982; Greeno, 1980; Glaser, 1981, 1990; Linder & Siegel, 1983; Mitchell, 1988; Underwood, 1975; Stevenson, 1983). Therefore, the dynamic approach to identify the functioning of attention in problems serves as a conceptual relation between the two areas of research.

In order to extend the dynamic approach explicitly across the study of infants and children with ADHD, use of the discrimination problem-solving task is warranted for several reasons. First, such a task is methodologically appropriate to the behavioral characteristics of the ages of the children. Whereas most of the tasks that are used to assess ADHD in older children rely upon verbal and/or reading skills (Mitchell et al., 1990), infants clearly do not have these abilities and would not be able to perform these tasks. The discrimination problem-solving task has been used successfully with subjects ranging from infancy to students in college (Gholson, 1980). Second, the discrimination problem-solving task is used to measure comparable attentional processes across the ages. Sustained attention may be indexed by the duration of time for children to solve the problems. Selective attention may be observed by the number of errors that are made while children isolate the relevant stimulus feature across the target pairs that is correct. And, third, this approach allows an investigator to simultaneously measure the operation of attentional components thought to be deficient in children with ADHD as they interact with task demands in order to solve a problem (Douglas & Benezra, 1990; Gholson, 1980; Reardon & Naglieri, 1992).

Although there have been some studies that have addressed the ability of children with ADHD to solve complex problems, only one to our knowledge is similar to the discrimination problem-solving task. In this one task, such children (then called hyperactive) performed as well as comparison children when given a concept-learning task in which they had to respond to the relevant feature in stimuli containing naturalistic objects or numerical concepts (Freibergs & Douglas, 1969).

A preliminary project was recently performed to directly apply the discrimination problem-solving task to identify the operation of attentional processes associated with ADHD with four children with the condition and four without it ranging from 5 to 7 years of age (Lucko, 1994). The task was extremely similar to that used with infants. Stimuli were presented on video screens and contained features that varied in four dimensions: color—black and white; form—square and circle; bar position—above and below; and side—left and right (as illustrated in Figure 7.1). The presentation of stimuli contained all combinations of features and varied across trials. In contrast to the procedure with infants, children were required to press one of two buttons located beneath pairs of stimuli. The child was instructed *to pick the one that always makes the music play,* that is, to find the feature that consistently was rewarded. Two problems were given, each containing a maximum of 48 trials. During the first problem, the picture containing the *square* was correct regardless of the variation of the other features. During the second problem, the same set of stimuli were presented; however, during this problem, the *black* feature was now correct regardless of the variation of the other features. If the child responded to the correct feature, a 1-second burst of music was immediately presented to the child. If the child responded to an incorrect feature, no music was presented. Once a child made a response, the trial ended and the next was initiated. The criterion for solving the problem was four correct responses in a row.

Visual inspection of these data reveal two primary findings. (1) Both groups of children appeared to solve the first problem easily and performed similarly with regard to the number of trials needed to reach criterion (see

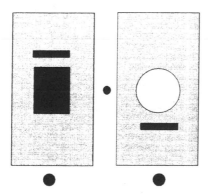

FIGURE 7.1. Example of stimulus presentation.

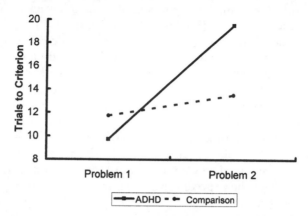

FIGURE 7.2. Trials to criterion for each discimination problem.

Figure 7.2) and the total duration of time to solution (see Figure 7.3). (2) Children with ADHD appeared to have difficulty in solving the second problem: The number of trials to criterion and the duration needed to solve the second problem increased dramatically for them. Although the comparison children experienced some difficulty, as evidenced by the slightly increased number of trials in the second problem, this problem is clearly more difficult for the children with ADHD.

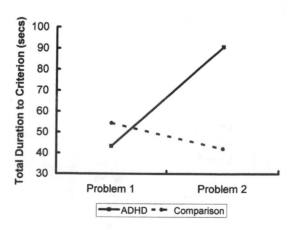

FIGURE 7.3. Total duration to criterion for each discrimination problem.

Thus, several interesting conclusions may be drawn about the attentional processing of children with ADHD in the discrimination problem-solving task. First, both groups of children were successfully able to solve both problems; however, there were differences in their performance of the problems leading to solution. Second, it is unclear whether children with ADHD have deficits in either sustained or selective attention because differences were found across problems; they took a longer duration to solve the second problem and made more errors in selecting the reinforced feature on that problem, but neither of these differences were found on the first problem. And, third, interpretations regarding the exclusive role of selective or sustained attention would be erroneous because they would fail to consider the interaction among attentional processes with the demands of responding to the individual problems. The observation of clear differences in the performance of the children with ADHD from the first problem to the second suggests some difficulty in responding across problems. The only difference between the two problems was in the reinforced (i.e., correct) feature; in the first problem children were required to respond to the square feature, whereas in the second problem they were required to respond to the black feature. If children with ADHD had difficulty in selective or sustained attention, differences should have been observed from the outset of the task in the first problem, but they were not. Thus, the observation of interproblem differences implies that another problem is involved, namely, that children with ADHD have trouble in switching their attentional responding to test a new stimulus feature when required to do so (e.g., Douglas & Peters, 1979; Schachar & Logan, 1990).

This process by which a subject selects and tests features during the learning sequence has been termed a *hypothesis* (Gholson, 1980; Levine, 1975). Gholson proposed that the manner in which such hypotheses were developed and tested in a discrimination problem-solving task was a function of a central processor and various cognitive subprocesses (Gholson, 1980; Gholson & Beilin, 1979). Further, children may use one of two systems to generate these hypotheses (Gholson, Levine, & Phillips, 1972). One system of hypotheses eventually leads to correct responding. The other system, that of stereotypes, never leads to solutions and is insensitive to feedback, even when it involves repeated disconfirmation. Given that children with ADHD have difficulty in switching responding from a previously correct response to the new correct answer, it is plausible that they use a deficient system to test their hypotheses. Specifically, it appears that children with ADHD generate hypotheses to solve the first problem but during the second problem they fail to revise their use of hypotheses and rely instead upon stereotypic responding.

USING THE DYNAMIC PROBLEM-SOLVING APPROACH TO EMPIRICALLY LINK ATTENTION DURING INFANCY AND CHILDHOOD ADHD: A RESEARCH AGENDA

To recap, several points have been discussed in order to consider cognitive antecedents of ADHD in infancy so as to eventually detect infants either with ADHD or at-risk for ADHD before the onset of developmental difficulties later during childhood. First, after a long and intensive course of study, investigators studying ADHD in children cannot specify whether sustained or selective attention is the primary cognitive problem. It has been concluded that attention should be considered as it is actually used in an active, problem-solving task. Second, from recent studies of attention in infants, it has been shown that a problem-solving approach using a discrimination task reveals that infants flexibly and actively use their attentional skills in order to solve a problem or reach a goal (e.g., Coldren & Colombo, 1994). Third, it appears that both areas of research share the use of a dynamic approach to assess attentional functioning instead of simple attentional competence. And, fourth, the discrimination problem-solving task is appropriate for both infants and older children to access their attentional performance in a dynamic problem-solving situation. The use of this task has revealed that children at both ages use hypotheses to guide their attention to solve the problems and that, in the case of children with ADHD, their hypothesis testing appears to be deficient.

Given this common conceptual basis between attention in infants and in children with ADHD, the first task in a research agenda to empirically relate attention between the two groups will be to replicate and extend the findings of the preliminary investigation using the discrimination problem-solving task with children with ADHD. Specific efforts will be made to discover the types of hypothesis that children with ADHD use to solve discrimination problems. Although there are suggestions that such children use a hypothesis-testing system of responding until they reach a solution, this cannot be confirmed directly until probes trials are inserted into the trials to monitor hypotheses and strategy deployment. For instance, it appears from the preliminary evidence that children with ADHD continued to respond to the previously reinforced feature from the first problem instead of inhibiting their response to that feature to select and test the new feature in the second problem. In other words, these children's performance could be interpreted as evidence that they are unable to eliminate the previously correct response to detect the new correct response in the second problem even given consistent evidence to the contrary (cf. Freibergs & Douglas, 1969). Whether or not this may be due to a failure in hypothesis testing by children with ADHD may be detected through the use of blank trials, which are simply one or more trials whereas the experimenter provides no feedback to the subject and which are interspersed systematically among feedback trials. These blank trials serve as probes to test for the subject's use of a particular hypothesis. The adoption of each hypothesis (e.g., *focus on form*) is indicated by a unique pattern of responses by the subject (Levine, 1975); if the subject shows a pattern of responding that does not correspond to any possible hypothesis, it may be concluded that the subject is responding randomly.

Just as we need to explore the manner by which children with ADHD test hypotheses, we also need to fully explore hypothesis testing in infants. From the examination of infants' pattern of responding prior to reaching a solution, they were found to be systematic and organized in their ability to locate and select the appropriate relevant feature or dimension in a changing stimulus array over trials. This pattern of organized and deliberate strategic responding may be interpreted as evidence that infants engage in a processes of forming and testing hypotheses to guide their attention to solve the problem (Coldren & Colombo, 1994). To strengthen these conclusions about whether infants are active in selecting stimuli and operating according to hypothesis-testing systems, we need designs in which probe trials are inserted into the problems (Levine, 1966). Whether infants adopt hypotheses to achieve task solutions would be indicated by a unique pattern of responses over the probe trials; if infants show a pattern of responding that does not correspond to any possible hypothesis, it would suggest that they are responding randomly.

Given knowledge of the hypotheses and types of responding that are used by infants and children, the next step is to determine how hypothesis testing develops between infancy and childhood. Because theoretical and empirical accounts of attention during task performance have been primarily confined to older ages (Enns & Cameron, 1987; Lane & Pearson, 1982; Well et al., 1980), failure to consider infants has resulted in a gap in our understanding of the development of these skills between infancy and childhood (Gholson, 1980; Siegler, 1983). Developmentally, Gholson's (1980) model specified that very young children's way of responding to discrimination problems consisted predominantly of response sets rather than true hypotheses because the former are not sensitive to feedback. For older children, however, response patterns conforming to the presence of hypotheses—and that are indeed sensitive to feedback—dominated their responding (Gholson et al., 1972). Therefore, we need to investigate how the types of hypothesis used by infants are related to the types of hypothesis used by children from approximately 4 to 6 years of age. There is the additional need to understand the types of hypotheses used by infants and relate them to the types of hypotheses used specifically by children with ADHD.

Once such information has been obtained using a similar task at both ages, efforts can then be directed at linking the two areas by searching for common indices or patterns of hypothesis testing between children with ADHD and infants. If we are able to accomplish this task, we will then be in the position discover which infants are prospectively at high risk for the development of ADHD (e.g., Carlson et al., 1995). Although it is not anticipated that the approach and research agenda that have been proposed in this chapter will be directly useful as an assessment for the diagnosis of the disorder (e.g., Gordon, 1987), it is expected that it will yield important and much needed developmental data to unite our understanding of attentional processes across children, thereby providing a basis for prediction of attentional disorders. As a result, investigators with both basic and applied interests in attention will gain insight into the nature and development of attentional processes in all children.

ACKNOWLEDGMENTS

We wish to thank the parents and children for their generous participation in the preliminary project. Appreciation is also given to Thomas Jennings, who helped design and build the experimental apparatus and collect data. Special thanks to Jeanne M. Funk, PhD, and the staff of the Department of Pediatrics at the Medical College of Ohio for their cooperation and assistance. An earlier version of this chapter was presented at the Conference on Human Development in Pittsburgh (1994).

REFERENCES

Achenbach, T. M. (1992). Developmental psychopathology. In M. H. Bornstein & M. E. Lamb (Eds.), *Developmental psychology: An advanced textbook* (pp. 629–675). Hillsdale, NJ: Erlbaum.

Baltes, P. B., Reese, H. W., & Nesselroade, J. R. (1977). *Life-span developmental psychology: Introduction to research methods.* Monterey, CA: Brooks/Cole.

Banks, M. S., & Salapatek, P. (1983). Infant visual perception. In M. M. Haith & J. J. Campos (Eds.), *Handbook of child psychology: Vol. 2. Infancy and developmental psychobiology* (pp. 435–571). New York: Wiley.

Barkley, R. A. (1989). Attention-deficit/hyperactivity disorder. In E. J. Mash & R. A. Barkley (Eds.), *Treatment of childhood disorders* (pp. 39–72). New York: Guilford Press.

Barkley, R. A. (1990). *Attention-deficit/hyperactivity disorder: A handbook for diagnosis and treatment.* New York: Guilford Press.

Barkley, R. A. (1991). Diagnosis and assessment of attention-deficit/hyperactivity disorder. *Comprehensive Mental Health Care, 1*(1), 27–43.

Bornstein, M. H., & Sigman, M. D. (1986). Continuity in mental development from infancy. *Child Development, 57,* 251–274.

Brown, A. (1982). Learning and development: The problems of compatibility, access, and induction. *Human Development, 25,* 89–115.

Burke, R. S. (1990). A cognitive-developmental approach to studying attention deficits. In J. T. Enns (Ed.), *The development of attention: Research and theory* (pp. 365–381). New York: Elsevier.

Campbell, S. B. (1985). Hyperactivity in preschoolers: Correlates and prognostic implications. *Clinical Psychology Review, 5,* 405–428.

Carlson, E. A., Jacobvitz, D., & Sroufe, L. A. (1995). A developmental investigation of inattentiveness and hyperactivity. *Child Development, 66,* 37–54.

Caron, R. F., & Caron, A. J. (1978). Effects of ecologically relevant manipulations on infant discrimination learning. *Infant Behavior and Development, 1,* 291–307.

Chee, P., Logan, G., Schachar, R., Lindsay, P., & Wachsmuth, R. (1989). Effects of event rate and display time on sustained attention in normal, hyperactive, and control children. *Journal of Abnormal Child Psychology, 17,* 371–391.

Cohen, L. B., & Salapatek, P. (Eds.). (1975). *Infant perception: From sensation to cognition: Vol. 1. Basic visual processes.* New York: Academic Press.

Coldren, J. T., & Colombo, J. (1994). The nature and processes of preverbal learning: Implications from nine month old infants' discrimination problem solving. *Monographs of the Society for Research in Child Development, 59*(4, Serial No. 241).

Colombo, J. (1993). *Infant cognition: Predicting later intellectual functioning.* Newbury Park, CA: Sage.

Colombo, J., Mitchell, D. W., Coldren, J. T., & Atwater, J. (1990). Discrimination learning during the first year: Stimulus and positional cues. *Journal of Experimental Psychology: Learning, Memory, and Cognition, 16*(1), 98–109.

Douglas, V. I. (1980). Higher mental processes in hyperactive children. In R. M. Knights & D. J. Bakker (Eds.), *Rehabilitation, treatment, and management of learning disorders* (pp. 65–92). Baltimore: University Park Press.

Douglas, V. I. (1983). Attentional and cognitive problems. In M. Rutter (Ed.), *Developmental neuropsychiatry* (pp. 280–328). New York: Guilford Press.

Douglas, V. I. (1988). Cognitive deficits in children with attention disorder with hyperactivity. In L. M. Bloomingdale & J. Sergeant (Eds.), *Attention deficit disorder: Criteria, cognition, and intervention* (pp. 65–81). New York: Pergamon Press.

Douglas, V. I., & Benezra, E. (1990). Supraspan verbal memory in attention deficit disorder with hyperactivity in normal and reading-disabled boys. *Journal of Abnormal Child Psychology, 18*(6), 617–638.

Douglas, V. I., & Peters, K. G. (1979). Toward a clearer definition of the attentional definition of hyperactive children. In G. Hale & M. Lewis (Eds.), *Attention and cognitive development* (pp. 173–247). New York: Plenum Press.

Enns, J. T. (1990). Relations between components of visual attention. In J. T.

Enns (Ed.), *The development of attention: Research and theory* (pp. 139–158). New York: Elsevier.

Enns, J. T., & Cameron, S. (1987). Selective attention in young children: The relations between visual search, filtering, and priming. *Journal of Experimental Child Psychology, 44,* 38–63.

Enns, J. T., & Girgus, J. S. (1985). Developmental changes in selective and integrative visual attention. *Journal of Experimental Child Psychology, 40,* 319–337.

Firestone, P., & Douglas, V. (1975). The effects of reward and punishment on reaction times and autonomic activity in hyperactive and normal children. *Journal of Abnormal Child Psychology, 3,* 201–216.

Freibergs, V., & Douglas, V. I. (1969). Concept learning in normal and hyperactive children. *Journal of Abnormal Psychology, 74,* 388–395.

Gholson, B. (1980). *The cognitive-developmental basis of human learning.* New York: Academic Press.

Gholson, B., & Beilin, H. (1979). A developmental model of human learning. In H. W. Reese (Ed.), *Advances in child development and behavior* (Vol. 13, pp. 47–81). New York: Academic Press.

Gholson, B., Levine, M., & Phillips, S. (1972). Hypotheses, strategies, and stereotypes in discrimination learning. *Journal of Experimental Child Psychology, 13,* 423–446.

Glaser, R. (1981). The future of testing: A research agenda for cognitive psychology and psychometrics. *American Psychologist, 36,* 923–936.

Glaser, R. (1990). The reemergence of learning theory within instructional research. *American Psychologist, 45*(1), 29–39.

Goodman, G., & Poillion, M. J. (1992). ADD: Acronym for any dysfunction or difficulty. *Journal of Special Education, 26*(1), 37–56.

Goodman, R., & Stevenson, J. (1989). A twin study of hyperactivity—II: The aetiological role of genes, family relationships and perinatal adversity. *Journal of Child Psychology and Psychiatry, 30*(5), 691–709.

Gordon, M. (1987). How is a computerized attention test used in the diagnosis of attention deficit disorder? *Journal of Children in Contemporary Society, 19,* 53–64.

Greeno, J. (1980). Psychology of learning, 1960–1980: One participant's observations. *American Psychologist, 35*(8), 713–728.

Guevremont, D. C., DuPaul, G. J., & Barkley, R. A. (1990). Diagnosis and assessment of attention-deficit–hyperactivity disorder in children. *Journal of School Psychology, 28,* 51–78.

Halperin, J. M., Newcorn, J. H., Sharma, V., Healey, J. M., Wolf, L. E., Pascualvaca, D. M., & Schwartz, S. (1990). Inattentive and nonattentive ADHD children: Do they constitute a unitary group? *Journal of Abnormal Psychology, 18*(4), 437–449.

Hartsough, C. S., & Lambert, N. M (1985). Medical factors in hyperactive and normal children: Prenatal, developmental, and health findings. *American Journal of Orthopsychiatry, 55*(2), 190–200.

Hayes, K. L. (1953). The backward curve: A method for the study of learning. *Psychological Review, 60,* 269–275.

Hooks, K., Milich, R., & Lorch, E. P. (1994). Sustained and selective attention in boys with attention-deficit–hyperactivity disorder. *Journal of Clinical Child Psychology, 23*(1), 69–77.

Horowitz, F. D., & Colombo, J. (1990). Future agendas and directions in infancy research. *Merrill-Palmer Quarterly, 36*(1), 173–178.

Hynd, G. W., Hern, K. L., Voeller, K. K., & Marshall, R. M. (1991). Neurobiological basis of attention-deficit–hyperactivity disorder. *School Psychology Review, 20*(2), 174–186.

Hynd, G. W., Nieves, N., Connor, R. T., Stone, P. Town, P., Becker, M. G., Lahey, B. B., & Lorys, A. R. (1989). Attention deficit disorder with and without hyperactivity: Reaction time and speed of cognitive processing. *Journal of Learning Disabilities, 22*(9), 573–580.

Jacobvitz, D., & Sroufe, L. A. (1987). The early caregiver–child relationship and attention-deficit disorder with hyperactivity in kindergarten: A prospective study. *Child Development, 58*, 1488–1495.

Kahneman, D. (1973). *Attention and effort.* Englewood Cliffs, NJ: Prentice-Hall.

Klee, S. H., & Garfinkel, B. D. (1983). The computerized continuous performance task: A new measure of inattention. *Journal of Abnormal Child Psychology, 11*, 487–496.

Korkman, M., & Peltomaa, K. (1991). A pattern of test findings predicting attention problems at school. *Journal of Abnormal Child Psychology, 19*(4), 451–467.

Lane, D. M., & Pearson, D. A. (1982). The development of selective attention. *Merrill-Palmer Quarterly, 28*(3), 317–337.

Levine, M. (1966). Hypothesis behavior by humans during discrimination learning. *Journal of Experimental Psychology, 71*, 331–338.

Levine, M. (1975). *A cognitive theory of learning.* Hillsdale, NJ: Erlbaum.

Linder, B. A., & Siegel, L. S. (1983). The learning paradigm as a technique for investigating cognitive development. In J. Bisanz, G. L. Bisanz, & R. Kail (Eds.), *Learning in children* (pp. 37–60). New York: Springer-Verlag.

Lucko, J. (1994). *Attentional capabilities in children with attention deficit hyperactivity disorder.* Unpublished honors thesis, University of Toledo.

Luk, S. (1985). Direct observations studies of hyperactive behaviors. *Journal of the American Academy of Child Psychiatry, 24*, 338–344.

McCall, R. B., & Carriger, M. S. (1993). A meta-analysis of infant habituation and recognition memory performance as predictors of later IQ. *Child Development, 64*, 57–79.

McGee, R., Williams, S., & Feehan, M. (1992). Attention-deficit disorder and age of onset of problem behaviors. *Journal of Abnormal Child Psychology, 20*(5), 487–502.

Mitchell, D. W. (1988). *Process and product: The assessment of individual differences in the psychometric and cognitive traditions.* Unpublished manuscript, University of Kansas, Department of Human Development.

Mitchell, W. G., Chavez, J. M., Baker, S. A. Guzman, B. L., & Azen, S. P. (1990). Reaction time, impulsivity, and attention in hyperactive children and control: A video game technique. *Journal of Child Neurology, 5*, 195–204.

Neill, W. T. (1977). Inhibitory and faciliatory processes in selective attention.

Journal of Experimental Psychology: Human Perception and Performance, 3, 444–450.

Olson, G., & Sherman, T. S. (1983). Attention, learning, and memory in infants. In M. M. Haith & J. J. Campos (Eds.), *Handbook of child psychology: Vol. 2. Infancy and developmental psychobiology* (pp. 1001–1080). New York: Elsevier.

Pearson, D. A., & Lane, D. M. (1990). Reorientation in hyperactive and non-hyperactive children: Evidence for developmentally immature attention? In J. T. Enns (Ed.), *The development of attention: Research and theory* (pp. 345–363). New York: Elsevier.

Prior, M., Sanson, A., Freethy, C., & Geffen, G. (1985). Auditory attentional abilities in hyperactive children. *Journal of Child Psychology and Psychiatry, 26,* 289–304.

Rapport, M. D., & Kelly, K. L. (1991). Psychostimulant effects on learning and cognitive function: Findings and implications for children with attention deficit hyperactivity disorder. *Clinical Psychology Review, 11,* 61–92.

Reardon, S. M., & Naglieri, J. A. (1992). PASS cognitive processing characteristics of normal and ADHD males. *Journal of School Psychology, 30,* 151–163.

Richards, J. E., & Casey, B. J. (1992). Development of sustained attention in the human infant. In B. A. Campbell, H. Hayne, & R. Richardson (Eds.), *Attention and information processing in infants and adults: Perspectives from human and animal research* (pp. 30–60). Hillsdale. NJ: Erlbaum.

Rosenthal, R. H., & Allen, T. W. (1978). An examination of attention, arousal, and learning dysfunctions of hyperactive children. *Psychological Bulletin, 85,* 689–715.

Rosenthal, R. H., & Allen, T. W. (1980). Intratask distractibility in hyperkinetic and nonhyperkinetic children. *Journal of Abnormal Child Psychology, 8,* 175–187.

Ross, D. M., & Ross, S. A. (1982). *Hyperactivity: Current issues, research, and theory.* New York: Wiley.

Rubenstein, R. A., & Brown, R. T. (1994). An evaluation of the validity of the diagnostic category of attention deficit disorder. *American Journal of Orthopsychiatry, 54*(3), 398–413.

Ruff, H. A. (1990). Individual differences in sustained attention during infancy. In J. Colombo & J. W. Fagen (Eds.), *Individual differences in infancy* (pp. 247–270). Hillsdale, NJ: Erlbaum.

Schachar, R., & Logan, G. (1990). Are hyperactive children deficient in attentional capacity? *Journal of Abnormal Child Psychology, 18*(5), 493–513.

Seidel, W. T., & Joschko, M. (1990). Evidence of difficulties in sustained attention in children with ADHD. *Journal of Abnormal Child Psychology, 18,* 217–229.

Sergeant, J. (1988). From DSM-III attention deficit disorder to functional defects. In L. M. Bloomingdale & J. Sergeant (Eds.), *Attention deficit disorder: Criteria, cognition, and intervention* (pp. 183–198). New York: Pergamon Press.

Sergeant, J., & van der Meere, J. (1990). Convergence of approaches in localizing the hyperactivity deficit. In B. B. Lahey & A. E. Kazdin (Eds.), *Advances in clinical child psychology* (Vol. 13, pp. 207–246). New York: Plenum Press.

Siegler, R. (1983). Information-processing approaches to development. In W. Kessen (Ed.), *Handbook of child psychology* (4th ed.): *Vol. 1. History, theory, and methods* (pp. 129–211). New York: Wiley.

Stevenson, H. (1983). How children learn: The quest for a theory. In P. H. Mussen (Series Ed.), W. Kessen (Ed.), *Handbook of child psychology* (4th ed.): *Vol. 1. History, theory, and methods* (pp. 213–236). New York: Wiley.

Strutt, G. F., Anderson, D. R., & Well, A. D. (1975). A developmental study of the effects of irrelevant information on speeded classification. *Journal of Experimental Child Psychology, 20,* 127–135.

Swanson, J. M., Posner, M., Potkin, S., Bonforte, S., Youpa, D., Fiore, C., Cantwell, D., & Crinella, F. (1991). Activating tasks for the study of visual–spatial attention in ADHD children: A cognitive anatomic approach. *Journal of Child Neurology, 6,* 119–127.

Swanson, J. M., Shea, C., McBurnett, K., Potkin, S. G., Fiore, C., & Crinella, F. (1990). Attention and hyperactivity. In J. T. Enns (Ed.), *The development of attention: Research and theory* (pp. 383–403). New York: Elsevier.

Tant, J. L., & Douglas, V. I. (1982). Problem solving in hyperactive, normal, and reading-disabled boys. *Journal of Abnormal Child Psychology, 10*(3), 285–306.

Tarnowski, K. J., Prinz, R. J., & Hay, S. M. (1986). Comparative analysis of attention deficits in hyperactive and learning-disabled children. *Journal of Abnormal Psychology, 95,* 341–345.

Thompson, L. A., Fagan, J. F., & Fulker, D. W. (1991). Longitudinal predictions of specific cognitive abilities from infant novelty preference. *Child Development, 62,* 530–538.

Underwood, B. J. (1975). Individual differences as a crucible in theory construction. *American Psychologist, 30*(2), 128–134.

van der Meere, J., & Sergeant, J. (1988a). Controlled processing and vigilance in hyperactivity: Time will tell. *Journal of Abnormal Child Psychology, 16,* 641–655.

van der Meere, J., & Sergeant, J. (1988b). Focused attention in persuasively hyperactive children. *Journal of Abnormal Child Psychology, 16,* 627–639.

Weissberg, R., Ruff, H., & Lawson, K. R (1990). The usefulness of reaction time tasks in studying attention and organization of behavior in young children. *Developmental and Behavioral Pediatrics, 11*(2), 59–64.

Well, A. D., Lorch, E. P., & Anderson, D. R. (1980). Developmental trends in distractibility: Is absolute or proportional decrement the appropriate measure of interference? *Journal of Experimental Child Psychology, 30,* 109–124.

Whalen, C. K., & Henker, B. (1980). The social ecology of psychostimulant treatment: A model for conceptual and empirical analysis. In C. K. Whalen & B. Henker (Eds.), *Hyperactive children: The social ecology of identification and treatment* (pp. 3–49). New York: Academic Press.

Wright, J. C., & Vlietstra, A. G. (1975). The development of selective attention: From perceptual exploration to logical search. In H. W. Reese (Ed.), *Advances in child development and behavior* (Vol. 10, pp. 195–239). New York: Academic Press.

Zeaman, D., & House, B. J. (1963). An attentional theory of retardate discrimination learning. In N. R. Ellis (Ed.), *Handbook of mental deficiency* (pp. 159–223). New York: McGraw-Hill.

SECTION IV
CHILDHOOD, ATTENTION, AND PSYCHOPATHOLOGY

Teratogenic Effects of Alcohol on Attention

Karen Kopera-Frye
Heather Carmichael Olson
Ann P. Streissguth

In the last two decades, it has become clear that alcohol is a teratogen. A teratogen is defined as any agent capable of inducing abnormal or atypical fetal development. Hundreds of carefully controlled animal studies have provided evidence that alcohol ingested during pregnancy readily crosses the placenta, enters the fetal circulatory system, and results in a wide range of adverse offspring effects, ranging from death to subtle effects on growth, body formation, and neurobehavioral function. Once an affected child is born, the teratogenic effects of alcohol can be seen in a variety of physical malformations, including flattening of the child's midface or growth retardation. There is evidence that alcohol exposure *in utero* can also cause diffuse brain damage through cell death and disruption of neuronal migration, although the mechanisms by which alcohol causes insult to the developing fetus are not yet clearly delineated. The resulting central nervous system (CNS) dysfunction in affected individuals can be manifested in a myriad of lasting and debilitating behavioral or learning problems, and especially in attentional deficits. Of course, these teratogenic effects depend on the dose, timing, and duration of the prenatal exposure to alcohol, and—as with other teratogens—not all exposed offspring are affected. Individual differences occur: Some fetuses are susceptible to the effects of alcohol, whereas others are resilient.

Disordered attention appears basic to many of the cognitive and behavioral difficulties observed among individuals who are affected by alcohol exposure before birth. This chapter is organized around the hypothesis that CNS dysfunction caused by prenatal exposure to alcohol results in attentional difficulties, which in turn impact higher-order cognitive processes and subsequently compromise intellectual, academic, neuropsychological, and adaptive functioning. The ongoing functional problems of the fetal alcohol-affected individual, or "secondary disabilities," are especially problematic if the environment does not provide ways to facilitate development or compensate for the problems. Such secondary disabilities can range from learning problems or attention deficit disorder (ADD) to more serious difficulties in adaptive functioning including school failure, joblessness, mental illness, and so forth.

Given the central role that attentional deficits are hypothesized to play in fetal alcohol effects, it is particularly important to study the relationship between prenatal alcohol exposure and disruptions in attention. Indeed, alcohol teratogenesis is a topic that could be of great interest to experts in the field of attention research, who could bring important insights and methods to the field. The study of alcohol effects on attention provides several unique research opportunities. First, theoretical models of attention can be expanded by examining ways in which the elements of attention are impacted by CNS dysfunction arising from prenatal alcohol exposure, as well as through study of developmental changes in the manifestations of disrupted attention in individuals with fetal alcohol effects. Second, knowledge of brain–behavior relationships can be advanced as the neural substrates of fetal alcohol effects on attention are delineated in both animal and human research. Third, study of the role that disrupted attention plays in the lives of alcohol-affected children can lead to clinical research on useful and specific approaches to prevention and intervention.

Research on alcohol teratogenesis formally began in 1973, when the teratogenic potential of alcohol was first suspected. The last two decades have been spent building evidence for the argument that alcohol is, in fact, a teratogen. Researchers and clinicians have been engaged in defining the full range of alcohol-related birth defects, from the striking and most serious manifestations of developmental disability seen in fetal alcohol syndrome (FAS) and possible fetal alcohol effects (FAE) to the more subtle functional learning and behavior deficits detected within groups of individuals who are exposed to lower levels of alcohol before birth. Researchers involved in the study of FAE have also faced the challenge of creating public health policy to prevent alcohol-related birth defects and have assisted in such efforts as the U.S. Surgeon General's warning against drinking during pregnancy, labeling of alcoholic beverage warnings, advocacy of alcohol/drug treatment for pregnant women, and public education about the consequences of drinking during pregnancy.

The field of alcohol teratogenesis is still in its infancy. Up to this point research has documented the presence of alcohol-related attentional difficulties and associated behavioral manifestations but has not specified how alcohol disrupts the attentional system. It is very difficult to unravel the links between a multifaceted construct such as attention and the often diffuse brain damage caused by prenatal alcohol exposure. However, recent advances in the study of alcohol effects suggest the need to move beyond simple description of effects to understanding the mechanisms producing such effects. To stimulate this move, the present chapter provides a careful review of convergent data on attentional problems and alcohol effects from several research areas and then suggests directions for future study.

It is important to note that research examining the effects of prenatal alcohol exposure on CNS dysfunction is guided by several general principles of behavioral teratology originally proposed by Wilson (1977) and later modified by Vorhees (1986). Applied to alcohol effects, these principles specify that the type and magnitude of the behavioral effect on the organism (the "response") depends on the prenatal "dose" of alcohol reaching the developing nervous system. The pattern, timing, and amount of alcohol exposure are important in defining the "dose." This important principle in behavioral teratology is known as the "dose–response relationship." To understand the full extent of gestational alcohol exposure effects, then, it is critical to study the dose–response relationship. We are able to do this by examining both children with FAS who were exposed to high levels of alcohol exposure and children not formally diagnosed as having FAS yet alcohol-exposed at lower levels before birth. In this way we can understand the full spectrum of prenatal alcohol effects on the CNS, from mental retardation to more subtle but debilitating attentional difficulties.

To fully consider fetal alcohol effects and their relationship with attention, we shall review four research areas in this chapter. First are clinical follow-up studies that describe the specific patterns of physical malformations and serious cognitive impairment seen in children with FAS or possible FAE. Second are more general clinical case studies of children born to alcoholic mothers yet not formally diagnosed with FAS or labeled as having possible fetal alcohol effects. Third are experimental studies on alcohol teratogenesis with animals that have been carried out concurrently with the clinical research on humans. These animal studies provide the definitive etiological link between alcohol as a teratogen and patterns of deficit in growth, morphology, learning, and behavior that are similar to those seen in humans who have been prenatally exposed. Fourth are large longitudinal prospective studies of the growth and behavioral and cognitive functioning of infants, children, and adolescents who were prenatally exposed to a full range of maternal alcohol use during pregnancy, including exposure at the level of social drinking. These epidemiological studies examine the impact of alcohol on behavior within the full context of human experience. To date, only one of these epidemiological studies has assessed prenatally alcohol-exposed children from birth through adolescence. Termed the Seattle Longitudinal Prospective Study on Alcohol and Pregnancy, that project has been carried out in our laboratory. Findings from the Seattle Study describe the enduring effects of alcohol exposure on the developing CNS, even at lower levels of exposure, and results of this study are highlighted in the present chapter.

In reviewing the four areas of research, it has become clear to us that alcohol-related attentional disruption has a variety of behavioral manifestations and that findings on attentional function must be placed within a developmental framework. Since teratogens such as alcohol produce brain damage prenatally by modifying the developing brain, it is also clear that a lifespan approach is necessary for a complete examination of alcohol effects. In studying the lives of alcohol-exposed children, it is necessary to look for signs of CNS dysfunction from birth onward, a rather different approach from the more familiar methods of the neuropsychologist or neuropathologist who looks for damage to the normal brain resulting from trauma or disease.

In the study of alcohol effects in animals, attention-related constructs to be reviewed include habituation, state regulation, response inhibition, overall activity level, and even learning deficits. In human studies on alcohol effects that are reviewed here, attention-related constructs differ according to developmental level. In infants, habituation, state regulation, sleep–wake cycling, and speed of information processing are seen as related to attention. In young children, naturalistic behavioral observations of activity level and attentional focus are accepted as evidence of attention-related constructs, while as children grow older, data on activity level, attention, and information processing are measured in the classroom situation, by parental report, or by self-report. From early childhood on, performance on laboratory tests of vigilance (sustained attention) are accepted as one assessment of attentional function. Other types of neuropsychological tasks, carried out in the laboratory and administered with paper and pencil or by computer, are used to tap other components of attention.

Following the literature on alcohol effects, this chapter touches on the limited evidence gathered in the search for structural and functional disruption in the brain that may be responsible for alcohol-related attentional deficits and for associated cognitive impairment. As the following sections will show, the need for further research in all these areas is very clear. To that end, a program of research on alcohol effects and attention will be outlined. These beginning research ideas are meant to intrigue researchers with a most important and interesting problem: the impact of prenatal alcohol exposure on attention.

CLINICAL STUDIES OF PATIENTS WITH FAS/FAE

The initial evidence of the teratogenic effects of alcohol came from recognition of cases of FAS, first identified in 1973. FAS is the diagnostic term for a birth defect caused by prenatal alcohol exposure. FAS is diagnosed when patients have three defining criteria: (1) growth deficiency of prenatal origin for height or weight; (2) a pattern of specific minor anomalies that includes characteristic facial features (e.g., short palpebral fissures, midface hypoplasia, thin upper lip, smooth and/or long philtrum); and (3) CNS dysfunction, including such manifestations as microcephaly, delayed development, hyperactivity, attention deficits, learning disabilities, intellectual deficits, and so forth (Clarren & Smith, 1978; Smith, 1982).

Since 1973, hundreds of cases of FAS have been documented. Currently FAS is recognized as the leading known cause of mental retardation in the United States (Abel & Sokol, 1987), surpassing the prevalence of Down syndrome and spina bifida. But FAS is only the tip of the iceberg. Patients who were exposed to alcohol *in utero* and who display several of the above characteristics (but do not show all of the hallmark features and so do not warrant a diagnosis of FAS) are described as having *possible FAE* (Clarren & Smith, 1978). While possible FAE is not a medical diagnosis, it is a useful clinical and research label. It describes a condition where clear prenatal alcohol exposure is identified as one of the possible causes of a patient's disability, and does not merely describe a milder form of FAS (Sokol & Clarren, 1989).

In patients with FAS/possible FAE, prenatal alcohol exposure is related to a wide spectrum of long-term physical and behavioral impairments, many related to attention (Smith, 1979; Streissguth et al., 1991; Streissguth, 1992; Coles, 1992; Spohr, Willms, & Steinhausen, 1993). The clinical literature is replete with behavioral observations of childhood attention deficits, impulsivity, hyperactivity, and disrupted state regulation, as well as related behavioral deficits that occur later in life. Among those with fetal alcohol effects, evidence of attentional difficulties may take different forms depending on the level of development, from infancy through adolescence. For example, hyperactivity, defined as observations of excessive gross motor activity in a young child, may be observed later in life as an inability to attend to classroom tasks.

Findings on Hyperactivity, Academics, and Adaptive Behavior

Hyperactivity, tremulousness, hypotonia, and hyperacusis (Pierog, Chandavasu, & Wexler, 1977), irritability (Lemoine, Harrousseau, Borteyru, & Menuet, 1968), weak sucking ability, feeding difficulties, and delayed development have all been observed in infants and young children with FAS/possible FAE (Jones & Smith, 1973; Streissguth, Herman, & Smith, 1978). Additionally, hyperactivity and attentional deficits characterized 89% of 41 children with FAS studied by Hanson, Jones, and Smith (1976) and 72% of those examined by Majewski and Majewski (1988). Iosub, Fuchs, Bingol, and Gromisch (1981) reported a variety of difficulties in a sample of 63 children with FAS, some raised with their biological parents and others in foster care. While a majority exhibited mental retardation and developmental delays (46% and 41%, respectively), the most common deficits in this group were hyperactivity (74%) and speech difficulties (80%). In a 10-year follow-up of 8 of the first 11 children diagnosed with FAS in 1973, 7 of them exhibited continued difficulties with attention; however of the 4 who presented as hyperactive at the age of 1–4 years only one remained hyperactive at age 10 years (Streissguth, Clarren, & Jones, 1985). Steinhausen, Nestler, and Spohr (1982) have documented hyperactivity, as well as eating and sleeping difficulties, speech impairment, clumsiness, difficulty with peers, and stereotyped behaviors, as significantly differentiating children with FAS from a group of controls. Spohr et al. (1993) reported that 71% of 60 patients with FAS/FAE were hyperactive (average age = 3 years), while 52% remained so 10 years later. Thus, these early studies of children with FAS demonstrate a host of behaviors indicating CNS difficulties, particularly hyperactivity, which later studies have linked to attentional difficulties.

Multiple, chronic academic difficulties have also been described in patients with FAS/possible FAE (Spohr & Steinhausen, 1987; Spohr et al., 1993; Streissguth et al., 1991). When patients were examined on the Wide Range Achievement Test—Revised (WRAT-R), which assesses school achievement in reading, spelling, and arithmetic, Streissguth et al. (1991) found arithmetic deficits to be the most pronounced in a group of 47 adolescents with FAS/possible FAE. Interestingly, this same relative weakness in mathematics was later found in a larger epidemiological sample of adolescents prenatally exposed to lower levels of alcohol (Sampson, Streissguth, Barr, & Bookstein, 1989).

Rating scales or structured interviews are frequently used to obtain standardized data from parents or caregivers on problems in adaptive function among older individuals exposed to alcohol in utero. Streissguth et al. (1991) measured level of adaptive functioning via the Vineland Adaptive Behavior Scales (VABS), a semistructured caretaker interview, among 31 nonretarded adolescents and adults with FAS/possible FAE. Frequently reported were difficulties with poor concentration and attention, social withdrawal, impulsivity, and periods of high anxiety. LaDue, Streissguth, and Randels (1992) found that 77% of 54 adolescents and adults with FAS/possible FAE exhibited poor concentration and attention as assessed by the VABS. Carmichael Olson, Feldman, Streissguth, Sampson, and Bookstein (1996) found problematic adaptive function in a group of nine teenagers with FAS using the VABS, and a variety of behavioral problems using the Child Behavior Checklist (CBCL/4-16; Achenbach & Edelbrock, 1983). Five of the nine showed clinical levels of internalizing and/or externalizing behavior problems. Many types of problems were reported, with immaturity and hyperactivity often part of the behavioral picture.

Neuropsychological Findings

Given the many alcohol-related behavioral difficulties observed in earlier clinical studies, the neuropsychological functioning of alcohol-affected individuals has recently become a focus of investigation. These studies have employed more sophisticated, controlled means of examining CNS dysfunction and attentional difficulties, rather than relying on informal behavioral observation techniques or caregiver interviews. Conry (1990) compared a sample of 19 school-age children with FAS/possible FAE to matched controls and found the children with FAS to be significantly more impaired on all neuropsychological measures relative to controls. Of special note was their slowed reaction time as measured by latency of responding (depression of a telegraph key) to a lighted stimulus, possibly due to distractibility impeding performance and resulting in sustained attention difficulties. Nanson and Hiscock (1990) compared equal numbers of young children with FAS/possible FAE, ADD, and controls on reaction time and vigilance tasks. Results indicated that children with FAS/possible FAE had slower response rates when compared to normals and children with ADD, yet exhibited errors similar to the ADD group, thus suggesting inability to inhibit impulsive responding.

Mattson et al. (1992) described below-norm performance in recall and recognition, as well as an excessive number of perseverative responses and intrusions, in two retarded adolescents with FAS on The California Verbal Learning Test—Research Edition (Delis, Kramer, Kaplan, & Ober, 1987), thus suggesting difficulties with auditory attention and memory, among other problems. Gray and Streissguth (1990) reported impaired performance on a spatial memory task requiring sustained attention in seven adolescents and adults with FAS compared to matched age and sex controls, although IQ was not controlled. Kodituwakku, Handmaker, Cutler, Weathersby, and Handmaker (1995) compared a sample of 10 higher-functioning individuals with FAS and FAE with controls having no known prenatal alcohol exposure. While several verbal and self-regulatory tasks did not differ between groups, alcohol-affected individuals did show specific difficulties on tasks tapping such skills as planning and auditory attentional capacity. In an exploratory study, Carmichael Olson et al. (1996)

administered tests of IQ, adaptive behavior, and neuropsychological tasks presumed sensitive to alcohol effects to nine nonretarded adolescents with FAS. Comparing their performance to psychometric norms and a comparison sample of adolescents with little or no prenatal alcohol exposure, the teenagers with FAS had typically poor school performance and adaptive behavior, and a wide range of cognitive and academic function. Though no single profile characterized all subjects, the FAS group as a whole showed significant neuropsychological deficits, with decrements in visual–spatial skills, difficulties in processing speed and accuracy, problems with attentional and memory tasks, and poor performance on tasks of cognitive flexibility and planning. Deficits of executive function and perseverative responding were found (despite average sustained and divided attention) among 16 nonretarded young adults with FAS (Kerns, Don, Mateer, & Streissguth, in press). In general, then, neuropsychological studies focusing on patients with FAS/possible FAE suggest particular problems with attention, as well as deficits in short- and long-term memory, spatial skills, executive function, and information processing.

CHILDREN OF ALCOHOLIC MOTHERS

Studies of children of alcoholic mothers provide information about the degree of behavioral and/or performance impairments observed in persons heavily exposed to alcohol *in utero,* but without regard to the diagnostic features of FAS or possible FAE. Estimates suggest that approximately one-third of the children of chronically alcoholic mothers who drank during pregnancy may potentially display FAS characteristics (Aronson, 1984; Jones, Smith, Streissguth, & Myrianthopoulos, 1974; Seidenberg & Majewski, 1978). However, it should be noted that chronicity or stage of maternal alcoholism, as well as pattern of exposure, are critical determinants in determining whether full manifestation of the FAS phenotype will occur (Majewski, 1993; Majewski & Majewski, 1988).

As with studies focusing only on children with FAS, some of the first studies of children born to alcoholic women were primarily concerned with describing the behaviors of the exposed children. One study compared the behavior of children born prior to and subsequent to maternal alcoholism and reported that children born prior to the onset of the mother's alcoholism were seen as having "vegetative, emotional, behavioral" disorders with onset at 9–10 years; those born after had "profound impairments of the CNS that were manifest early in infancy" (Shruygin, 1974). This early study is important in that it points out potential differences in the postnatal versus the prenatal impact of maternal alcoholism on the offspring. Additionally, a study by Jones et al. (1974) and Streissguth

(1976) found borderline-to-moderate mental deficiency in 44% of 23 children of alcoholic mothers, as compared to less than 5% of the controls matched on 12 variables reflecting sociodemographic background. This study was important because both cases and controls were selected from a pool of 55,000 families participating in the Collaborative Perinatal Project of the National Institute of Neurological Diseases and Stroke, thus allowing a degree of covariate control and follow-up across 7 years that is difficult to achieve in smaller studies.

Later studies replicated these results and extended the findings to other types of behavioral difficulties as well. Aronson (1984) and Aronson, Kyllerman, Sable, Sandin, and Olegard (1985) found that 50% of 99 children of alcoholic mothers had borderline or retarded intellectual ability and 49% exhibited neuropsychological symptoms defined as hyperactivity, impulsivity, difficulties with concentration, or perseveration. A follow-up study with a subsample of the children revealed impairment on visual–spatial tasks, reasoning, and continued behavioral difficulties (Aronson et al., 1985). Similarly, Larsson and Bohlin (1987) reported that 80% of 15 children of alcoholic mothers exhibited behavioral difficulties (e.g., hyperactivity and short attention span) at the 2-year follow-up. Despite their normal IQ scores, Shaywitz, Cohen, and Shaywitz (1980) found behavioral and learning difficulties in all of the children of alcoholic mothers that they studied. Hyperactivity and school failure were noted in 14 of the 15 children. Steinhausen, Nestler, and Huth (1982) found that 19 children of alcoholic mothers exhibited a greater degree of psychiatric symptoms (e.g., impaired concentration and stereotypic behaviors) that did a control group matched by sex and age.

In summary, several studies now highlight the long-term CNS risks to children of alcoholic mothers. Problems include developmental delays, hyperactivity, and fine motor problems, in addition to compromised intellectual and academic functioning. Of all of these, attentional difficulties (including hyperactivity, impulsivity, poor concentration) are among the most frequently reported and are even evident in children with average intellectual capacity.

PARALLEL FINDINGS
IN EXPERIMENTAL ANIMAL MODELS

It is the animal studies that provide the irrefutable link between gestational alcohol exposure and offspring deficits. Animal models are particularly useful, as they allow for manipulation of timing and exposure levels, as well as control of nutrition and the postnatal environment. Animal research delineates the range and specific patterns of alcohol effects using tightly controlled experiments that would not be ethical in human studies. It is striking how findings from animal studies parallel those described in the less controlled studies of alcohol-affected humans (Driscoll, Streissguth, & Riley, 1990; West, 1986).

When exposed to high doses of alcohol, animals exhibit structural brain malformations such as decreased neuronal migration and atypical cell proliferation (Miller, 1992), delayed myelination of the fetal brain (Phillips, 1992), and permanent cell loss in the hippocampus and cerebellum (Goodlett, Bonthius, Wasserman, & West, 1992; Goodlett & West, 1992). Studies of state regulation or neurobehavioral integrity in alcohol-exposed rats have found a failure to habituate (ability to "tune out" redundant stimuli) and longer latency to habituate (Barron, Gagnon, & Riley, 1986), decreased inhibitory capability (Goodlett et al., 1992; Riley, Lochry, & Shapiro, 1979), and increased level of exploratory behaviors and overall activity (Abel, 1982; Bond, 1986; Mattson, Carlos, & Riley, 1993).

Alcohol-exposed rats are also more likely to exhibit learning deficits that may well be associated with underlying attentional deficits. Poorer associative learning (Barron et al., 1988; Goodlett et al., 1992), impaired radial arm maze performance (Reyes, Wolf, & Savage, 1989), inefficient passive–avoidance learning, impaired acquisition of single-pattern alternation tasks (Greene, Diaz-Granados, & Amsel, 1992), disruption in reversal learning in discrimination tasks, and deficits in cliff avoidance learning tasks (Riley, Lochry, Shapiro, & Baldwin, 1979; Duffy & Leonard, 1991; Driscoll, Chen, & Riley, 1982) have all been documented. An intriguing recent study (La Fiette, Carlos, & Riley, 1994) revealed that alcohol-exposed rats were able to learn the pattern in a serial task, yet unable to inhibit increased running tendencies in response to differential rewards relative to controls. While the exposed rats were able to perform the correct response (run to the pellets), they were unable to adjust their response rate according to different reinforcement conditions (number of pellets) relative to controls, possibly due to overactivity and inability to inhibit responding. Martin, Martin, Sigman, and Radow (1978) found that exposed rats were unable to learn reinforcement schedules but performed more efficiently on schedules requiring a slower response. Alcohol-related learning deficits have also been demonstrated in nonhuman primates; Clarren, Astley, Gunderson, and Spellman (1992) found that alcohol-exposed macaques exhibited deficient performance on object permanence tasks and tasks measuring memory and learning. To successfully perform these types of tasks, the animal must remember the specific task events as well as the relationships among the events. Thus, efficient learning in the animal involves visual tracking of the stimuli and learning the rules of the reinforcement schedule, processes shown to be impaired in hippocampal-lesioned animals. One possible explanation for the impaired task performance may be presence of a general deficit in response inhibition (La Fiette et al., 1994).

Prenatal alcohol exposure has been shown to affect a wide range of behaviors in humans, with larger effects typically associated with greater exposure. Alcohol effects seen in animal studies on measures of attentional and associated behaviors such as activity level, learning, and inhibition corroborate earlier clinical studies of individuals with FAS/possible FAE. Findings from animal studies are also in accord with those from recent epidemiological longitudinal studies of children exposed to the full range of maternal alcohol use, including lower levels of exposure.

EPIDEMIOLOGICAL/POPULATION-BASED STUDIES

Population-based studies are concerned with effects of prenatal alcohol exposure on CNS dysfunction at lower levels of exposure and can trace the course of alcohol effects over time. Such studies draw subjects from the entire exposure range and do not focus only on those individuals formally diagnosed with FAS. Indirect evidence for a dose–response effect between alcohol and attention lies in the congruence in findings of behavioral difficulties and impairment in epidemiological studies with those from clinical investigations of more heavily alcohol-exposed individuals. Epidemiological studies have several advantages in the study of alcohol-related attentional difficulties: They typically involve research designs that provide experimental and statistical control for potential confounders; they employ more sophisticated means of measuring attentional disturbance in exposed persons than do clinical studies; and they allow the dose–response relationship between prenatal alcohol exposure and behavioral outcome, the crux of teratogenic research, to be examined within the full context of human experience.

In this section, data from longitudinal prospective population-based studies of alcohol teratology will be considered across the lifespan from infancy to adolescence, highlighting attention-related findings. In particular, three issues need to be considered as we interpret the collective findings of these epidemiological studies. First, unlike animal studies that explicitly control the amount of gestational alcohol exposure, the degree of exposure to alcohol in epidemiological studies is defined by maternal self-report, which has inherent limitations. Second, design characteristics influence the ability of a study to detect the presence of any offspring effects of fetal alcohol exposure. Important design characteristics include: recruitment procedures (who gets into the study initially); the precision with which alcohol exposure is assessed; the reliability of alcohol and outcome measurement; sensitivity of outcome measures to alcohol effects; ages when data are collected; and sample size. Third, methods of data reduction and transformation, choice of statistical techniques, and the capability within a study design to adjust for potentially confounding variables are critical considerations in the interpretation of study findings. Differences in research design and methods may be primarily responsible for differing results across studies.

State Regulation and Other Attentional-Related Outcomes in Infancy

In epidemiological research, studies in the neonatal period (often within the first day or two of life) are of interest since the behavioral effects of teratogens can be demonstrated with minimal environmental influence. Indicators of neurophysiological development, such as sleep cycles, have been studied in alcohol-exposed infants. Early findings indicated that neonates of heavy-drinking mothers had poorer state regulation (increased disruption of the sleep–wake cycle), showed decreased quality of quiet sleep, and spent less time sleeping (Rosett et al., 1979; Sander et al., 1977). Ten years later, corroborating studies reported sleep disturbances in larger samples of neonates exposed to lower levels of prenatal alcohol exposure (Scher, Richardson, Coble, Day, & Stoffer, 1988; Stoffer, Scher, Richardson, Day, & Coble, 1988). Such disruption in state regulation among alcohol-exposed infants is an early sign of faulty self-regulation abilities and a potential harbinger of attentional and other self-regulatory deficits at later ages.

Some studies have employed the Neonatal Behavioral Assessment Scale (NBAS) to measure components of neurobehavioral integrity among alcohol-exposed infants. Two measures, habituation and arousal (both measuring responsiveness to environmental stimuli), have shown particularly important alcohol-related effects. In the Seattle Longitudinal Prospective Study on Alcohol and Pregnancy carried out in our laboratory, Streissguth, Barr, and Martin (1983) examined 417 infants with the NBAS at 1 day of age. They found an increased level of difficulty in habituating to auditory and visual stimuli and lower levels of arousal to be related to increased levels of alcohol exposure. Similarly, Jacobson, Fein, Jacobson, Schwartz, and Dowler (1984) found increased prenatal exposure to be related to lower levels of arousal (decreased range of state) on the NBAS in 173 3-day-old infants exposed to differing levels of alcohol. Coles, Smith, Fernhoff, and Falek (1985) reported that alcohol-exposed infants exhibited alterations in reflexive behavior, immature motoric behavior, and increased activity level when compared to nonexposed infants. Using the NBAS, Smith, Coles, Lancaster, Fernhoff, and Falek (1986) found that individual differences in orientation (ability to attend to stimuli and remain alert) were due to the duration of exposure, whereas differences in autonomic regulation (presence of startles and tremors) were primarily due to duration and level of exposure. In contrast, some researchers have not found a relationship between alcohol exposure and NBAS performance (Ernhart et al., 1985; Richardson, Day, & Taylor, 1989). Such discrepancies in study results probably reflect variation in study procedures, differences in infant state during test administration (in at least one study), and a significant amount of missing data on the habituation tests in the second study.

With older infants, researchers have used the Bayley Scales of Infant Development. Some epidemiological studies, including the Seattle Study, have found poorer performance with increased prenatal alcohol exposure (Streissguth, Barr, Martin, & Herman, 1980; Coles, Smith, & Falek, 1987; J. L. Jacobson et al., 1993), whereas some have not (Ernhart et al., 1985; Richardson & Day, 1991). More recently, an information-processing paradigm that employs the Fagan Visual Recognition Test and the Cross-Modal Transfer Task has been used with a sample of 403 alcohol-exposed infants less than 1 year of age. S. W. Jacobson and colleagues (Jacobson, Jacobson, Sokol, Martier, & Ager, 1993) found that prenatal alcohol exposure was significantly related to a developmentally lower level of infant play and to longer fixation duration on visual recognition and cross-modal transfer tasks. These findings reflect difficulties with the ability to imitate modeled behavior and decreased speed of information processing, and suggest an inability to effectively disengage attention in response to subsequent stimuli (S. W. Jacobson et al., 1993).

Neuropsychological Findings in the Preschool Years

Several prospective studies have gone beyond the period of infancy into the preschool years to examine the effects of prenatal alcohol exposure on attention, among other areas of deficit. Their findings are important in that evidence of inattention has been reported in alcohol-exposed children after infancy, together with behavioral descriptions of poor self-control and internal regulation, suggesting pervasiveness of exposure effects. Inattention has been documented via naturalistic observation in the child's home, by performance on laboratory tests of attention, and by independent examiner ratings during standardized testing in the laboratory.

Landesman-Dwyer, Ragozin, and Little (1981) examined attentional behaviors of 128 children studied in their homes during mealtime and storytime. Mothers were recruited prenatally for all levels of alcohol use, but those reporting high levels were excluded from subsequent analysis. Thus, the study sample included children with histories of moderate to no alcohol exposure but excluded those with environmental risk factors that might be confounded with maternal alcoholism. Even after adjusting for covariates such as prenatal maternal smoking and the quality of the postnatal home environment, Landesman-Dwyer et al. found that prenatal alcohol exposure was related to shortened attentional episodes, more frequent disruptions of attention, increased fidgety behaviors, and a higher proportion of intervals of inattention.

In the Seattle Study, several controlled laboratory measures of attention and vigilance were obtained when the 465 children reached 4 years of age. A vigilance test was used in which the child watched a large model of a Victorian house and was instructed to press a telegraph key whenever a kitten appeared in a window (at irregular intervals). Increased prenatal alcohol exposure was related to increased errors of omission, commission, longer reaction time, and less accurate responding, despite the fact that the children were physically oriented to the display panel (Streissguth et al., 1984). Additionally, slower information processing was manifested among children in the Seattle Study on the Wisconsin Fine Motor Steadiness Battery (Matthews & Klöve, 1978). Increased prenatal exposure was related to longer "time in error," reflecting the time it takes the child to move the stylus away from the edge of the maze in response to an auditory stimulus signaling an error (Barr, Streissguth, Darby, & Sampson, 1990). Boyd, Ernhart, Greene, Sokol, and Martier (1991) used a paradigm similar to that used in the Seattle study to measure vigilance in 245 4-year-olds but did not find an impact of prenatal alcohol exposure on attention. However, there were differences in sample recruitment criteria, prenatal alcohol measures, treatment of covariates, and administration of the vigilance test in the home (as opposed to administration in the lab, as in the Seattle Study); these differences may account for the discrepant findings between studies. Within the Seattle Study, there is clear evidence of attentional difficulties across situations, even when different procedures are used for assessing attention. The congruence of findings across situations lends support to the idea that a stable central attentional deficit exists among alcohol-affected preschool children.

Attentional Findings during Middle Childhood: Focus on the Seattle Study

Several longitudinal prospective studies have been extended to follow up the effects of prenatal alcohol exposure on attentional development in school-age children. Typically, vigilance tasks such as the Continuous Performance Test (CPT) have been used (Rosvold, Mirsky, Sarason, Bransome, & Beck, 1956). In the Atlanta study (Brown et al., 1991), 68 children (mean age = 6 years) were administered a CPT, and behavioral checklists and videotaped play sessions were employed. Children of mothers who drank throughout their pregnancy exhibited an inability to sustain attention across trials on the CPT yet no difficulties with impulsivity. Various modifications of CPT-type tasks are frequently used as laboratory measures of attentional problems (Boyd et al., 1991; Greene et al., 1991), and false-alarm errors are reported at increased levels among hyperactive children (O'Dougherty, Nuechterlein, & Drew, 1984) and learning-disabled, nonhyperactive children up through 15 years of age (Swanson, 1983).

Detailed description of the CPT used in the longitudinal Seattle Study is given here, since it was employed with slight modification at both the 7- and 14-year assessments, with important and consistent findings. In the Seattle Study CPT, omission and commission errors are measured in both an X-Task and an AX-Task. In the X-Task, the child is asked to push the button each time the letter "X" appears in a string of letters that are presented one at a time for brief regular intervals. In the AX-Task, the subject must respond to the letter "X" only when it has been preceded in sequence by the letter "A." Errors of omission (failing to press the button when the target appears) and errors of commission (or "false alarms," pressing the button in the absence of the target) are scored.

At age 7 years, the Seattle Study CPT was an 8-minute task involving sequential presentation of 360 single letters (of which 60 were targets) for both the X and the AX conditions. Multiple regression analyses data revealed that prenatal alcohol exposure was significantly related to vigilance scores, even after adjusting for many potential covariates including other prenatal exposures, postnatal conditions, experience with computer equipment, and demographics. Although all three CPT scores (errors of commission, omission, and mean reaction time) were significantly related to prenatal alcohol exposure, errors of commission in the AX-Task showed the strongest linear relationship. Commission errors suggest impulsivity by reflecting the child's difficulty in withholding a response. Impulsive children often press the button to the "A" without waiting to see if it is followed by an "X," or they select "X's" that have not been preceded by "A's." Performance on this task was quite well correlated with independent, "blinded" examiner behavior ratings of child impulsivity, organization, and endurance during the laboratory session (Streissguth et al., 1986). Although it was clear that prenatal alcohol exposure was related to disruptions in attention at age 7 years, the use of traditional multiple regression techniques (characteristic of Seattle Study methods of statistical analysis in the early 1980s) did not permit fine-grained analyses of the "dose" (prenatal alcohol exposure) or the "response" (attentional problems).

Attentional Findings during Middle Childhood:
Partial-Least-Squares Analysis in the Seattle Study

Understanding the effects of prenatal alcohol exposure on child development requires statistical methodology that can effectively assess the dose–response relationship between multiple measures of alcohol exposure and multiple measures of child performance, and evaluate this relationship over time. For this purpose, the Seattle group has been developing the application of a latent variable modeling procedure, based on the partial-least-squares (PLS) statistical methods developed by Wold and colleagues (e.g., Jöreskog & Wold, 1982), to the Seattle data. PLS techniques have the advantage of avoiding the multiple significance tests that are a problem in dealing with complex longitudinal data sets, while permitting detection of the basic association between multiple constructs. The aim of these PLS methods in research on alcohol teratology is to analyze and explain the varying ability of the multiple (correlated) measures of alcohol exposure to predict multiple correlated measures of child performance, and similarly to describe the salience of these child performance measures for prenatal alcohol. PLS involves fitting a simple least-squares model to the nonblock correlation matrix, the way most other methods fit to actual data values instead.

In the Seattle Study, 13 alcohol consumption scores (which reflect quantity, pattern, and timing of alcohol consumption) are represented as a block of variables providing a multifaceted assessment of alcohol "dose," while a block of child performance measures constitutes the "response." Explicit linear combinations of the alcohol scores and the performance measures are computed as "latent variables" (LVs) that "explain" the entries in the correlation matrix between the individual alcohol scores and response measures. The analysis has two primary components: the interpretation of the saliences of the alcohol scores (the coefficients defining the "Alcohol LV") together with the corresponding saliences of performance measures (the coefficients defining the "Performance LV"); and the examination of the individual scores on the Alcohol and Performance LVs (and their correlation). The reader is referred to Bookstein, Streissguth, Sampson, and Barr (1990) and Streissguth, Bookstein, Sampson, and Barr (1993) for a more extensive discussion of the PLS analytic technique. In 1987, researchers working on the Seattle Study began to utilize PLS techniques for establishing the relationship between prenatal alcohol exposure and child outcome. Discussed here are PLS analyses that specifically focus on alcohol-related attentional outcomes for children at 7 and 11 years of age, and (in the next subsection) for adolescents at 14 years of age.

Laboratory measures have revealed important information about alcohol effects on attention in middle childhood. For the 7-year-olds, PLS analysis of CPT scores identified the AX-Task, and primarily the number of commission errors, as the score most highly associated with prenatal alcohol exposure (Sampson et al., 1989). Also for the 7-year-olds, PLS analysis of subtest scores from the Wechsler Intelligence Scale for Children–Revised (WISC-R) and the WRAT-R showed that the Arithmatic scores were the most salient for prenatal alcohol exposure. This corroborated early clinical case study findings in patients with FAS/possible FAE. Interestingly, increased alcohol exposure was also related to poorer functioning on the WISC-R Digit Span subtest, suggesting difficulties with auditory attention (Streissguth, Barr, & Sampson, 1990). In the Seattle Study, children's behaviors in the classroom at the age of 7 years were rated by teachers on the Myklebust Pupil Rating Scale (Myklebust, 1981). Greater prenatal alcohol exposure was significantly related to reports of decreased ability to retain information and with problems in cooperation, impulsivity, and organization (Sampson et al., 1989). Additionally, independent "blinded" examiner behavior ratings in the laboratory revealed increased distractibility, overpersistence, and poor organization within the same group of children.

In behavioral teratology research it is important to study the effects of teratogens in various settings to understand the generalizability of alcohol-related deficits. Observations of similar behavior problems across different settings and by different raters strengthen the conclusion that these alcohol-related attentional deficits are stable, and not simply transient phenomena occurring because of situational characteristics, such as a particular test setting. Continued follow-up of 458 children participating in the Seattle Study at the age of 11 years revealed findings consistent with the longitudinal data at 7 years of age. PLS analysis showed that increased prenatal alcohol exposure was significantly related to higher teacher questionnaire ratings of such problem behaviors as distractibility, restlessness, lack of persistence, and reluctance to meet challenges using the Multigrade Inventory for Teachers (Shaywitz, 1986). Higher prenatal exposure was also associated with teacher ratings of the children's learning difficulties, including information processing and reasoning problems, and deficits in academic function across the domains of reading, spelling, and mathematics. Finally, greater prenatal exposure was also related to evidence of subtle academic difficulties (especially on Mathematics and Total Achievement), as indexed by scores on standardized national achievement tests administered by the schools. These results again corroborated earlier clinical findings and suggest difficulties with abstraction and cognitive processing, presumably associated with alcohol-related attentional difficulties (Carmichael Olson, Sampson, Barr, Streissguth, & Bookstein, 1992).

Attentional Findings in Adolescence: Recent Information from the Seattle Study

To date, the Seattle Study is the only project that has followed a sample of moderately alcohol-exposed children from birth to the age of 14 years. Given the enduring attentional difficulties evident at earlier ages in the Seattle Study, coupled with clinical research highlighting neuropsychological deficits among older patients with FAS, attention was a critical variable of interest when the Seattle sample was assessed in adolescence. Attention tests selected for inclusion in the 14-year battery were based on notions put forth by Mirsky and colleagues suggesting that attentional processes consist of separate elements including the abilities to *encode, shift, focus,* and *sustain* attention (Mirsky, Anthony, Duncan, Ahearn, & Kellam, 1991). Among others, the following tests were administered in the Seattle Study to 462 adolescents: the Digit Span and Arithmetic subtests from the WISC-R (hypothesized measures of *encoding*); the Wisconsin Card Sorting Test (a concept-identification task thought to measure the ability to *shift* attention); the Talland Letter Cancellation Test (a perceptual–motor speed test thought to tap the ability to *focus* attention); and the CPT (a hypothesized measure of the ability to *sustain* attention over time). Two measures of reaction time were derived from the CPT: standard deviation of reaction time (SDRT) and mean reaction time (MRT). PLS analyses indicated that prenatal alcohol exposure was salient for SDRT (a measure of individual variability in reaction time thought to measure fluctuating attentional states) but not for MRT (a measure of reaction time averaged over all trials during the CPT). Presumed problems with inhibition of response (assessed by increased commission errors on the CPT AX-Task and Talland Letter Cancellation Test) and observed spatial learning deficits (assessed by a computerized version of the Stepping Stone Maze) were also related to prenatal alcohol exposure. Overall, difficulties in the *focus* and *sustain* elements of attention were those most salient for prenatal alcohol exposure whereas weaker alcohol effects were seen on tasks tapping the *shift* and *encoding* elements.

Longitudinal Nature of the Seattle Study Findings with Respect to Attention

In the Seattle Study, analyses of attentional measures at the 4-, 7-, and 14-year examinations reveal robust continuities in alcohol-related attentional deficits across this 10-year span (Streissguth, Bookstein, Sampson, & Barr, 1995). For example, the correlation of the Vigilance LV with the Alcohol LV at each of the three ages is between .20 and .22, and the correlation of the 7-year Vigilance LV with the 14-year Vigilance LV is .49.

The Seattle data indicate that the measure of individual variability of reaction time (SDRT) as assessed by the vigilance tasks at the ages of 4, 7, and 14 years capture an important dimension of this enduring alcohol effect on attention. In contrast, the measure of MRT grows less salient for prenatal alcohol exposure as the children age. At each age, despite differences in the vigilance tasks used, SDRT is the vigilance measure most strongly associated with gestational alcohol exposure (Streissguth et al., 1995). This finding suggests that inconsistency in speed or response (assessed by SDRT), rather than average mean performance (assessed by MRT), may be a sensitive indicator of alcohol-related brain dysfunction over time. Interestingly, SDRT has been described as representing "microlapses in attention" in studies of focal epilepsy (Mirsky & Cardon, 1962; Mirsky & Van Buren, 1965), and this deficit in consistency of response speed may be associated with hippocampal damage. Poor performance on a noncomputerized version of the Stepping Stone Maze and the CPT, measures similar to those on which alcohol-exposed individuals show problems, has been found with patients evidencing several forms of brain dysfunction such as hippocampal lesions (Milner, 1964) and traumatic brain injury (Stuss et al., 1989).

Another longitudinal finding in the Seattle data indicates that the 19 "worst performers" on the 14-year Vigilance LV had all performed below average on tests given at the age of 7 years. Although these 19 teenagers represented only 10% of the subjects who performed below average on the vigilance task at 7 years of age, they are of great interest. For these adolescents, problems in vigilance and sustained attention appear to be a persistent and pervasive problem, evident over time in spite of special education and other forms of intervention. Such long-term findings of individual differences go beyond the correlational analyses of group differences discussed earlier and suggest that alcohol-related attentional deficits reflect ongoing compromise of the CNS that may not be ameliorated by ordinary remedial programming (Streissguth et al., 1995).

In the Seattle Study, both examiner and teacher ratings of alcohol-exposed children also demonstrated attentional deficits. Examiner ratings of distractibility, impulsivity, disorganization, and impersistence from both the 4- and 7-year exams were moderately predictive of poor overall performance on the 14-year vigilance measure (CPT). Of all the behavioral ratings obtained, some of the strongest predictive correlations over time were between the 7-year Vigilance LV and the 11-year teacher rating of "Attention" ($r = -.36$), and the 11-year teacher rating of "Attention" and the 14-year Vigilance LV ($r = -.42$). These longitudinal findings highlight the enduring effects of prenatal alcohol exposure, which appear to last well into adolescence, and suggest future avenues to be explored in elucidating the breakdown of attentional processes among prenatally alcohol-exposed individuals.

RESEARCH ON
BRAIN–BEHAVIOR RELATIONSHIPS

At the cutting edge of research in alcohol teratology is the effort to identify anatomical and/or biochemical mechanisms responsible for the enduring teratogenic effects of prenatal alcohol exposure on function (Goodlett
& West, 1992; Ward & West, 1992). Tracing brain–behavior relationships is best accomplished by synthesizing findings from animal studies
(which allow for rigorous experimental manipulation) and results of longitudinal natural "life experiments" among alcohol-affected individuals. So
far, research has described certain structural malformations and biochemical differences in alcohol-exposed animals that may be tied to functional
deficits in response inhibition, motor, and visual spatial reasoning seen
clinically among alcohol-affected individuals. An important focus in this
research domain will be on the disruption caused by prenatal alcohol exposure of neural substrates underlying the complex construct of attention.

The hippocampus is one of the most widely investigated brain structures thought to be sensitive to the teratogenic effects of alcohol. According to Ward and West (1992), this structure is of research interest because
(1) the hippocampus is composed of relatively simple structural layers of
pyramidal cells and granule cells; (2) it has been shown to be affected by
long-term alcohol use in adult rodents (Phillips, 1989); and (3) lesions
in this area are known to be associated with the types of behavioral deficits
observed among alcohol-exposed offspring, for example, poor response
inhibition and increased perseverative responding (Goodlett et al., 1992;
Wigal & Amsel, 1990). Alcohol-exposed rats make repetitive incorrect
choices or errors in a 12-arm radial maze (Goodlett et al., 1992). These
errors are similar to both the classic "hippocampal errors" seen in patients
with hippocampal lesions (Milner, 1964) and to the errors made by
alcohol-affected individuals on a maze test in the longitudinal Seattle Study
(Streissguth et al., 1994).

Another brain structure that appears sensitive to the effects of prenatal alcohol exposure is the cerebellum. Studies have shown decreased
Purkinje cell growth as a function of ethanol exposure in rats (Bonthius
& West, 1990; Phillips & Cragg, 1982). Since these cells are generated
prenatally, reduction in their number following postnatal exposure suggests that the reduction occurs via cell death and not retarded cell generation (Ward & West, 1992). Disruption in cerebellar maturation is
associated with findings among exposed rats of poor motor coordination
and altered gait patterns (Meyer, Kotch, & Riley, 1990), as the cerebellum is responsible for functions of equilibrium, muscle tonicity, and the
coordination of motoric activity. Interestingly, similar problems with
balance and gait (Marcus, 1987), clinical observations of delayed motor-

ic development (Jones, Smith, Ulleland, & Streissguth, 1973), and fine motor problems (Barr et al., 1990) have been observed among alcohol-exposed humans.

The neocortex has also been examined in prenatally exposed rats; findings indicate that alcohol decreases the number and size of cell bodies (Miller & Potempa, 1990) and redistributes neocortical neurons (Miller, Chiaia, & Rhoades, 1990). Impaired neuronal migration in humans, as evidenced by the presence of ectopic sheets in the cortex, has been found in autopsied brains of children with FAS (Clarren, Alvord, Sumi, Streissguth, & Smith, 1978). Prenatal alcohol exposure has been reported to delay the start of neocortical neurogenesis and extend cell proliferation by 2 days in rats (Miller, 1986, 1989). Areas corresponding to the somatosensory and motor cortices appear to be more sensitive to the effects of ethanol in rats as compared to the auditory area (Miller & Dow-Edwards, 1988; Miller & Potempa, 1990). This finding may shed light on the deficits in visual–spatial abilities often seen in alcohol-affected patients, as these areas appear critical to adequate performance on visual–spatial tasks.

Additional structures of interest in brain–behavior research on fetal alcohol effects include the basal ganglia and corpus callosum. Cellular damage and shrinkage in size of the basal ganglia have been documented in individuals with FAS in addition to an atrophied or absent corpus callosum (Mattson & Riley, 1995). The reader is referred to Mattson, Jernigan, and Riley (1994) and Mattson and Riley (1996) for interesting overviews of work on brain–behavior research in alcohol teratogenesis.

Results of studies on the impact of ethanol exposure on neurotransmitter systems (seratonin, dopamine) have complemented findings of the structural studies described above. In general, neurotransmitter studies in rats suggest that prenatal alcohol exposure leads to deficient levels of seratonin in the brainstem (Druse, Kuo, & Tajuddin, 1991) and decreased levels of dopamine in the hypothalamus and striatum (Cooper & Rudeen, 1988; Druse, Tajuddin, Kuo, & Connerty, 1990). Additionally, Clarren et al. (1990) found decreased dopamine levels in the striatum among exposed pig-tailed macaques. Other neurotransmitter systems have been less adequately studied (e.g., gamma-aminobutyric acid, histamine). It is plausible that nonoptimal levels of neurotransmitters present in the brain impede communication between respective brain synapses, thus indirectly affecting performance.

FUTURE DIRECTIONS AND SUMMARY

Overall, the clinical, experimental animal, and epidemiological findings discussed in this chapter clearly support the notion that alcohol exposure before birth can have teratogenic effects that result in long-term CNS compromise. There is convincing evidence that attentional difficulties starting in early infancy and still detectable in adolescence are an important manifestation of alcohol-related CNS dysfunction. Since attentional processes are involved in many aspects of daily function, there is great potential for debilitating ongoing secondary disabilities associated with prenatal alcohol exposure. Such secondary disabilities have certainly been found in clinical studies of individuals with FAS and possible FAE, and in a subtler form are even demonstrated as alcohol-related behavior problems in epidemiological group studies of alcohol teratogenesis (e.g., Carmichael Olson et al., in press).

But there is still much to learn about the extent, pattern, and underlying neural substrates of alcohol-related attentional deficits, how these deficits contribute to the occurrence of debilitating secondary disabilities, and what are worthwhile approaches to prevention and intervention. Programmatic research is needed. The first step is continued careful description of alcohol-related attention problems; such findings must be replicated in several laboratories with clinical, animal, and epidemiological data. Of special importance is the need to document the long-term nature of alcohol-related attentional deficits and associated problems in daily function from infancy to adolescence, and into adulthood, as is being done in the Seattle Study.

Another important research step is to specify attentional functions that are disrupted due to prenatal alcohol exposure. A step in this direction is offered by recent cognitive theories of attention that have proven to be productive in the study of assorted disease entities. For example, Mirsky and colleagues (1991) used the National Institute of Mental Health Attention Battery and found deficits in the *focus* and *sustain* elements of attention in clinical groups of adult epileptics and schizophrenics. Interestingly, these were the same two elements of attention found to be the most disrupted among alcohol-affected adolescents in the Seattle Study using the same research battery. The models of attention proposed by Mirsky et al. (1991) or Posner and Petersen (1990) might be useful applications to research directed at understanding the attentional deficits typical among fetal alcohol-affected patients (e.g., see the exploratory study of Carmichael Olson et al., 1996). Such research can be a rich source of information on the development of the attentional system and disruptions of this system, if maturational changes are taken into account.

Comparison research involving other disordered groups is another fruitful research direction. Researchers have compared the attention deficits of prenatally alcohol-exposed children with those of children diagnosed with ADD (with and without hyperactivity) and have found both similarities and differences (Coles, 1992; Coles et al., 1993; Nanson & Hiscock,

1990). The comparison research can be expanded to include patients with fetal alcohol effects and those with other disorders involving impaired attention, such as autism (Ciesielski, Courchesne, & Elmasian, 1990), schizophrenia (Nuechterlein, 1983), lead intoxication (Needleman et al., 1979), affective disorders (American Psychiatric Association, 1987), and petit mal epilepsy (Mirsky, Primac, Ajmone Marsan, Rosvold, & Stevens, 1960). Such studies should move beyond mere description and focus on the mechanisms responsible for disrupted attention, discovering useful techniques for the assessment of attentional problems, as well as examining the role of disrupted attention in the lives of alcohol-affected individuals, and designing possible intervention strategies for use with alcohol-affected persons.

The use of innovative psychophysiological techniques may increase our understanding of alcohol teratogenesis and tie together alcohol-related biochemical and structural anomalies with functional deficits. This may pave the way for better medication management of individuals with FAS, or provide new and more reliable assessment of CNS dysfunction. In a pioneering study, Mattson et al. (1992) employed neuropsychological assessment, magnetic resonance imaging (MRI), and electroencephalogram (EEG) recording in 2 patients with FAS and found abnormalities of the corpus callosum, moderate EEG anomalies, and deficits in neuropsychological functioning. Ongoing research is now focusing on concurrent neuropsychological assessment and MRI studies of larger samples of alcohol-affected individuals. Studies of cerebral blood flow (using techniques such as positron emission tomography) and electrical activity in the brain (examining, for instance, event-related potentials) may shed light on the areas of the brain engaged in information processing during various neuropsychological tasks.

One of the most critical issues in research with alcohol-affected individuals lies in the fact that birth defects such as FAS are *totally preventable*. Alcohol-related attentional difficulties and attendant secondary disabilities will not occur if a fetus is not exposed to alcohol before birth. Various approaches to prevention are under development, and research on their effectiveness is essential. Legislative actions have been undertaken (e.g., warning labels on alcoholic beverages and warning signs at points of liquor purchase). Screening and identification systems are being developed to locate women at high risk for producing children with FAS or possible FAE. These include such strategies as community-based FAS diagnostic clinics (Clarren & Astley, 1997), using appropriate assessment techniques in prenatal health care settings, or empowering counselors who directly work with substance-using women (Kopera-Frye, Tswelnaldin, Streissguth, & LaDue, 1994). The goal of FAS prevention can also be addressed as part of the treatment for chemically dependent women who are pregnant or parenting. One interesting approach designed to do this pairs paraprofessional advocates with the very highest-risk substance-abusing women from late pregnancy through the child's 3rd birthday (Grant, Ernst, Streissguth, Phipps, & Gendler, 1996).

Of course, a final research direction lies in the need to develop and test effective intervention techniques for remediating attentional and other behavioral deficits among alcohol-affected individuals. Suggested interventions based on case studies and clinical experience have been published (e.g., Burgess, Lasswell, & Streissguth, 1993; Streissguth & Novick, 1995; Streissguth & Kanter, 1997; Novick & Streissguth, 1996; Carmichael Olson & Burgess, 1997; Carmichael Olson, 1994; Weiner & Morse, 1994; Streissguth & Finnegan, 1996; Klinefeld & Wescott, 1993), and a variety of FAS curricula, newsletters, and resource guides are now available (e.g., Streissguth & Little, 1994; Morse & Weiner, 1993; *Iceberg*). Neuropsychological and speech/language research is beginning to describe the deficits resulting from prenatal alcohol exposure, and naturally occurring "protective factors" have been identified in the lieves of fetal-alcohol-affected individuals (Streissguth, Barr, Kogan, & Bookstein, 1996). Interventions can be constructed to target these deficits, enhance important protective factors, and systematically test the intervention strategies clinical wisdom suggests.

In summary, there are compelling theoretical and practical reasons to pursue study on alcohol-related attentional deficits, in particular, and on alcohol teratogenesis, in general. Researchers in the field of attention are essential to this endeavor, given the hypothesis that disruption in attention underlies many of the debilitating problems seen in alcohol-affected individuals. Attention researchers can specify the elements and underlying neural substrates of the attentional system, thereby advancing study of the ways in which alcohol disrupts attention at different points in development. Researchers in the field can increase understanding of the relationship between disrupted attention and serious problems in daily living among alcohol-affected individuals. In sum, they can do much to articulate brain–behavior relationships, and further the prevention, assessment, and remediation of the major public health problem of alcohol-related birth defects.

ACKNOWLEDGMENTS

The research reported here was supported in part by a U.S. Public Health Service grant from the National Institute on Alcohol Abuse and Alcoholism (AA01455-01-18) and by a Centers for Disease Control grant (R04/CCR008515-01) to Ann P. Streissguth. We wish to express our gratitude to Maria Lingat-Collier for technical assistance in preparation of this manuscript. We thank the editors, Jim Enns and Jake Burack, for their helpful comments, and Allan Mirsky and

Paul Sampson for their valuable insights. Above all, we acknowledge the loyal participation of the Seattle Study families and patients of the Fetal Alcohol and Drug Unit who have taught us a great deal.

REFERENCES

Abel, E. L. (1982). In utero alcohol exposure and developmental delay of response inhibition. *Alcoholism: Clinical and Experimental Research, 6,* 369–376.

Abel, E. L., & Sokol, R. J. (1987). Incidence of fetal alcohol syndrome and economic impact of FAS-related anomalies. *Drug and Alcohol Dependence, 19,* 51–70.

Achenbach, T. M., & Edelbrock, G. (1983). *Manual for the Behavior Checklist and Revised Child Behavior Profile.* Burlington, VT: University of Vermont, Department of Psychiatry.

American Psychiatric Association. (1987). *Diagnostic and statistical manual of mental disorders* (3rd ed., rev.). Washington, DC: Author.

Aronson, M. (1984). *Children of alcoholic mothers.* Unpublished doctoral dissertation, Departments of Pediatrics and Psychology, University of Göteberg, Sweden.

Aronson, M., Kyllerman, M., Sabel, K. G., Sandin, B., & Olegard, R. (1985). Children of alcoholic mothers: Developmental, perceptual and behavioural characteristics as compared to matched controls. *Acta Paediatrica Scandinavica, 74,* 27–35.

Barr, H. M., Streissguth, A. P., Darby, B. L., & Sampson, P. D. (1990). Prenatal exposure to alcohol, caffeine, tobacco, and aspirin: Effects on fine and gross motor performance in 4-year old children. *Developmental Psychology, 26,* 339–348.

Barron, S., Gagnon, W. A., Mattson, S. N., Kotch, L. E., Meyer, L. S., & Riley, E. P. (1988). The effects of prenatal alcohol exposure on odor associative learning in rats. *Neurotoxicology and Teratology, 10,* 333–339.

Barron, S., Gagnon, W. A., & Riley, E. P. (1986). The effects of prenatal alcohol exposure on respiration rate and response to a novel odor in neonatal rats. *Society for Neuroscience Abstracts, 12,* 51.

Bond, N. W. (1986). Fetal alcohol exposure and hyperactivity in rats: The role of the neurotransmitter systems involved in arousal and inhibition. In J. R. West (Ed.), *Alcohol and brain development* (pp. 45–70). New York: Oxford University Press.

Bonthius, D. J., & West, J. R. (1990). Alcohol-induced neuronal loss in developing rats: Increased brain damage with binge exposure. *Alcoholism: Clinical and Experimental Research, 14,* 107–118.

Bookstein, F. L., Streissguth, A. P., Sampson, P. D., & Barr, H. M. (1996). Exploiting redundant measurement of dose and behavioral outcome: New methods from the teratology. *Developmental Psychology, 32,* 404–415.

Boyd, T. A., Ernhart, C. B., Greene, T. H., Sokol, R. J., & Martier, S. (1991). Prenatal alcohol exposure and sustained attention in the preschool years. *Neurotoxicology and Teratology, 13,* 49–55.

Brown, R. T., Coles, C. D., Smith, I. E., Platzman, K. A., Silverstein, J., Erick son, S., & Falek, A. (1991). Effects of prenatal alcohol exposure at school age—II: Attention and behavior. *Neurotoxicology and Teratology, 13,* 369–376.

Burgess, D. M., Lasswell, S. L., & Streissguth, A. P. (1993). *Educating children prenatally exposed to alcohol and other drugs* [Brochure]. Seattle: Fetal Alcohol and Drug Unit, University of Washington.

Carmichael Olson, H. (1994). The effects of prenatal alcohol exposure on child development. *Infants and Young Children, 6,* 10–25.

Carmichael Olson, H., & Burgess, D. M. (1997). Early intervention for children prenatally exposed to alcohol and other drugs. In M. J. Guralnick (Ed.), *The effectiveness of early intervention* (pp. 109–145). Baltimore, MD: Brookes.

Carmichael Olson, H., Feldman, J. J., Streissguth, A. P., Sampson, P. D., & Bookstein, F. L. (1996). *Neuropsychological deficits in adolescents with fetal alcohol syndrome* (Tech. Rep. No. 96-17). Seattle: University of Washington, Fetal Alcohol and Drug Unit.

Carmichael Olson, H., Sampson, P. D., Barr, H. M., Streissguth, A. P., & Bookstein, F. L. (1992). Prenatal exposure to alcohol and school problems in late childhood: A longitudinal prospective study. *Development and Psychopathology, 4,* 341–359.

Carmichael Olson, H., Streissguth, A. P., Sampson, P. D., Barr, H. M., Bookstein, F. L., & Thiede, K. (in press). Association of prenatal alcohol exposure with behavioral and learning problems in adolescence. *Journal of the American Academy of Child and Alolescent Psychiatry.*

Ciesielski, K. T., Courchesne, E., & Elmasian, R. (1990). Effects of focused selective attention tasks on event-related potentials in autistic and normal individuals. *Electroencephalography and Clinical Neurophysiology, 75,* 207–220.

Clarren, S. K., Alvord, E. C., Sumi, S. M., Streissguth, A. P., & Smith, D. W. (1978). Brain malformations related to prenatal exposure to ethanol. *Journal of Pediatrics, 92,* 64–67.

Clarren, S. K., & Astley, S. J. (1997). The development of the fetal alcohol syndrome diagnostic and prevention network in Washington state. In A. P. Streissguth & J. Kanter (Eds.), *The challenge of fetal alcohol syndrome: Overcoming secondary disabilities.* Seattle: University of Washington Press.

Clarren, S. K., Astley, S. J., Bowden, D. M., Lai, H., Milam, A. H., Rudeen, P. K., & Shoemaker, W. J. (1990). Neuroanatomic and neurochemical abnormalities in non-human primate infants exposed to weekly doses of ethanol during gestation. *Alcoholism: Clinical and Experimental Research, 14,* 674–683.

Clarren, S. K., Astley, S. J., Gunderson, V. M., & Spellman, D. (1992). Cognitive and behavioral deficits in nonhuman primates associated with very early embryonic binge exposure to ethanol. *Journal of Pediatrics, 121,* 789–796.

Clarren, S. K., & Smith, D. W. (1978). The fetal alcohol syndrome. *New England Journal of Medicine, 298,* 1063–1067.

Coles, C. D. (1992). Prenatal alcohol exposure and human development. In M. W. Miller (Ed.), *Development of the central nervous system: Effects of alcohol and opiates* (pp. 9–36). New York: Wiley-Liss.

Coles, C. D., Brown, R. T., Raskind-Hood, C. L., Platzman, K. A., Smith, I. E., & Falek, A. (1993, March). *A comparative study of neurocognitive func-*

tioning in fetal alcohol syndrome (FAS) and attention deficit hyperactivity disorder (ADHD). Paper presented at the biennial meeting of the Society for Research in Child Development, New Orleans, LA.

Coles, C. D., Smith, I. E., & Falek, A. (1987). A neonatal marker for cognitive vulnerability to alcohol's teratogenic effects. *Alcoholism: Clinical and Experimental Research, 11,* 197.

Coles, C. D., Smith, I., Fernhoff, P. M., & Falek, A. (1985). Neonatal neurobehavioral characteristics as correlates of maternal alcohol use during gestation. *Alcoholism: Clinical and Experimental Research, 9,* 1–7.

Conry, J. (1990). Neurophysiological deficits in fetal alcohol syndrome and fetal alcohol effects. *Alcoholism: Clinical and Experimental Research, 14,* 650–655.

Cooper, J. D., & Rudeen, P. K. (1988). Alterations in regional catecholamine content and turnover in the male rat brain in response to in utero ethanol exposure. *Alcoholism: Clinical and Experimental Research, 12,* 282–285.

Delis, D. C., Kramer, J. H., Kaplan, E., & Ober, B. A. (1987). *The California Verbal Learning Test: Research Edition.* New York: Psychological Corporation.

Driscoll, C. D., Chen, J. S., & Riley, E. P. (1982). Passive avoidance performance in rats prenatally exposed to alcohol during various periods of gestation. *Neurobehavioral Toxicology, 2,* 207–211.

Driscoll, C. D., Streissguth, A. P., & Riley, E. P. (1990). Prenatal alcohol exposure: Comparability of effects in humans and animal models. *Neurotoxicology and Teratology, 12,* 231–237.

Druse, M. J., Kuo, A., & Tajuddin, N. (1991). Effects of in utero ethanol exposure on the developing serotonergic system. *Alcoholism: Clinical and Experimental Research, 15,* 678–684.

Druse, M. J., Tajuddin, N., Kuo, A. P., & Connerty, M. (1990). Effects of in utero ethanol exposure on the developing dopaminergic system in rats. *Journal of Neuroscience Research, 27,* 233–240.

Duffy, O., & Leonard, B. E. (1991). Changes in behaviour and brain neurotrans mitters following pre- and post-natal exposure of rats to ethanol. *Medical Science Research, 19,* 279–280.

Ernhart, C. B., Wolf, A. W., Linn, P. L., Sokol, R., Kennard, M., & Filipovich, H. F. (1985). Alcohol-related birth defects: Syndromal anomalies, intrauterine growth retardation and neonatal behavioral assessment. *Alcoholism: Clinical and Experimental Research, 9,* 447–453.

Goodlett, C. R., Bonthius, D. J., Wasserman, E. A., & West, W. R. (1992). An animal model of CNS dysfunction associated with fetal alcohol exposure: Behavioral and neuroanatomical correlates. In I. Gormezano & E. A. Wasserman (Eds.), *Learning and memory: The behavioral and biological substrates* (pp. 183–208). Englewood, NJ: Erlbaum.

Goodlett, C. R., & West, J. R. (1992). Fetal alcohol effects: Rat model of alcohol exposure during the brain growth spurt. In I. S. Zagon & T. A. Slotkin (Eds.), *Maternal substance abuse and the developing nervous system* (pp. 45–75). San Diego, CA: Academic Press.

Grant, T. M., Ernst, C. C., Streissguth, A. P., Phipps, P., & Gendler, B. (1996). When case management isn't enough: A model of paraprofessional advocacy for drug- and alcohol-abusing mothers. *Journal of Case Management, 5*(1), 3–11.

Gray, J. K., & Streissguth, A. P. (1990). Memory deficits and life adjustment in adults with fetal alcohol syndrome: A case-control study. *Alcoholism: Clinical and Experimental Research, 14,* 294.

Greene, P. L., Diaz-Granados, J. L., & Amsel, A. (1992). Blood ethanol concentration from early postnatal exposure: Effects on memory-based learning and hippocampal neuroanatomy in infant and adult rats. *Behavioral Neuroscience, 106,* 51–61.

Greene, T., Ernhart, C. B., Ager, J., Sokol, R., Martier, S., & Boyd, T. (1991). Prenatal alcohol exposure and cognitive development in the preschool years. *Neurotoxicology and Teratology, 13,* 57–68.

Halgren, E., Squires, N. K., Wilson, C. L., Rohrbaugh, J. W., Babb, T. L., & Crandall, P. H. (1980). Endogenous potentials generated in the human hippocampal formation and amygdala by infrequent events. *Science, 210,* 803–805.

Hanson, J. W., Jones, K. L., & Smith, D. W. (1976). Fetal alcohol syndrome: Experience with 41 patients. *Journal of the American Medical Association, 235,* 1458–1460.

Iceberg. [Quarterly newsletter published by Fetal Alcohol Syndrome Information Service; PO Box 95597, Seattle, WA 98145-2597.]

Iosub, S., Fuchs, M., Bingol, N., & Gromisch, D. S. (1981). Fetal alcohol syndrome revisited. *Pediatrics, 68,* 475–479.

Jacobson, J. L., Jacobson, S. W., Sokol, R. J., Martier, S. S., Ager, J. W., & Kaplan-Estrin, M. G. (1993). Teratogenic effects of alcohol on infant development. *Alcoholism: Clinical and Experimental Research, 17,* 174–183.

Jacobson, S. W., Fein, G. G., Jacobson, J. L., Schwartz, P. M., & Dowler, J. K. (1984). Neonatal correlates of prenatal alcohol exposure to smoking, caffeine, and alcohol. *Infant Behavior and Development, 7,* 253–265.

Jacobson, S. W., Jacobson, J. L., Sokol, R. J., Martier, S. S., & Ager, J. W. (1993). Prenatal alcohol exposure and infant information processing ability. *Child Development, 64,* 1706–1721.

Jagust, W. J. (1992). PET and SPECT imaging in cognitive disorders of aging and alcoholism. In S. Zakhari & E. Witt (Eds.), *Imaging in alcohol research* (Monograph No. 21, pp. 333–357). Rockville, MD: National Institute on Alcohol Abuse and Alcoholism.

Jones, K. L., & Smith, D. W. (1973). Recognition of the fetal alcohol syndrome in early infancy. *Lancet, 2,* 999–1001.

Jones, K. L., Smith, D. W., Streissguth, A. P., & Myrianthopoulos, N. C. (1974). Outcome in offspring of chronic alcoholic women. *Lancet, 1,* 1076–1078.

Jones, K. L., Smith, D. W., Ulleland, C. N., & Streissguth, A. P. (1973). Patterns of malformation in offspring of chronic alcoholic mothers. *Lancet,* 1267–1271.

Jöreskog, K. G., & Wold, H. (Eds.). (1982). *Systems under indirect observation: Causality–structure–prediction* (Pts. 1 and 2). Amsterdam: North-Holland.

Kerns, K., Don, A., Mateer, C. A., & Streissguth, A. P. (in press). Cognitive deficits in non-retarded adults with fetal alcohol syndrome. *Journal of Learning Disabilities.*

Klinefeld, J., & Wescott, S. (Eds.). (1993). *Fantastic Antone succeeds! Experiences in educating children with fetal alcohol syndrome.* Fairbanks: University of Alaska Press.

Kodituwakku, P. W., Handmaker, N. S., Cutler, S. K., Weathersby, E. K., & Handmaker, S. D. (1995). Specific impairments in self-regulation in children exposed to alcohol prenatally. *Alcoholism: Clinical and Experimental Research, 19,* 1558–1564.

Kopera-Frye, K., Tswelnaldin, P., Streissguth, A. P., & LaDue, R. A. (1994). Preventing FAS by empowering Native American chemical dependency counselors. *The IHS Primary Care Provider, 19,* 66–69.

LaDue, R. A., Streissguth, A. P., & Randals, S. P. (1992). Clinical considerations pertaining to adolescents and adults with fetal alcohol syndrome. In T. B. Sonderegger (Ed.), *Perinatal substance abuse: Research findings and clinical implications* (pp. 104–131). Baltimore: John Hopkins University Press.

La Fiette, M. H., Carlos, R., & Riley, E. P. (1994). Effects of prenatal alcohol exposure on serial pattern performance in the rat. *Neurotoxicology and Teratology, 16,* 41–46.

Landesman-Dwyer, S., Ragozin, A. S., & Little, R. E. (1981). Behavioral correlates of prenatal alcohol exposure: A four-year follow-up study. *Neurobehavioral Toxicology and Teratology, 3,* 187–193.

Larsson, G., & Bohlin, A. B. (1987). Fetal alcohol syndrome and preventative strategies. *Pediatrician, 14,* 51–56.

Lemoine, P., Harrousseau, H., Borteyru, J. P., & Menuet J. C. (1968). Les enfants de parents alcooliques: Anomalies observées à propos de 127 cas. *Ouest Médical, 8,* 476–482.

Majewski, F. (1993). Alcohol embryopathy: Experience in 200 patients. *Brain Dysfunction 6,* 248–265.

Majewski, F., & Majewski, B. (1988). Alcohol embryopathy: Symptoms, auxological data, frequency, among the offspring and pathogenesis. *Excerpta Medica International Conference Series, 805,* 837–841.

Marcus, J. C. (1987). Neurological findings in the fetal alcohol syndrome. *Neuropediatrics, 18,* 158–160.

Martin, J. C., Martin, D. C., Sigman, G., & Radow, B. (1978). Maternal ethanol consumption and hyperactivity in cross-fostered offspring. *Physiological Psychology, 6,* 362–365.

Matthews, C. G., & Klöve, H. (1978). *Wisconsin Fine Motor Steadiness Battery: Administration manual for child neuropsychological battery.* Madison: Neuropsychological Laboratory, University of Wisconsin Medical School.

Mattson, S. N., Carlos, R., & Riley, E. P. (1993). The behavioral teratogenicity of alcohol is not affected by pretreatment with aspirin. *Alcohol, 10,* 51–57.

Mattson, S. N., Jernigan, T. L., & Riley, E. P. (1994). MRI and prenatal alcohol exposure: Images provide insight into FAS. *Alcohol Health and Research World, 18,* 49–52.

Mattson, S. N., & Riley, E. P. (1995). Prenatal alcohol exposure to alcohol: What the images reveal. *Alcohol Health and Research World, 19*(4), 273–278.

Mattson, S. N., Riley, E. P., Jernigen, T. L., Ehlers, C. L., Delis, D. C., Jones, K. L., Stern, C., Johnson, K. A., Hesselink, J. R., & Bellugi, U. (1992). Fetal alcohol syndrome: A case report of neuropsychological, MRI, and EEG assessment of two children. *Alcoholism: Clinical and Experimental Research, 16,* 1001–1003.

Meyer, S. N., & Riley, E. P. (1996). In E. L. Abel (Ed.), *Fetal alcohol syndrome: From mechanisms to prevention.* Boca Raton, FL: CRC Press.

Meyer, L. S., Kotch, L. E., & Riley, E. P. (1990). Alterations in gait following ethanol exposure during the brain growth spurt in rats. *Alcoholism: Clinical and Experimental Research, 14,* 23–27.

Miller, M. W. (1986). Effects of alcohol on the generation and migration of cerebral cortical neurons. *Science, 233,* 1308–1311.

Miller, M. W. (1989). Effects of prenatal exposure to ethanol on neocortical development—II: Cell proliferation in the ventricular zones of the rat. *Journal of Comparative Neurology, 287,* 326–338.

Miller, M. W. (1992). Effects of prenatal exposure to ethanol on cell proliferation and neuronal migration. In M. W. Miller (Ed.), *Development of the central nervous system: Effects of alcohol and opiates* (pp. 47–69). New York: Wiley-Liss.

Miller, M. W., Chiaia, N. L., & Rhoades, R. W. (1990). An intracellular recording and injection study of corticospinal neurons in rat somatosensory cortex: Effect of prenatal exposure to ethanol. *Journal of Comparative Neurology, 297,* 91–105.

Miller, M. W., & Dow-Edwards, D. L. (1988). Structural and metabolic alterations in rat cerebral cortex induced by prenatal exposure to ethanol. *Brain Research, 474,* 316–326.

Miller, M. W., & Potempa, G. (1990). Numbers of neurons and glia in mature rat somatosensory cortex: Effects of prenatal exposure to ethanol. *Journal of Comparative Neurology, 293,* 92–102.

Milner, B. (1964). Some effects of frontal lobectomy in man. In J. M. Warren & K. Akert (Eds.), *The frontal granular cortex and behavior* (pp. 313–334). New York: McGraw-Hill.

Mirsky, A. F. (1987). Behavioral and psychophysiological markers of disordered attention. *Environmental Health Perspectives, 74,* 191–199.

Mirsky, A. F., Anthony, B. J., Duncan, C. C., Ahearn, M. B., & Kellam, S. G. (1991). Analysis of the elements of attention: A neuropsychological approach. *Neuropsychology Review, 2,* 109–145.

Mirsky, A. F., & Cardon, P. V. (1962). A comparison of the behavioral and physiological changes accompanying sleep deprivation and chlorpromazine in man. *Electroencephalography and Clinical Neurophysiology, 14,* 1–10.

Mirsky, A. F., Primac, D. W., Ajmone Marsan, C., Rosvold, H. E., & Stevens, J. A. (1960). A comparison of the psychological test performance of patients with focal and nonfocal epilepsy. *Experimental Neurology, 2,* 75–89.

Mirsky, A. F., & Van Buren, J. M. (1965). On the nature of the "absence" in centerncephalic epilepsy: A study of some behavioral, electroencephalic, and autonomic factors. *Electroencephalography and Clinical Neurophysiology, 18,* 334–348.

Morse, B. A., & Weiner, L. (1993). *FAS: Parent and child* [Brochure]. Brookline, MA: Boston University School of Medicine, Fetal Alcohol Education Program.

Myklebust, H. R. (1981). *The Pupil Rating Scale Revised: Screening for learning disabilities.* San Antonio: Psychological Corporation.

Nanson, J. L., & Hiscock, M. (1990). Attention deficits in children exposed to alcohol prenatally. *Alcoholism: Clinical and Experimental Research, 14,* 656–661.

Needleman, H. L., Gunnol, C., Leviton, A., Reed, R., Peresie, H., Maher, C., & Barrett, P. (1979). Deficits in psychologic and classroom performance of children with elevated dentine lead levels. *New England Journal of Medicine, 13,* 689–695.

Novick, N. J., & Streissguth, A. P. (1996, Winter). Thoughts on treatment of adults and adolescents impaired by fetal alcohol exposure. *Treatment Today, 20–21.*

Nuechterlein, K. H. (1983). Signal detection in vigilance tasks and behavioral attributes among offspring of schizophrenic mothers and among hyperactive children. *Journal of Abnormal Psychology, 92,* 4–28.

O'Dougherty, M., Nuechterlein, K. H., & Drew, B. (1984). Hyperactive and hypoxic children: Signal detection, sustained attention, and behavior. *Journal of Abnormal Psychology, 93,* 178–191.

Phillips, D. E. (1992). Effects of alcohol on the development of glial cell and myelin. In R. R. Watson (Ed.), *Alcohol and neurobiology: Brain development and hormone regulation* (pp. 83–108). Boca Raton, FL: CRC Press.

Phillips, S. C. (1989). The threshold concentration of dietary ethanol necessary to produce toxic effects on hippocampal cells and synapses in the mouse. *Experimental Neurology, 104,* 68–72.

Phillips, S. C., & Cragg, B. G. (1982). Change in susceptibility of rat cerebellar Purkinje cells to damage by alcohol during fetal, neonatal, and adult life. *Neuropathology and Applied Neurobiology, 8,* 441–454.

Pierog, S., Chandavasu, O., & Wexler, I. (1977). Withdrawal symptoms in infants with the fetal alcohol syndrome. *Journal of Pediatrics, 90,* 630–633.

Posner, M. I., & Petersen, S. E. (1990). The attention system of the human brain. *Annual Review of Neuroscience, 13,* 25–42.

Reyes, E., Wolfe, J., & Savage, D. D. (1989). The effects of prenatal alcohol exposure on radial arm maze performance in adult rats. *Physiology and Behavior, 46,* 45–48.

Richardson, G. A., & Day, N. L. (1991). Prenatal exposure to alcohol, marijuana, and tobacco: Effects on infant mental and motor development. *Abstracts of the Society for Research in Child Development, 8,* 421.

Richardson, G. A., Day, N. L., & Taylor, P. M. (1989). The effect of prenatal alcohol, marijuana, and tobacco exposure on neonatal behavior. *Infant Behavior and Development, 12,* 199–209.

Riley, E. P., Lochry, E. A., & Shapiro, N. R. (1979). Lack of response inhibition in rats prenatally exposed to alcohol. *Psychopharmocology (Berlin), 62,* 47–52.

Riley, E. P., Lochry, E. A., Shapiro, N. R., & Baldwin, J. (1979). Response perseveration in rats exposed to alcohol prenatally. *Psychopharmacology (Berlin), 10,* 255–259.

Rosett, H., Snyder, P., Sander, L., Lee, A., Cook, P., Weiner, L., & Gould, J.

(1979). Effect of maternal drinking on neonate state regulation. *Developmental Medicine and Child Neurology, 21,* 464–473.

Rosvold, H. E., Mirsky, A. F., Sarason, I., Bransome, E. D., & Beck, L. N. (1956). A continuous performance test of brain damage. *Journal of Consulting Psychiatry, 20,* 343–350.

Sampson, P. D., Streissguth, A. P., Barr, H. M., & Bookstein, F. L. (1989). Neurobehavioral effects of prenatal alcohol. Part II: Partial least squares analysis. *Neurotoxicology and Teratology, 11,* 477–491.

Sander, L. W., Snyder, P., Rosett, H. L., Lee, A., Gould, J. B., & Ouelette, F. (1977). Effects of alcohol intake during pregnancy on newborn state regulation: A progress report. *Alcoholism: Clinical and Experimental Research, 1,* 233–241.

Scher, M. S., Richardson, G. A., Coble, P. A., Day, N., & Stoffer, D. (1988). The effects of prenatal alcohol and marijuana exposure: Disturbances in neonatal sleep cycling and arousal. *Pediatric Research, 24,* 101–105.

Seidenberg, J., & Majewski, F. (1978). Zur Häufigkeit der Alkoholembryopathie in den verschiedenen Phasen der mutterlichen Alkoholkrankheit. *Hamburg Suchtgefahren, 24,* 63–75.

Shaywitz, S. E. (1986). *Early recognition of educational vulnerability—EREV* (Tech. rep.). Hartford, CT: State Department of Education.

Shaywitz, S. E., Cohen, D. J., & Shaywitz, B. A. (1980). Behavioral and learning difficulties in children with normal intelligence born to alcoholic mothers. *Journal of Pediatrics, 96,* 978–982.

Shruygin, G. I. (1974). Ob osobennostyakh psikhicheskogo razvitiya detei ot materei, stradayushchikh khronicheskim alkogolizmom [Characteristics of the mental development of children of alcoholic mothers]. *Pediatriya (Moskva), 11,* 71–73.

Smith, D. W. (1979). Fetal drug syndromes: Effects of ethanol and hydantoins. *Pediatrics in Review, 1,* 165–172.

Smith, D. W. (1982). *Recognizable patterns of human malformation: Genetic, embryologic and clinical aspects.* Philadelphia: Saunders.

Smith, I. E., Coles, C. D., Lancaster, J., Fernhoff, P. M., & Falek, A. (1986). The effect of volume and duration of prenatal ethanol exposure on neonatal physical and behavioral development. *Neurobehavioral Toxicology and Teratology, 8,* 375–381.

Sokol, R. J., & Clarren, S. K. (1989). Guidelines for use of terminology describing the impact of prenatal alcohol on the offspring. *Alcoholism: Clinical and Experimental Research, 13,* 597–598.

Spohr, H. L., & Steinhausen, H. C. (1987). Follow-up studies of children with FAS. *Neuropediatrics, 18,* 13–17.

Spohr, H. L., Willms, J., & Steinhausen, H. C. (1993). Prenatal alcohol exposure and long-term developmental consequences. *Lancet, 341,* 907–910.

Steinhausen, H. C., Nestler, V., & Huth, H. (1982). Psychopathology and mental functions in the offspring of alcoholic and epileptic mothers. *Journal of the American Academy of Child Psychiatry, 21,* 268–273.

Steinhausen, H. C., Nestler, V., & Spohr, H. L. (1982). Development and psychopathology of children with fetal alcohol syndrome. *Journal of Developmental and Behavioral Pediatrics, 3,* 49–54.

Stoffer, D. S., Scher, M. S., Richardson, G. A., Day, N. L., & Coble, P. (1988). A Walsh–Fourier analysis of the effects of moderate alcohol consumption on neonatal sleep-state cycling. *Journal of the Statistician Association, 83,* 954–963.

Streissguth, A. P. (1976). Psychologic handicaps in children with fetal alcohol syndrome. *Annals of the New York Academy of Sciences, 273,* 140–145.

Streissguth, A. P. (1992). Fetal alcohol syndrome and fetal alcohol effect: A clinical perspective of later developmental consequences. In I. S. Zagon & T. A. Slotkin (Eds.), *Maternal substance abuse and the developing nervous system* (pp. 5–25). San Diego: Academic Press.

Streissguth, A. P., Aase, J. M., Clarren, S. K., Randals, S. P., LaDue, R. A., & Smith, D. W. (1991). Fetal alcohol syndrome in adolescents and adults. *Journal of the American Medical Association, 265,* 1961–1967.

Streissguth, A. P., Barr, H. M., Kogan, J., & Bookstein, F. L. (1996). *Understanding the occurrence of secondary disabilities in clients with fetal alcohol syndrom (FAS) and fetal alcohol effects (FAE).* Seattle: University of Washington, Fetal Alcohol and Drug Unit.

Streissguth, A. P., Barr, H. M., & Martin, D. C. (1983). Maternal alcohol use and neonatal habituation assessed with the Brazelton Scale. *Child Development, 54,* 1109–1118.

Streissguth, A. P., Barr, H. M., Martin, D. C., & Herman, C. S. (1980). Effects of maternal alcohol, nicotine, and caffeine use during pregnancy on infant motor development at 8 months. *Alcoholism: Clinical and Experimental Research, 4,* 152–164.

Streissguth, A. P., Barr, H. M., & Sampson, P. D. (1990). Moderate prenatal alcohol exposure: Effects on child IQ and learning problems at age 7½ years. *Alcoholism: Clinical and Experimental Research, 14,* 662–669.

Streissguth, A. P., Barr, H. M., Sampson, P. D., Parrish-Johnson, J. C., Kirchner, G. L., & Martin, D. C. (1986). Attention, distraction, and reaction time at age 7 years and prenatal alcohol exposure. *Neurobehavioral Toxicology and Teratology, 8,* 717–725.

Streissguth, A. P., Bookstein, F. L., Sampson, P. D., & Barr, H. M. (1993). *The enduring effects of prenatal alcohol exposure on child development, birth through 7 years: A partial least squares solution.* Ann Arbor: University of Michigan Press.

Streissguth, A. P., Bookstein, F. L., Sampson, P. D., & Barr, H. M. (1995). Attention: Prenatal alcohol and continuities of vigilance and attentional problems from 4 through 14 years. *Development and Psychopathology, 7,* 419–446.

Streissguth, A. P., Clarren, S. K., & Jones, K. L. (1985). Natural history of Fetal Alcohol Syndrome: A follow-up of eleven patients. *Lancet, 2,* 85–92.

Streissguth, A. P., & Finnegan, L. P. (1996). Effects of prenatal alcohol and drugs. In J. Kinney (Ed.), *Clinical manual of substance abuse* (2nd ed., pp. 254–271). St. Louis: Mosby-Year Book.

Streissguth, A. P., Herman, C. S., & Smith, D. W. (1978). Intelligence, behavior, and dysmorphogenesis in the fetal alcohol syndrome: A report on 20 patients. *Journal of Pediatrics, 92,* 363–367.

Streissguth, A. P., & Kanter, J. (Eds.). (1997). *The Challenge of fetal alcohol syndrome: Overcoming secondary disabilities.* Seattle: University of Washington Press.

Streissguth, A. P., & Little, R. E. (1994). Unit 5: Alcohol, pregnancy, and the fetal alcohol syndrome (2nd ed.). In Project Cork Institute Medical School Curriculum, *Biomedical education: Alcohol use and its medical consequences.* [Slide/teaching unit available from Milner-Fenwick, Inc., 2125 Greenspring Drive, MD 21093; 1-800-432-8433.]

Streissguth, A. P., Martin, D. C., Barr, H. M., Sandman, B. M., Kirchner, G. L., & Darby, B. L. (1984). Intrauterine alcohol and nicotine exposure: Attention and reaction time in 4-year-old children. *Developmental Psychology, 20,* 533–541.

Streissguth, A. P., & Novick, N. J. (1995, Fall). Fetal alcohol syndrome and fetal alcohol effects in the treatment setting. *Treatment Today,* 14–15.

Streissguth, A. P, Sampson, P. D., Carmichael Olson, H., Bookstein, F.L., Barr, H. M., Scott, M., Feldman, J., & Mirsky, A. F. (1994). Maternal drinking during pregnancy: Attention and short-term memory in 14-year-old offspring: A longitudinal prospective study. *Alcoholism: Clinical and Experimental Research, 18,* 202–218.

Stuss, D. T., Stethem, L. L., Hugenholtz, H., Picton, T. W., Pivik, J., & Richard, M. T. (1989). Reaction time after head injury: Fatigue, divided and focused attention, and consistency of performance. *Journal of Neurology, Neurosurgery, and Psychiatry, 52,* 742–748.

Swanson, H. L. (1983). A developmental study of vigilance in learning-disabled and nondisabled children. *Journal of Abnormal Child Psychology, 11,* 415–429.

Vorhees, C. V. (1986). Principles of behavioral teratology. In E. P. Riley & C. V. Vorhees (Eds.), *Handbook of behavioral teratology* (pp. 23–46). New York: Plenum Press.

Ward, G. R., & West, J. R. (1992). Effects of ethanol during development on neuronal survival and plasticity. In M. W. Miller (Ed.), *Development of the central nervous system: Effects of alcohol and opiates* (pp. 109–138). New York: Wiley-Liss.

Weiner, L., & Morse, B. A. (1994). Intervention and the child with FAS. *Alcohol Health and Research World, 18*(1), 67–72.

West, J. R. (Ed.). (1986). *Alcohol and brain development.* New York: Oxford University Press.

Wigal, T., & Amsel, A. (1990). Behavioral and neuroanatomical effects of prenatal, postnatal, or combined exposure to ethanol in weanling rats. *Behavioral Neuroscience, 104,* 116–126.

Wilson, J. G. (1977). Current status of teratology: General principles and mechanisms derived from animal studies. In J. G. Wilson & F. C. Fraser (Eds.), *Handbook of teratology: General principles and etiology* (Vol. 1, pp. 47–74). New York: Plenum Press.

Attention-Deficit/ Hyperactivity Disorder in Mental Retardation

NATURE OF ATTENTION DEFICITS

Deborah A. Pearson
Amy M. Norton
Ellen C. Farwell

In recent years, a wide body of literature has been amassed that is strongly suggestive of developmental gains in attention throughout childhood (Brodeur, Trick, & Enns, Chapter 4, this volume; Hagen & Hale, 1973; Lane & Pearson, 1982), yet relatively little is known about how attention is manifested in children whose developmental course is affected by syndromes such as attention-deficit/hyperactivity disorder (ADHD [DSM-IV: 314.01]; American Psychiatric Association, 1994) or mental retardation (MR).

The choice of these dual diagnoses is of particular interest because both of them are inherently linked to attentional difficulties. Although a rich literature has been amassed in both of these areas, with very few exceptions researchers have gone to great lengths to exclude children with MR from studies of ADHD and vice versa. As a result, the relationship between these syndromes has never been explored; that is, we do not know what the impact of ADHD is on children with MR. It may be the case that these two syndromes are entirely independent of each other, in which case the differences between children with and without ADHD who have MR would parallel the differences between children with and without ADHD in the general school-age population. Or it may be the case that there is a certain amount of overlap between the syndromes of MR and ADHD such that ADHD is manifested somewhat differently in children with MR (relative to their peers with MR but without ADHD) than it is in children in the general school-age population (relative to their peers without ADHD in the general school-age population).

The purpose of this chapter will be to explore the attention deficits that are associated with ADHD in children with MR and to examine the developmental issues surrounding the relationship between these two syndromes. The attention deficits associated with ADHD in the general population will be discussed initially, followed by the nature of attention deficits associated with ADHD in MR.

ATTENTION DEFICITS ASSOCIATED WITH ADHD IN THE GENERAL POPULATION

ADHD is manifested in terms of three major clusters of symptoms: inattention, overactivity, and impulsivity (American Psychiatric Association, 1987, 1994). Within the cognitive domain, children with ADHD have been shown to have significant deficits in sustained attention, impulsivity, and some areas of visual and auditory selective attention (Barkley, 1990, 1991; Douglas, 1983; Ross & Ross, 1982).

Sustained Attention

Sustained attention, or the ability to remain on task, has traditionally been assessed using vigilance tasks that require subjects to sustain performance over a period of time. Many of these tasks are modifications of the Continuous Performance Test (CPT), which was developed by Rosvold, Mirsky, Sarason, Bransome, and Beck (1956). The CPT, originally designed to detect brain damage in children and adults, has become one of the most reliable measures used to differentiate children with ADHD from children without ADHD (Barkley, 1991; Sykes, Douglas, & Morgenstern, 1973). The CPT requires the child to monitor a computer screen for the occurrence of a predetermined target or target sequence. Other instruments frequently used to assess sustained attention are paper and pencil tasks in which subjects search rows of figures or letters for prearranged target figures. In these tasks, correct targets are "canceled," or crossed out, upon detection.

Children with decrements in sustained attention often begin a test session performing in a manner similar to that of their peers without such decrements, but their performance typically declines the longer they remain on task. As a result, their response latencies become longer, they make fewer correct detections, and respond to more nontargets as time on task lengthens. Using a variety of paradigms, a number of studies (e.g., Aman & Turbott, 1986; Barkley, DuPaul, & McMurray, 1990; Sykes et al., 1973) have found that children with ADHD are not able to sustain their attention as well as their peers without ADHD.

However, caution should be used when interpreting findings from tasks such as the CPT because there are many extraneous factors that can significantly affect performance. Variables affecting performance outcome include task length, the child's reaction to an artificial setting (e.g., the clinic or laboratory), the examiner's presence or absence in the testing room, that is, children with ADHD perform better in the presence of an examiner (Draeger, Prior, & Sanson, 1986), and the intrinsic appeal of the task (children with ADHD perform better on tasks that appeal to them; Barkley, 1991; Klee & Garfinkel, 1983; Pelham, 1981; Power, 1992). Thus, when different vigilance studies are compared, it is necessary to closely examine specific task characteristics.

Selective Attention

Selective attention, or the ability to focus attention on relevant stimuli while ignoring irrelevant stimuli, has been extensively studied in children with ADHD with both visual and auditory measures. Visual selective attention is often assessed by using distraction tasks, in which performance in nondistracting conditions is compared with performance in distracting conditions. The most effective measures of selective attention ability are tasks that have little reliance on memory ability, such as the Speeded Classification Task (Strutt, Anderson, & Well, 1975), in which subjects sort stimuli in the presence or absence of distracting dimensions. Similarly, auditory selective attention is often measured using dichotic listening tasks, which also carry minimal memory loads. In this type of task, subjects must disregard items (e.g., tones, words) that are sent to one ear and attend to those heard in the other ear (Zekulin-Hartley, 1982). Typically, when distracting messages or visual stimuli are introduced into a task, children with a deficit in selective attention show decrements in performance, relative to nondistracting conditions. These decrements are manifested as longer reaction times and higher error rates. Using a variety of paradigms, a number of studies have shown that children with ADHD, relative to children without ADHD, are less able to selectively allocate their attention to relevant stimuli while ignoring irrelevant distractors. For a review please see Pearson and Lane (1990). It should be noted that these decrements (in distracting conditions relative to nondistracting conditions) occur in tasks of short duration; thus, these deficits are not simply manifestations of deficits in sustained attention.

Impulsivity

Impulsivity, or the tendency to respond without reflection, has also been compared in children with ADHD, and their peers without ADHD. Tests of impulsivity have often used tasks in which a child must match a sample stimulus with one of several alternatives or must wait for a predetermined delay period before responding. In the match-to-sample tasks, impulsive children typically respond without scanning all of their alternatives, resulting in short latencies of response and high error rates. One widely used match-to-sample task is the Matching Familiar Figures Test (Kagan, Rosman, Day, Albert, & Phillips, 1964). In this test, children with ADHD have been shown to be more impulsive in their response style (Campbell, Douglas, & Morgenstern, 1971). Although match-to-sample tasks have been found to differentiate children with ADHD from children without ADHD in the general population (Campbell et al., 1971), other investigators have found no evidence of differences in performance on these tasks between children with and without ADHD (Barkley et al., 1990).

Other tasks used to measure impulsivity are delay of gratification tasks, in which the child must wait a predetermined period of time in order to obtain an award or to win points. This type of task uses the method of differential reinforcement of low rate responding, in which reinforcement is given after a prearranged time interval has elapsed since the last reinforcement (Skinner, 1938). Impulsive children have more difficulty in waiting the appropriate length of time before responding, which results in lower scores on the task (Gordon, 1983). Using a variety of paradigms, several studies have demonstrated that, when compared to children without ADHD, children with ADHD have performance decrements on delay of gratification measures (Gordon, 1979; Gordon & Mettelman, 1988; McClure & Gordon, 1984). These studies provide support for Douglas's widely noted characterization of children with ADHD as having difficulty with the ability to "stop, look, and listen" (Douglas, 1972).

It should be noted that some investigations have revealed inconsistencies among different measures of impulsivity. Most importantly, there is a low intercorrelation among different instruments (e.g., the delay of gratification measures and the Matching Familiar Figures Test) that supposedly measure impulsivity (Milich & Kramer, 1985). Furthermore, while performance on match-to-sample tasks has a high correlation with age (Cairns & Cammock, 1978; Sandberg, Rutter, & Taylor, 1978), performance on delay of gratification tasks has not been found to be related to age (McClure & Gordon, 1984). These inconsistent findings suggest that perhaps these different tasks tap different facets of impulsivity. For instance, it may be the case that some instruments tap impulsivity that is related to motoric channels whereas other instruments tap more "cognitive" aspects of impulsivity (McClure & Gordon, 1984). Of course, task characteristics, such as the length of time that an individual must wait on the delay of gratification task, the degree of complexity in the match-to-sample stimuli, and the nature of reinforcement, may also play a role in the differences noted between studies (Barkley, 1991; Klee & Garfinkel, 1983; Pelham, 1981; Power, 1992). These factors suggest that the concept of "impulsivity" requires considerably more investigation.

As can be seen from this brief summary, attention deficits and impulsivity have been widely studied in children with ADHD in the general population. In the next section, the nature of attention deficits in children and adults with MR will be explored, followed by a discussion of the attention deficits associated with ADHD in persons with MR.

ATTENTION DEFICITS ASSOCIATED WITH MR

It has long been suggested that some degree of attention deficit is associated with MR (Zeaman & House, 1963). In order to more fully understand the nature of the deficits underlying global attention difficulties, specific components of attention in MR such as sustained attention, selective attention, breadth of attention, and impulsivity have been examined.

Sustained Attention

Sustained attention is frequently studied in individuals with MR by using vigilance tasks such as the CPT. Although the vigilance performance of children with MR has been found to be inferior to that of children of the same chronological age who do not have MR (Jones, 1971; Semmel, 1965), when the former group are matched to children of a similar mental age these differences disappear (Crosby, 1972). Thus, these studies suggest that simple vigilance performance is not deficient in children with MR when mental age is controlled, although it is deficient with respect to children of the same chronological age.

By adolescence and young adulthood, few differences remain between individuals with and without MR on simple vigilance performance (Jones, 1971; Ware, Baker, & Sipowicz, 1962). However, on more complicated vigilance tasks requiring more effortful cognitive processing, adults with MR miss more targets and respond inappropriately to nontargets more often than do their peers without MR (Tomporowski, 1990; Tomporowski, Hayden, & Applegate, 1990). Furthermore, even within the population of individuals with MR, individuals with severe retardation perform worse than individuals with mild retardation on a complex vigilance task (Das, 1970). Overall, these studies suggest that when simple vigilance tasks are administered, younger children with MR demonstrate performance decrements but older individuals with MR only show these decrements when more effortful processing is required.

Other studies of sustained attention have found that although children with MR can sustain attention for equal or even longer periods than children without MR, they are not as efficient at exploring stimuli or as flexible in response style (Krakow & Kopp, 1982, 1983; Loveland, 1987). It has been suggested that these long periods of sustained attention by individuals with MR may actually represent a "failure to lose interest," as opposed to an ability to sustain interest. Evidence for this hypothesis has been provided by Shafer and Peeke (1982), who found that adults with MR failed to habituate to repetitive auditory stimuli whereas subjects without MR did so quickly.

Thus, the individual with MR who is "sustaining attention" may not be involved in an active process of sustaining a directed focus of attention, but instead may be engaging in an undirected response style. For instance, Ellis, Woodley-Zanthos, Dulaney, and Palmer (1989) found that individuals with MR persisted in using an attentional strategy that was no longer adaptive. These studies suggest that some instances in which individuals with MR appear to be adequately sustaining attention may instead be manifestations of cognitive inertia, that is, persistence in an automatic response when it is no longer appropriate. This finding has been noted in individuals with MR of differing etiologies, including Down syndrome (Krakow & Kopp, 1982, 1983; Loveland, 1987) and familial retardation (Dulaney & Ellis, 1994; Ellis et al., 1989).

Selective Attention

Selective attention in individuals with MR has been studied extensively using distractibility studies. Many of these studies have repeatedly used distractors that are intrinsic to the task at hand; that is, they are embedded within the context of the task. For instance, children with MR have been found to be less capable of attending to relevant cues in a discriminant learning task than their mental-age-matched peers without MR (Ullman & Routh, 1971). Additionally, in the presence of distractors, children with MR have more difficulty remembering information (Holowinsky & Farrelly, 1988) and in inhibiting responses caused by distracting dimensions of task stimuli (Ellis et al., 1989). When attention was artificially drawn to relevant cues by increasing their salience, the performance of subjects with MR improved significantly (Ager, 1983). Using a metronome beat as a distractor, Follini, Sitkowski, and Stayton (1969) found that children with MR had more difficulty ignoring an auditory distractor than their same-aged peers without MR. Taken collectively, these studies suggest that children with MR have more difficulty than their peers without MR in controlling the focus of their attention and that at least part of this difficulty can be traced to deficits in selectively attending to relevant cues.

Not all studies using intrinsic distractors (i.e., distractors embedded within a task) have found evidence of deficits in selective attention in individuals with MR. For example, when mental age was controlled, children with and without MR performed similarly on studies using visual search tasks (Das, 1971; Spitz & Borland, 1971). Furthermore, when subjects were matched on mental age, no significant differences emerged between individuals with and without MR on dichotic listening performance (Zekulin-Hartley, 1982), incidental learning performance (Hagen & Huntsman, 1971), or forced-choice reaction time performance (Burack, 1994).

Other studies of selective attention in individuals with MR have used extrinsic distractors, or distractors that were external to the experimental task. For example, it has been found that, even when matched for mental age, subjects with MR spent more time glancing off task, thus making them appear more distractible than their peers without MR (Turnure, 1970; Turnure & Zigler, 1964). Furthermore, the susceptibility of persons with MR to distraction has been shown to be related to the level of task difficulty. For example, Sen and Clarke (1968) found that although adults with MR were distracted by extraneous stimulation during a difficult task, they were unaffected by the same distractors when the task was easy. Furthermore, adults with lower mental ages were more distracted by the extraneous stimulation than were adults with higher mental ages.

On the other hand, Baumeister and Ellis (1963) found that adults with MR actually made more correct responses and had shorter response latencies on a delayed match-to-sample task in the presence of extraneous visual stimulation, relative to a nondistracting condition. They hypothesized that the extrinsic distraction raised the arousal level of subjects, which in turn facilitated enhanced alertness. In a later study, Belmont and Ellis (1968) found that adults with MR were not more distractible than adults of similar chronological age without MR. They suggested that some forms of distraction may have no effect or even a facilitative effect upon performance in a learning situation because they act as general arousers, resulting in greater alertness and concomitant improvements in attention.

Although there appears to be some inconsistency between studies, one pattern emerges that may help to explain these differences. Specifically, it may be that in tasks in which distractors are similar to the central task stimuli (i.e., the task requires more effortful processing) persons with MR show decrements in performance, whereas in tasks in which the distractors are easily distinguished from the central task stimuli, no such performance decrements are produced. Taken collectively, these studies suggest that in some instances, persons with MR have more difficulty than individuals in the general population in attending selectively to relevant cues.

Breadth of Attention/Immediate Memory

In addition to problems with distractibility, persons with MR have also been shown to have deficiencies in "breadth of attention" tasks requiring short-term memory. Breadth-of-attention tasks assess the ability to process more than one dimension of a stimulus at the same time. In this type of task, subjects are asked to abstract information and retain it over a period of time. Mackie and MacKay (1982) found that young adults with MR were able to discern a relevant dimension as well as could their mental-age-matched peers without MR, but they could not retain it as long. In a task requiring subjects to verbally label a target stimulus, individuals with MR showed performance decrements relative to individuals without MR when matched for mental age in both immediate memory and retention aspects of the task (Whiteley, Zaparniuk, & Asmundson, 1987). These studies suggest that although persons with MR seem to be able to discern relevant information as well as subjects without MR do when a task uses little effortful processing, they are differentially sensitive to interference such as verbal labeling.

It is difficult to ascertain the reason for this apparent deficit in selective attention. It may be the case that persons with MR are not as capable of flexibly filtering information from the environment as their peers without MR. Specifically, when little effort is required to distinguish targets and distractors, little interference is noted in persons with MR. However, in situations that perhaps require more active filtering, persons with MR may be unable to flexibly allocate attention in accordance with task demands. As a result, attention is "sucked in" by stimulus characteristics, rather than being actively directed.

On the other hand, this deficit in selective attention may be related to less overall attentional capacity in persons with MR. In this model of attention (Kahneman, 1973), attention is seen as consisting of a limited "pool" of cognitive capacity that can be allocated to perform mental work. In situations that require little cognitive effort, such as distinguishing between targets and distractors that are very dissimilar, the more limited attentional capacity of persons with MR is not exceeded and performance shows little decrement, if any. However, in situations requiring more cognitive effort, this limited capacity would be exceeded and performance decrements would be noted.

Impulsivity

Impulsivity (as defined earlier) has not been studied as extensively as have other facets of cognition in persons with MR. Rotundo and Johnson (1981) characterized half of their sample of children with MR (including organic, familial, and Down syndrome etiologies) as being impulsive, as compared to 20% of their sample of children without MR. Within the group with MR, the level of impulsivity varied according to etiology of MR. Children with an organic basis for their MR were the most impulsive (59%), followed by children with familial MR (45%), followed by children with Down syndrome (37%). Similar problems with impulsivity have been found in adolescents with mild to borderline MR (Leff & Meyer, 1984), and in children and adults with fragile X syndrome (Bregman, Leckman, & Ort, 1988; Dykens, Hodapp, & Leckman, 1989). These findings strongly suggest that children with MR may have an increased vulnerability toward impulsivity and that this vulnerability is linked to etiology.

Hyperactivity/Activity Level

Hyperactivity, or excessive activity level, has also been studied in persons with MR. Payne (1968) found that 18% of individuals with MR had clinically significant levels of hyperactivity. Other researchers have examined whether or not activity level is associated with cognitive performance. For example, Foshee (1958) found that adults with MR with either high or low levels of activity (as rated by their caregivers) performed similarly on easy and complex learning tasks. In a follow-up study, Gardner, Cromwell, and Foshee (1959) found that increased visual stimulation decreased activity level in both "hypoactive" and "hyperactive" adults with MR, although the hyperactive group demonstrated a greater reduction in activity during the stimulation. However, other investigations by this group were not suggestive of changes in activity level in adults with MR (who were not classified as "hyperactive" or "hypoactive") when extraneous noise or visual stimulation was introduced (Cromwell & Foshee, 1960; Spradlin, Cromwell, & Foshee, 1960). Overall, these studies suggest that although persons with MR are more vulnerable to difficulties with excessive activity, under most circumstances, excessive activity is not always associated with performance decrements per se.

Although the literature examining attention, impulsivity, and activity level in persons with MR is somewhat inconsistent, it clearly provides evidence that persons with MR exhibit some degree of difficulties in these areas (particularly attentional difficulties), relative to persons without MR, especially in childhood and when effortful attentional strategies are needed. Therefore, although attention deficits appear to accompany MR, not all persons with MR have clinically significant attention deficits that are associated with ADHD, because their attention is usually commensurate with what would be expected on the basis of their mental age. On the other hand, there are some individuals whose attention skills are impaired even when their mental age is taken into account. It is these individuals—whose attention skills are significantly more impaired than what would be expected on the basis of their developmental level—who should be viewed as carrying the dual diagnoses of MR and ADHD.

ADHD IN MR

Although there is an extensive literature on both attention in children with MR and on the attention deficits associated with ADHD, there is relatively little known about the syndrome of ADHD in children with MR. Indeed, subaverage intelligence (IQ level < 80) has traditionally been used as an exclusion criterion in studies of ADHD (Barkley, 1990; Douglas, 1983) in order to study "pure" ADHD, that is, ADHD not confounded by the presence of another syndrome. The relationship between the syndromes ADHD and MR will be explored next.

Prevalence

Using the Behavior Problem Checklist (Quay, 1977), Epstein, Cullinan, and Polloway (1986) compared students in regular education classrooms with students in classrooms serving children with mild MR and found evidence of elevated problems with inattention in the latter group. In a survey of classrooms, Epstein, Cullinan, and Gadow (1986), using the Abbreviated Conners Teacher Rating Scale (Conners, 1973), found that the prevalence of ADHD (as defined by the percentage of children exceeding the common clinical cutoff score of 15 on the Conners Scale) was five times higher in children with mild MR, as compared to children from regular education classrooms. Similarly, Das and Melnyk (1989) found the prevalence of ADHD, as screened using a cutoff of 15 on the Conners Teacher Rating Scale, to be 33% of junior and senior high school students with mild MR. Ando and Yoshimura (1978) noted that younger children and children with lower IQs had a high prevalence of symptoms of hyperactivity, as assessed by teachers using a checklist of maladaptive behaviors, as compared to the general population. However, Fee, Matson, Moore, and Benavidez (1993) have more recently demonstrated that these problems of attention deficits and hyperactivity were not as closely associated with maladaptive behaviors such as conduct problems in children with MR as they were in children of normal intelligence.

These studies suggest that the prevalence of attention disorders is significantly higher in individuals with MR than it is in the general school-age population. Conservative estimates suggest that approximately 10% of children with MR warrant a diagnosis of ADHD (Hunt & Cohen, 1988), as compared with 3–5% in the general school-age population (American Psychiatric Association, 1994). In addition to familial retardation, the prevalence of ADHD has also been examined in children having genetic etiologies of MR. For example, it has been suggested that ADHD is a common behavioral problem in children with Down syndrome (Gath & Gumley, 1986; Myers & Pueschel, 1991; Patterson, 1992; Pueschel, Bernier, & Pezzullo, 1991). Symptoms of ADHD, such as severe inattention and impulsivity, have also been associated with fragile X syndrome (Bregman et al., 1988; Dykens et al., 1989).

When the prevalence rates of ADHD in MR are translated into actual numbers of individuals, the magnitude of this problem — and its impact upon society — become apparent. According to the U.S. Bureau of the Census, the population in the United States in 1992 was approximately 255 million. Given that approximately 3% (7.65 million) of Americans carry a diagnosis of MR (American Association on Mental Retardation, 1992), the prevalence estimates of 10% of individuals with MR having ADHD suggest that approximately 765,000 Americans carry these dual diagnoses. It has been suggested that ADHD is actually underdiagnosed in the population of individuals with MR because the symptoms may be less obvious than other disorders such as psychosis (Fisher, Burd, Kuna, & Berg, 1985). Furthermore, psychiatric and behavioral disturbances also suffer from "diagnostic overshadowing" (Reiss, Levitan, & Szyszko, 1982), or the tendency by clinicians to overlook additional psychiatric diagnoses once a diagnosis of MR is made. As such, these estimates of the prevalence of ADHD in MR may actually be conservative.

As previously noted, the study of symptoms associated with ADHD in persons with MR actually dates back several decades (Gardner et al., 1959; Spradlin et al., 1960; Tizard, 1968a, 1968b). However, it should be noted that these early investigations studied issues such as general activity level and social behavior in this population and typically used subjective staff ratings (rather than normed behavior scales) to label subjects as "overactive"; hence, it is not possible to determine whether or not these individuals would have met the formal diagnostic criteria for ADHD. In recent years, however, investigators have used more specific diagnostic criteria to study individuals whose symptomatology is consistent with a formal diagnosis of ADHD. The majority of these studies have focused on inattention, given that this symptom is the hallmark of ADHD. The attention deficits in children with MR and ADHD will be reviewed next.

Associated Attention Deficits

To date, only a few researchers have investigated the attentional deficits associated with ADHD in children with MR. Green, Dennis, and Bennets (1989) examined the behavioral patterns of toddlers with Down syndrome during standard developmental testing. They identified a subgroup of children who were distinctly elevated from the rest of the group with respect to hyperactivity and inattentive behaviors while performing these tests. These children showed particular deficits in the area of investment (the ability to organize and maintain attention) and in the ability to continue holding their attention when the tasks became more difficult.

Another study of inattention in MR (Melnyk & Das, 1992) used laboratory measures to directly compare children with MR and symptoms of ADHD to children with MR who did not have attention problems. They compared these "poor attenders" and "good attenders" on an auditory sustained attention task and a visual selective attention task, and found evidence of deficits in visual selective attention in the group of "poor attenders," relative to the other group. Although there no overall significant differences emerged between the two groups on the sustained attention measure, they did note that the "poor attenders" tended to show a decrement in performance as time on task progressed. It should be noted, however, that the "poor attenders" in this study did not carry a formal diagnosis of ADHD.

A more recent study examined cognition in children with MR who met the formal diagnostic criteria for ADHD (DSM-III-R; American Psychiatric Association, 1987). In this study, Pearson, Yaffee, Loveland, and Lewis (1996) compared school-age children with mild-to-moderate MR and ADHD to school-age children with mild-to-moderate MR who did not have ADHD on laboratory tasks that assess sustained and selective attention. These measures were adapted from the developmental attention literature to be appropriate to the developmental level of the children participating in this project.

Sustained attention was studied by Pearson et al. (1996) using an adaptation of the traditional Continuous Performance Test (CPT). In this adaptation, pictures were used instead of letters, and the target was a single picture (a witch), rather than a sequence of stimuli (e.g., an "A" followed by an "X"). Other pictures used as stimuli included a flag, a crescent moon and stars, a heart, a house, a child, a die, a checker board, a flower pot with flowers, a star, a teepee, and a wagon. The children were instructed to press a response button each time they saw the witch in order to protect the child from the witch. Although the picture of the child was androgynous, boys were told that they were protecting a boy, and girls were told that they were protecting a girl. (This difference in instructions was necessary because it was found in piloting that little girls declined to protect a boy from the witch.) The results indicated that the children with MR and ADHD detected fewer targets and responded to more non-targets than did their peers in the non-ADHD group. Interestingly, although the children with MR and ADHD made more omissions and more commissions than did their peers in the MR/nonADHD group, there was no evidence of a true deficit in sustained attention because their performance did not tend to decline as time on task lengthened. This finding is inconsistent with a deficit in sustained attention in children with MR and ADHD. However, the elevated commission rate was suggestive of a greater degree of impulsive responding in the MR/ADHD group.

Selective attention was assessed by Pearson et al. (1996) using the Speeded Classification Task (Strutt et al., 1975), in which the child sorts cards on the basis of two values of a relevant dimension (e.g., the presence of a horizontal line or a vertical line). This relevant condition can be presented by itself (the no-distraction condition) or else in the presence of one or two additional irrelevant dimensions (the distracting conditions). The results suggested that the sorting time of children with MR and ADHD was more slowed in the presence of distractors than that of their peers in the non-ADHD group, especially when they were sorting cards in the presence of highly salient distractors (i.e., distractors that were more difficult to ignore). The children with MR and ADHD also made approximately two times as many errors as did their peers in comparison group. This finding is consistent with a deficit in selective attention in children with MR and ADHD.

Thus, like Melnyk and Das (1992), Pearson et al. (1996) found evidence that children with MR and ADHD have deficits in visual selective attention but did not find evidence for deficits in sustained attention. These deficits were especially apparent when the children were sorting stimuli in a speeded classification task in the presence of highly salient distractors. As with previous investigations, this finding provided further evidence for the frequent observation that differences between children with and without ADHD are most likely to occur when more effortful processing (i.e., ignoring highly salient distractors) is needed for task performance. Although little evidence was found for deficits in sustained attention, the children with MR and ADHD did make significantly more errors in responding to nontargets than did their peers with MR but without ADHD.

In a recent study related to attention and cognition in children with MR and ADHD, Handen, McAuliffe, Janosky, Feldman, and Breaux (1994) examined differences in classroom behavior between children with MR and ADHD and children with MR who did not have ADHD. Using direct observation measures, the investigators found children with MR and ADHD to have lower levels of on-task behavior and elevated levels of fidgitiness, relative to the MR/non-ADHD group. Interestingly, both parents and teachers of children in the MR/ADHD group rated these children as having more problematic behaviors than their peers in the MR/non-ADHD group on behavioral scales tapping inattention, hyperactivity, and conduct problems. Thus, parent and teacher ratings of behavior appeared to be consistent with direct observations of classroom behavior in these children.

These two studies examining attention and classroom behavior in children carrying the formal diagnoses of MR and ADHD are the only studies in this area of which we are aware. Given the extensive literature examining attention deficits in children with ADHD in the general school-age population, it is clear that this area of inquiry needs significant further investigation in order to more clearly elucidate the nature of the attention deficits associated with ADHD in MR at a variety of levels of severity of MR (i.e., mild, moderate, severe). As has been noted by Einfeld and Aman (1993) and others (e.g., Pearson, 1993), ADHD may be manifested differently in individuals with milder versus more severe levels of MR. For instance, ADHD may be manifested in individuals with mild-to-moderate MR in a more "cognitive" manner (i.e., symptoms such as inattention may be more prominent), but in individuals with more severe levels of retardation the more motoric/organic features of ADHD (such as excessive movement) appear to be more prominent.

In order to compare ADHD in individuals of differing functional levels, it will be necessary to address the issue of appropriate diagnostic criteria for ADHD in children who have more severe levels of MR. Although traditional diagnostic instruments such as the Conners Scales are appropriate for children with mild levels of MR, the use of these instruments becomes increasingly suspect at more severe levels of MR (Aman, 1991). This is thought to be the case because the overlap in the typical behavioral repertoire of persons of normal IQ and persons with MR becomes smaller as the level of MR becomes more severe, and unfortunately most widely used diagnostic instruments are geared toward assessing behaviors seen in the normal IQ range. Thus, such instruments would not adequately assess behavior in persons with severe or profound MR, whose behavioral patterns are often very disparate from behaviors seen in the general population. Aman (1991) notes a variety of specialized instruments appropriate for such individuals.

In concluding this section on attention deficits associated with ADHD in MR, we note that the emerging literature on this topic suggests that attention deficits seen in children with MR and ADHD have some similarity to those seen in children with ADHD but of normal IQ. This similarity apparently is more clearly seen in the area of selective attention (Melnyk

& Das, 1992; Pearson et al., 1996) and in global impressions of attentional skills (Handen, McAuliffe, Janosky, Feldman, & Breaux, 1994). However, these studies suggest that there are other abilities in which children with MR and ADHD (relative to children with MR who do not have ADHD) do not seem to have the deficits associated with ADHD in children of normal IQ, such as sustained attention. Specifically, compared to children with MR but no ADHD, children with MR/ADHD do not show a decrement over time on task, although they may show inferior levels of absolute task performance (e.g., making more omissions or commissions).

It is possible to speculate that this discrepancy in sustained attention abilities in children with ADHD but of normal IQ and children with MR and ADHD may be related to the "cognitive inertia" phenomenon seen in persons with MR. To the extent that this phenomenon is operating in children with MR and ADHD, it may in an artificial sense "protect" them from the decrement in performance over time that is seen in children with ADHD of normal IQ (who would not have cognitive inertia). As a result, these children with MR and ADHD do not have the appearance of having a deficit in sustained attention.

However, in areas such as selective attention, children with MR and ADHD appear to have attention deficits over and above the level of their peers who have MR without ADHD. As with ADHD children of normal IQ, children with MR and ADHD appear to be more vulnerable, relative to their peers with MR but without ADHD, when they are doing tasks requiring more effortful processing (e.g., classifying stimuli in the presence of distractors, relative to conditions with no distractor).

In both of these situations, the syndromes of MR and ADHD appear to be additive in the sense that the child with MR and ADHD first has the fundamental cognitive characteristics associated with MR (such as cognitive inertia) and then has symptoms of ADHD overlaid upon that foundation. In the case of vigilance tasks, their underlying profile of cognitive inertia "insulates" them from attention decrements over time. In the case of selective attention, the underlying inefficient filtering and/or limited attentional capacity associated with their MR is magnified by the decrements in selective attention associated with ADHD.

FUTURE RESEARCH EXAMINING
THE RELATIONSHIP BETWEEN ADHD AND MR

Of central interest for future research will be the issue of how ADHD impacts the cognitive profile of children with MR. From the literature reviewed in this chapter, it has been hypothesized that ADHD is overlaid upon the basic foundation of MR, creating some situations in which the attention deficits associated with ADHD seem to be similar in children with and without MR, and creating other situations in which it is dissimilar. However, despite this divergence, Handen and his colleagues (Handon, Breaux, Golsing, Ploof, & Feldman, 1990; Handen et al., 1992; Handen, McAuliffe, Janosky, Feldman, & Breaux, 1995) have suggested that children with MR and ADHD respond in a similar manner to methylphenidate as do children with ADHD in the general population — although children in the former group are dissimilar from those in the latter in that they may be more vulnerable to medication side effects (Handon, Feldman, Golsing, Breaux, & McAuliffe, 1991). It appears that considerable work will be necessary in order to more fully elucidate the relationship between the syndromes of MR and ADHD.

Many factors will need to be considered in this future research. Future investigators should refine their studies by including tighter experimental control, double-blind placebo medication trials, and a wider range of dependent measures (Handen et al., 1992). Aman's work (e.g., Aman, 1982; Aman, Marks, Turbott, Wilsher, & Merry, 1991a, 1991b; Aman, Kern, McGhee, & Arnold, 1993a, 1993b) suggests that stimulants may not improve all symptoms associated with ADHD in these children, and it will be essential to examine a variety of dimensions of response to treatment in order to identify the domain of effectiveness of these treatments in this population. Furthermore, because stimulants such as methylphenidate have not been shown to improve all symptomatology associated with ADHD, it is crucial to consider other forms of accompanying treatment in developing treatment plans for children with MR and ADHD.

Clearly, as with children in the general population with ADHD, there is no one ultimate treatment to ameliorate the behavioral and attention problems encountered by children with MR and ADHD. For this reason, a multifaceted approach to intervention should be implemented for each individual. For example, stimulant medication may not improve social interactions, and therefore a child might benefit from receiving therapy in order to assist him/her in developing more appropriate interpersonal skills (Handen et al., 1990). Of course, as with all children with MR, appropriate special education services, in the least restrictive environment, should be implemented as soon as any cognitive deficit is noted. Ideally, this intervention would begin with infant stimulation programs, continue on into early childhood education programs, and then make the transition into traditional special education classrooms in the elementary school years. As with children with ADHD but without MR, children with MR and ADHD are likely to respond most favorably to structured classroom situations that feature as much one-on-one instruction as possible.

When assessing children with MR, researchers must consider the etiology of their participants' MR. Although many studies investigating the abilities of children with MR do not distinguish between subjects having different etiologies of MR, children with organic and familial MR perform differently on cognitive tasks and behavioral measures (Burack & Zigler, 1990; Burack, Hodapp, & Zigler, 1988; Zigler, 1967). Additionally, others have found differences between subjects with organic and familial MR in relation to activity level and time on task: while subjects with familial retardation became more active across trials, individuals with organic MR had a tendency to become less active as time on task progressed (Cromwell & Foshee, 1960). These studies suggest that when conducting research with individuals with MR, researchers must pay more attention to the effects of etiology of MR on performance.

Along those lines, the literature suggests that there is some degree of attention deficit that accompanies MR, so that when screening is being done on children with MR, assessments of individuals must follow standard diagnostic principles prior to their being classified ADHD. Since it has been found that the relationship is weak between teachers' ratings of inattention and inattention as defined by laboratory tasks (Pelham, 1981), a single rating scale should not be used as the only measure for assessment. In order to make a careful diagnosis of ADHD, it is necessary that scores on standardized parent and teacher rating scales, clinical impressions, and psychological testing be obtained.

As has been previously mentioned, a significant problem for clinicians and researchers seeking to make an accurate diagnosis of ADHD in MR is that there are relatively few tools for psychometric assessment of children and adults with MR, especially for individuals with a lower level of functioning. Although there are instruments that are being used to assess ADHD in children with MR, the majority of these instruments have been normed on individuals without MR (Handen et al., 1992). It is clear that behavioral instruments should be developed that would more appropriately tap the behavioral repertoire of children with MR, especially those individuals who are lower-functioning. Diagnostic tools such as the Reiss Scales for Children's Dual Diagnoses (Reiss & Valenti-Hein, 1990) are promising developments in this field; however, further studies will be necessary in order to elucidate the diagnostic effectiveness of such scales across various subgroups of individuals with MR.

A recent investigation by Pearson and Aman (1994) has provided some clarification as to the use of behavioral questionnaires in children with MR. Clinicians have been traditionally advised to correct for mental age when assessing the severity of behavioral ratings on such instruments (e.g., Barkley, 1990). Although this approach is intuitively appealing, we were aware of no previous data supporting this suggested interpretation of behavioral instruments. In order to examine the issue of whether or not it is necessary to correct for mental age in interpreting the severity of behavioral problems, behavioral ratings on the subscales of a number of instruments used to assess ADHD (e.g., the Conners Scales) were compared to both mental age and chronological age. The results of this investigation suggested that behavioral ratings were highly correlated with chronological age; however, there was no relationship between these ratings and mental age when the effect of chronological age was controlled for statistically. Thus, this study strongly suggests that there is little or no relationship between mental age and behavioral ratings in children with MR. For this reason, it does not appear to be necessary—or even appropriate—to interpret behavioral scales on the basis of mental age.

Further refinement is also necessary in the development and utilization of laboratory measures of attention—such as those used by Melnyk and Das (1992) and Pearson and her colleagues (1996)—that are sometimes used to clarify a diagnosis of ADHD. For instance, measures such as a CPT task that employs letter stimuli as targets may not be valid in children with MR because many children may not have the reading skills necessary for automatic processing of letter stimuli. In this circumstance, attentional deficits and simple floor effects due to inefficient processing of the test stimuli would be indistinguishable. For this reason, future researchers must make the appropriate developmental adaptations on laboratory measures when testing children with MR.

Another question to be addressed in future research concerns the effects of gender on attentional style in children with MR and ADHD. Previous cognitive research (Ackerman, Dykman, & Oglesby, 1983; Berry, Shaywitz, & Shaywitz, 1985) has suggested that the cognitive profile of girls with ADHD (without MR) may be different from that of boys with ADHD. Similarly, psychopharmacological research (e.g., Pelham, Walker, Sturges, & Hoza, 1989) has suggested that boys and girls with ADHD (without MR) may respond differently to methylphenidate, at least for some tasks. Interestingly, Pearson et al. (1996) noted that the ratio of boys to girls in the ADHD groups for each of these experiments was approximately 2:1. This ratio stands in contrast to the ratio of 4–9 boys to 1 girl (in clinical samples, the ratio is approximately 9 boys to 1 girl; in community samples, the ratio is approximately 4 boys to 1 girl) seen in ADHD children in the general population noted in DSM-IV (American Psychiatric Association, 1994). This finding is consistent with those of Tizard (1968a, 1968b), who found even closer male:female ratios (1.25:1). These studies suggest that girls with MR may have a higher risk for ADHD than girls in the general population, and it will be important to ascertain any underlying attentional differences between boys and girls with ADHD in order to plan for the most effective intervention for children of both genders.

It will also be interesting to explore why girls with MR appear to have a greater vulnerability to ADHD. Perhaps the greater prevalence of ADHD in girls with MR might have something to do with MR acting as an "environmental adversity," or stressor, that allows for greater vulnerability to an underlying ADHD gene, whereas girls in the general population (i.e., who do not have MR) may also have a gene for ADHD, but one that is dormant (does not get expressed) due to the lack of such stressor (B. L. Handen & M. G. Aman, personal communication, January 12, 1993). This hypothesis is consistent with the genetic segregation studies that have found that the "genetic substrate" for ADHD lies dormant in some children who carry it but that this biological vulnerability is only expressed following exposure to environmental adversity (Faraone et al., 1992, 1993).

Another issue to be addressed is comorbidity of ADHD with other psychiatric diagnoses in children with MR. For instance, children with ADHD in general school-age populations often carry concomitant diagnoses such as oppositional defiant disorder, conduct disorder, and learning disabilities (Barkley, 1990; Keller et al., 1992). There is also an extensive comorbidity between ADHD and major depression (Biederman, Newcorn, & Sprich, 1991; Keller et al., 1992). Although little is known about the comorbidity of ADHD with other psychiatric diagnoses in children with MR, if it is the case that the pattern of comorbidity is similar in this population, then future researchers will need to select homogeneous research populations that are free from the contributing symptomatology of other disorders. This contributing symptomatology could be seriously confounded with the symptoms of ADHD; for example, it has been well documented that depression is associated with significant deficits in problem solving and attention processes (Kaslow, Tanenbaum, Abramson, Peterson, & Seligman, 1983; McGee, Anderson, Williams, & Silva, 1986; Roy-Byrne, Weingartner, Bierer, Thompson, & Post, 1986), deficits that are also associated ADHD.

In conclusion, the investigation of the nature of and treatment for ADHD in MR has only just begun. The challenge for researchers investigating these dual diagnoses will be to address the issues raised here in order to close the significant gap in our understanding of knowledge in this area. A collaborative multicenter approach may prove to be an effective means of exploring these issues in an efficient and cost-effective manner. This approach would facilitate the blending of different areas of professional expertise (e.g., clinical psychology, psychopharmacology, neuropsychology) in order to provide a better perspective of the characteristics of the entire individual carrying the dual diagnoses of ADHD and MR, rather than the current focus on isolated pieces of information that cannot integrate function within the individual. This multicenter approach would also facilitate more powerful examinations of cultural and demographic factors that might interact with the manifestations of these dual diagnoses (e.g., would a child from a Mexican-American background in Texas have different environmental influences than those experienced by a child from an Anglo background in the Midwest, and would these influences impact cognitive style?) Such an approach might serve to considerably enhance our understanding of the nature of ADHD in MR, enabling more effective interventions to be devised for children carrying these dual diagnoses.

REFERENCES

Ackerman, P. T., Dykman, R. A., & Oglesby, D. M. (1983). Sex and group differences in reading and attention disordered children with and without hyperkinesis. *Journal of Learning Disabilities, 16,* 407–415.

Ager, A. (1983). An analysis of learning and attentional processes in mentally handicapped individuals. *International Journal of Rehabilitation Research, 6*(3), 369–370.

Aman, M. G. (1982). Stimulant drug effects in the developmental disorders and hyperactivity: Toward a resolution of disparate findings. *Journal of Autism and Developmental Disorders, 12,* 385–398.

Aman, M. G., Kern, R. A., McGhee, D. E., & Arnold, L. E. (1993a). Fenfluramine and methylphenidate in children with MR and ADHD: Clinical side effects. *Journal of the American Academy of Child and Adolescent Psychiatry, 32,* 851–859.

Aman, M. G., Kern, R. A., McGhee, D. E., & Arnold, L. E. (1993b). Fenfluramine and methylphenidate in children with MR and attention deficit hyperactivity disorder: Laboratory effects. *Journal of Autism and Developmental Disorders, 23,* 491–506.

Aman, M. G., Marks, R. E., Turbott, S. H., Wilsher, C. P., & Merry, S. N. (1991a). Clinical effects of methylphenidate and thioridazine in intellectually subaverage children. *Journal of the American Academy of Child and Adolescent Psychiatry, 30*(2), 246–256.

Aman, M. G., Marks, R. E., Turbott, S. H., Wilsher, C. P., & Merry, S. N. (1991b). Methylphenidate and thioridazine in the treatment of intellectually subaverage children: Effects on cognitive–motor performance. *Journal of the American Academy of Child and Adolescent Psychiatry, 30*(5), 816–824.

American Association on Mental Retardation. (1992). *Mental retardation: Definition, classification, and systems of supports* (9th ed.). Washington, DC: Author.

American Psychiatric Association. (1987). *Diagnostic and statistical manual of mental disorders* (3rd ed., rev.). Washington, DC: Author.

American Psychiatric Association. (1994). *Diagnostic and statistical manual of mental disorders* (4th ed.). Washington, DC: Author.

Ando, H., & Yoshimura, I. (1978). Prevalence of maladaptive behavior in retarded children as a function of IQ and age. *Journal of Abnormal Child Psychology, 6,* 345–349.

Barkley, R. A. (1990). *Attention-deficit hyperactivity disorder: A handbook for diagnosis and treatment.* New York: Guilford Press.

Barkley, R. A. (1991). Diagnosis and assessment of attention deficit–hyperactivity disorder. *Comprehensive Mental Health Care, 1,* 27–43.

Barkley, R. A., DuPaul, G. J., & McMurray, M. D. (1990). Comprehensive evaluation of attention deficit disorder with and without hyperactivity as defined by research criteria. *Journal of Consulting and Clinical Psychology, 58,* 775–789.

Baumeister, A. A., & Ellis, N. R. (1963). Delayed response performance of retardates. *American Journal of Mental Deficiency, 67,* 714–722.

Belmont, J. M., & Ellis, N. R. (1968). Effects of extraneous stimulation upon discrimination learning in normals and retardates. *American Journal of Mental Deficiency, 72,* 525–532.

Berry, C. A., Shaywitz, S. E., & Shaywitz, B. A. (1985). Girls with attention deficit disorder: A silent minority? A report on behavioral and cognitive characteristics. *Pediatrics, 76,* 801–809.

Biederman, J., Newcorn, J. H., & Sprich, S. (1991). Co-morbidity of attention deficit hyperactivity disorder and other major affective disorders. *Archives of General Psychiatry, 48,* 633–642.

Bregman, J. D., Leckman, J. F., & Ort, S. I. (1988). Fragile X syndrome: Genetic predisposition to psychopathology. *Journal of Autism and Developmental Disorders, 18,* 343–354.

Burack, J. A. (1994). Selective attention deficits in persons with autism: Preliminary evidence of an inefficient attentional lens. *Journal of Abnormal Psychology, 103,* 535–543.

Burack, J. A., Hodapp, R. M., & Zigler, E. (1988). Issues in the classification of MR: Differentiating among organic etiologies. *Journal of Child Psychology and Psychiatry, 29,* 765–779.

Burack, J. A., & Zigler, E. (1990). Intentional and incidental memory in organically mentally retarded, familial retarded, and nonretarded individuals. *American Journal on Mental Retardation, 94,* 532–540.

Cairns, E., & Commock, T. (1978). Development of a more reliable version of the Matching Familiar Figures Test. *Developmental Psychology, 14,* 555–560.

Campbell, S. B., Douglas, V. I., & Morgenstern, G. (1971). Cognitive styles in hyperactive children and the effect of methylphenidate. *Journal of Child Psychology and Psychiatry, 12,* 55–67.

Conners, C. K. (1973). Rating scales for use in drug studies in children. *Psychopharmacology Bulletin* (Special Issue: Pharmacotherapy), *126,* 24–28.

Cromwell, R. L., & Foshee, J. G. (1960). Studies in activity level: IV. Effects of visual stimulation during task performance in mental defectives. *American Journal of Mental Deficiency, 65,* 248–251.

Crosby, K. G. (1972). Attention and distractibility in mentally retarded and intellectually average children. *American Journal of Mental Deficiency, 77,* 46–53.

Das, J. P. (1970). Vigilance and verbal conditioning in the mildly and severely retarded. *American Journal of Mental Deficiency, 75,* 253–259.

Das, J. P. (1971). Visual search, stimulus density, and subnormal intelligence. *American Journal of Mental Deficiency, 76,* 357–361.

Das, J. P., & Melnyk, L. (1989). Attention checklist: A rating scale for mildly mentally handicapped adolescents. *Psychological Reports, 64,* 1267–1274.

Douglas, V. I. (1972). Stop, look, and listen: The problem of sustained attention and impulse control in hyperactive and normal children. *Canadian Journal of Behavioral Science, 4,* 259–282.

Douglas, V. I. (1983). Attentional and cognitive problems. In M. Rutter (Ed.), *Developmental neuropsychiatry* (pp. 280–329). New York: Guilford Press.

Draeger, S., Prior, M., & Sanson, A. (1986). Visual and auditory attention performance in hyperactive children: Competence or compliance. *Journal of Abnormal Child Psychology, 14,* 411–424.

Dulaney, C. L., & Ellis, N. R. (1994). Automatized responding and cognitive inertia in individuals with mental retardation. *American Journal on Mental Retardation, 99,* 8–18.

Dykens, E. M., Hodapp, R. M., & Leckman, J. F. (1989). Adaptive and maladaptive functioning of institutionalized and noninstitutionalized Fragile X males. *Journal of the American Academy of Child and Adolescent Psychiatry, 28,* 427–430.

Einfeld, S. L., & Aman, M. G. (1995). Issues in the taxonomy of psychopathology in MR. *Journal of Autism and Developmental Disorders, 25,* 143–167.

Ellis, N. R., Woodley-Zanthos, P., Dulaney, C. L., & Palmer, R. L. (1989). Automatic–effortful processing and cognitive inertia in persons with MR. *American Journal of Mental Retardation, 93,* 412–423.

Epstein, M. H., Cullinan, D., & Gadow, K. D. (1986). Teacher ratings of hyperactivity in learning-disabled, emotionally disturbed, and mentally retarded children. *Journal of Special Education, 22,* 219–229.

Epstein, M. H., Cullinan, D., & Polloway, E. A. (1986). Patterns of maladjustment among mentally retarded children and youth. *American Journal of Mental Deficiency, 91,* 127–134.

Faraone, S. V, Biederman, J., Chen, W. J., Krifcher, B., Keenan, K., Moore, D., Sprich, S., & Tsuang, M. (1992). Segregation analysis of attention deficit hyperactivity disorder: Evidence for a single gene transmission. *Psychiatric Genetics, 2,* 257–275.

Faraone, S. V., Biederman, J., Lehman, B. K., Spencer, T., Norman, D., Seidman, L. J., Kraus, I., Perrin, J., Chen, W. J., & Tsuang, M. T. (1993). Intellectual performance and school failure in children with attention deficit hyperactivity disorder and in their siblings. *Journal of Abnormal Psychology, 102,* 616–623.

Fee, V. E., Matson, J. L., Moore, L. A., & Benavidez, D. A. (1993). The differential validity of hyperactivity/attention deficits and conduct problems among mentally retarded children. *Journal of Abnormal Child Psychology, 21,* 1–11.

Fisher, W., Burd, L., Kuna, D. P., & Berg, D. (1985). Attention deficit disorders and the hyperactivities in multiply disabled children. *Rehabilitation Literature, 46,* 250–254.

Follini, P., Sitkowski, C. A., & Stayton, S. E. (1969). The attention of retardates and normals in distraction and non-distraction conditions. *American Journal of Mental Deficiency, 74,* 200–205.

Foshee, J. G. (1958). Studies in activity level: I. Simple and complex task performance in defectives. *American Journal of Mental Deficiency, 62,* 882–886.

Gardner, W. I., Cromwell, R. L., & Foshee, J. G. (1959). Studies in activity level: II: Effects of distal visual stimulation in organics, familials, hyperactives, and hypoactives. *American Journal of Mental Deficiency, 63,* 1028–1033.

Gath, A., & Gumley, D. (1986). Behavior problems in retarded children with special reference to Down's syndrome. *British Journal of Psychiatry, 149,* 156–161.

Gordon, M. (1979). The assessment of impulsivity and mediating behaviors in hyperactive and nonhyperactive boys. *Journal of Abnormal Child Psychology, 7,* 317–326.

Gordon, M. (1983). *The Gordon Diagnostic System.* Boulder: Clinical Diagnostic Systems.

Gordon, M., & Mettelman, B. B. (1988). The assessment of attention: I. Standardization and reliability of a behavior-based measure. *Journal of Clinical Psychology, 44,* 682–690.

Green, J. M., Dennis, J., Bennets, L. A. (1989). Attention deficit disorder in a group of young Down syndrome children. *Journal of Mental Deficiency Research, 32,* 501–505.

Hagen, J. W., & Hale, G. A. (1973). The development of attention in children. In A. Pick (Ed.), *Minnesota symposia on child development* (Vol. 7, pp. 117–140). Minneapolis: University of Minnesota Press.

Hagen, J. W., & Huntsman, N. J. (1971). Selective attention in mental retardates. *Developmental Psychology, 5,* 151–160.

Handen, B. I., Breaux, A. M., Gosling, A., Ploof, D. L., & Feldman, H. (1990). Efficacy of methylphenidate among mentally retarded children with attention deficit hyperactivity disorder. *Pediatrics, 86,* 922–930.

Handen, B. L., Breaux, A. M., Janosky, J., McAuliffe, S., Feldman, H., & Gosling, A. (1992). Effects and noneffects of methylphenidate in children with MR and ADHD. *Journal of the American Academy of Child and Adolescent Psychiatry, 31*(3), 455–461.

Handen, B. L., Feldman, H., Gosling, A., Breaux, A. M., & McAuliffe, S. (1991). Adverse side effects of methylphenidate among mentally retarded children with ADHD. *Journal of the American Academy of Child and Adolescent Psychiatry, 30*(2), 241–245.

Handen, B. L., McAuliffe, S., Janosky, J., Feldman, H., & Breaux, A. M. (1994). Classroom behavior and children with mental retardation: Comparison of children with and without ADHD. *Journal of Abnormal Child Psychology, 22,* 267–280.

Handen, B. L., McAuliffe, S., Janosky, J., Feldman, H., & Breaux, A. M. (1995). Methylphenidate in children with mental retardation and ADHD: Effects on independent play and academic functioning. *Journal of Developmental and Physical Disabilities, 7,* 91–103.

Holowinsky, I. V., & Farrelly, J. (1988). Intentional and incidental visual memory as a function of cognitive level and color of the stimulus. *Perceptual and Motor Skills, 66,* 775–779.

Hunt, R. D., & Cohen, D. J. (1988). Attentional and neurochemical components of MR: New methods for an old problem. In J. A. Stark, F. J. Menolascino, Albarelli, M. H., & Gray, V. C. (Eds.), *MR and mental health: Classification, diagnosis, treatment, services* (pp. 90–97). New York: Springer-Verlag.

Jones, F. L. (1971). *Vigilance performance of normals and mental retardates: The effects of age and extraneous stimulation.* Unpublished doctoral dissertation, University of Cincinnati, OH.

Kagan, J., Rosman, B. L., Day, D., Albert, J., & Phillips, W. (1964). Information processing in the child: Significance of analytic and reflective attitudes. *Psychological Monographs, 78,* 1–37.

Kahneman, D. (1973). *Attention and effort.* Englewood Cliffs, NJ: Prentice-Hall.

Kaslow, N. J., Tanenbaum, R. L., Abramson, L. Y., Peterson, C., & Seligman, M. (1983). Problem-solving deficits and depressive symptoms among children. *Journal of Abnormal Child Psychology, 11,* 497–501.

Keller, M. B., Lavore, P. W., Beardslee, W. R., Wunder, J., Schwartz, C. E., Roth, J., & Biederman, J. (1992). The disruptive behavioral disorders in children and adolescents: Comorbidity and clinical course. *Journal of the Academy of Child and Adolescent Psychiatry, 31,* 204–209.

Klee, S. H., & Garfinkel, B. D. (1983). The computerized continuous performance task: A new measure of inattention. *Journal of Abnormal Child Psychology, 11,* 487–496.

Krakow, J. B., & Kopp, C. B. (1982). Sustained attention in young Down syndrome children. *Topics in Early Childhood Special Education, 2,* 32–42.

Krakow, J. B., & Kopp, C. B. (1983). The effects of developmental delay on sustained attention in young children. *Child Development, 54,* 1143–1155.

Lane, D. M., & Pearson, D. A. (1982). The development of selective attention. *Merrill–Palmer Quarterly, 28,* 317–337.

Leff, R. M., & Meyer, J. D. (1984). Highly structured social skills training: A group case study. *The Behavior Therapist, 7,* 167–168.

Loveland, K. A. (1987). Behavior of young children with Down syndrome before the mirror: Exploration. *Child Development, 58,* 768–778.

Mackie, R., & Mackay, C. K. (1982). Attention vs. retention in discrimination learning of low-MA retarded adults and MA-matched nonretarded children. *American Journal of Mental Deficiency, 86,* 543–547.

McClure, D. F., & Gordon, M. (1984). Performance of disturbed hyperactive and nonhyperactive children on an objective measure of hyperactivity. *Journal of Abnormal Child Psychology, 12,* 561–572.

McGee, R., Anderson, J., Williams, S., & Silva, P. A. (1986). Cognitive correlates of depressive symptoms in 11-year-old children. *Journal of Abnormal Child Psychology, 14,* 517–524.

Melnyk, L., & Das, J. P. (1992). Measurement of attention deficit: Correspondence between rating scales and tests of sustained and selective attention. *American Journal on MR, 96,* 599–606.

Milich, R., & Kramer, J. (1985). Reflections on impulsivity: An empirical investigation of impulsivity as a construct. In K. Gadow & I. Bialer (Eds.), *Advances in learning and behavioral disabilities* (Vol. 3, pp. 57–94). Greenwich, CT: JAI Press.

Myers, B. A., & Pueschel, S. M. (1991). Psychiatric disorders in persons with Down syndrome. *Journal of Nervous and Mental Disease, 179,* 609–613.

Patterson, B. (1992, November). Attention deficit hyperactivity disorder and Down syndrome. *Down Syndrome News,* 119–120.

Payne, R. (1968). Regional cooperation in MR data collection. *MR, 6,* 52–53.

Pearson, D. A. (1993). Dual diagnosis in children: Attention deficit hyperactivity disorder. *Southwest Quarterly Review, 1,* 1–3.

Pearson, D. A., & Aman, M. G. (1994). Ratings of hyperactivity and developmental indices: Should clinicians correct for developmental level? *Journal of Autism and Developmental Disorders, 24,* 395–411.

Pearson, D. A., & Lane, D. M. (1990). Reorientation in hyperactive and non-hyperactive children: Evidence for developmentally immature attention? In J. T. Enns (Ed.), *The development of attention: Research and theory* (pp. 345–363). Amsterdam: Elsevier.

Pearson, D. A., Yaffee, L. S., Loveland, K. A., & Lewis, K. R. (1996). Sustained and selective attention in children with mental retardation: A comparison of children with and without ADHD. *American Journal on Mental Retardation, 100,* 592–607.

Pelham, W. E. (1981). Attention deficits in hyperactive and learning-disabled children. *Exceptional Education Quarterly, 2,* 13–23.

Pelham, W. E., Walker, J. L., Sturges, J., & Hoza, J. (1989). Comparative effects of methylphenidate on ADD girls and ADD boys. *Journal of the American Academy of Child and Adolescent Psychiatry, 28,* 773–776.

Pueschel, S. M., Bernier, J. C., & Pezzullo, J. C. (1991). Behavioral observations in children with Down's syndrome. *Journal of Mental Deficiency Research, 35,* 502–511.

Power, T. J. (1992). Contextual factors in vigilance testing of children with ADHD. *Journal of Abnormal Child Psychology, 20,* 579–592.

Quay, H. (1977). Measuring dimensions of deviant behavior: The Behavior Problem Checklist. *Journal of Abnormal Child Psychology, 5,* 277–287.

Reiss, S., Levitan, G., & Szyszko, J. (1982). Emotional disturbance and MR: Diagnostic overshadowing. *American Journal of Mental Deficiency, 86,* 567–574.

Reiss, S., & Valenti-Hein, D. (1990). *Reiss Scales for Children's Dual Diagnosis: Test Manual.* Chicago: International Diagnostic Systems.

Ross, D. M., & Ross, S. A. (1982). *Hyperactivity: Current issues, research, and theory* (2nd ed.). New York: Wiley.

Rosvold, H. E., Mirsky, A. F., Sarason, I., Bransome, E. D., & Beck, L. H. (1956). A continuous performance test of brain damage. *Journal of Consulting Psychology, 20,* 343–350.

Rotundo, N., & Johnson, E. G. (1981). Verbal control of motor behaviour in mentally retarded children: A re-examination of Luria's theory. *Journal of Mental Deficiency Research, 25,* 281–290.

Roy-Byrne, P. P., Weingartner, H., Bierer, L. M., Thompson, K., & Post, R. M. (1986). Effortful and automatic cognitive processes in depression. *Archives of General Psychiatry, 43,* 265–267.

Sandberg, S. T., Rutter, M., & Taylor, E. (1978). Hyperkinetic disorder in psychiatric clinic attenders. *Developmental Medicine and Child Neurology, 20,* 279–299.

Schafer, E. W. P., & Peeke, H. V. S. (1982). Down syndrome individuals fail to habituate cortical evoked potentials. *American Journal of Mental Deficiency, 87,* 332–337.

Semmel, M. I. (1965). Arousal theory and vigilance behavior of educable mentally retarded and average children. *American Journal of Mental Deficiency, 70,* 38–47.

Sen, A., & Clarke, A. M. (1968). Some factors affecting distractibility in the mental retardate. *American Journal of Mental Deficiency, 73,* 50–60.

Skinner, B. F. (1938). *The behavior of organisms.* New York: Appleton-Century-Crofts.

Spitz, H. H., & Borland, M. D. (1971). Effects of stimulus complexity on visual search performance of normals and educable retardates. *American Journal of Mental Deficiency, 75,* 724–728.

Spradlin, J. E., Cromwell, R. L., & Foshee, J. G. (1960). Studies in activity level—III: Effects of auditory stimulation in organics, familials, hyperactives and hypoactives. *American Journal of Mental Deficiency, 64,* 754–757.

Strutt, G. F., Anderson, D. R., & Well, A. D. (1975). A developmental study of the effects of irrelevant information on speeded classification. *Journal of Experimental Child Psychology, 20,* 127–135.

Sykes, D. H., Douglas, V. I., & Morgenstern, G. (1973). Sustained attention in hyperactive children. *Journal of Child Psychology and Psychiatry, 14,* 213–220.

Tizard, B. (1968a). Observations of over-active imbecile children in controlled and uncontrolled environments—I: Classroom studies. *American Journal of Mental Deficiency, 72,* 540–547.

Tizard, B. (1968b). Observations of over-active imbecile children in controlled and uncontrolled environments—II: Experimental studies. *American Journal of Mental Deficiency, 72,* 548–553.

Tomporowski, P. D. (1990). Sustained attention in mentally retarded persons. In W. I. Fraser (Ed.), *Key issues in MR research* (pp. 262–269). New York: Routledge.

Tomporowski, P. D., Hayden, A., & Applegate, B. (1990). Effects of background event rate on sustained attention of mentally retarded and nonretarded adults. *American Journal on Mental Retardation, 94,* 499–508.

Turnure, E. (1970). Distractibility in the mentally retarded: Negative evidence for an orienting inadequacy. *Exceptional Children, 37,* 181–186.

Turnure, J., & Zigler, E. (1964). Outer-directedness in the problem solving of normal and retarded children. *Journal of Abnormal and Social Psychology, 69,* 427–436.

Ullman, D. G., & Routh, D. K. (1971). Discriminant learning in mentally retarded and nonretarded children as a function of the number of relevant dimensions. *American Journal of Mental Deficiency, 86,* 560–566.

Ware, J. R., Baker, R. A., & Sipowicz, R. R. (1962). Performance of mental deficients on a simple vigilance task. *American Journal of Mental Deficiency, 66,* 647–650.

Whiteley, J. H., Zaparniuk, J., & Asmundson, G. J. G. (1987). Mentally retarded adolescents' breadth of attention and short-term memory processes during matching-to-sample discriminations. *American Journal of Mental Deficiency, 92,* 207–212.

Zeaman, D., & House, B. J. (1963). The role of attention in retardate discrimination learning. In N. R. Ellis (Ed.), *Handbook of mental deficiency* (pp. 159–223). New York: McGraw-Hill.

Zekulin-Hartley, X. Y. (1982). Selective attention to dichotic input of retarded children. *Cortex, 18,* 311–316.

Zigler, E. (1967). Familial MR: A continuing dilemma. *Science, 155,* 292–298.

A Componential View of Executive Dysfunction in Autism

REVIEW OF RECENT EVIDENCE

Susan E. Bryson
Reginald Landry
J. Ann Wainwright

Despite the tremendous growth in research, autism remains one of the most enigmatic disorders of childhood. The syndrome is defined formally by impairments in socialization, communication, and imagination, and by the presence of repetitive and ritualistic behavior (American Psychiatric Association, 1994; Wing & Gould, 1979). These typically coexist with varying degrees of intellectual impairment but are also found in people of normal or near-normal intelligence (Bryson, Clark, & Smith, 1988; Lotter, 1966). Perhaps most striking is the children's failure to relate to other people. The so-called classic child with autism is aloof, showing little interest in, and even rejecting, the overtures of others. Even in the most capable, described as socially passive or "active-but-odd" (Wing & Attwood, 1987), interactions are stilted and lack reciprocity.

In addition to the social-communicative impairment, autism is distinguished by an impoverished imagination and by a restricted, repetitive, and inflexible repertoire of behaviors. Symbolic play is typically absent, and even functional play is limited in scope and frequency (Sigman & Ungerer, 1984). Rather, children with autism tend to engage in repetitive behaviors such as spinning the wheel of a toy car or being unduly absorbed by timetables or birthdates. Repetitive behaviors are manifested at all levels of functioning: at the motoric level by perseverative and stereotypic movements, at the sensory–perceptual level by a fascination with particular stimuli, and at the cognitive level by recurrent thoughts, the pervasiveness of which suggests a common underlying mechanism (Frith & Frith, 1991).

The behavioral inflexibility of people with autism has received relatively little attention over the past several years. The psychological literature has focused instead on the communicative impairment (both verbal and nonverbal) and more recently on the social and emotional features of autism. One of the most influential views is that a failure in metarepresentation precludes the development of a "theory of mind," that is, the capacity to attribute thoughts, feelings, and desires to oneself and other people (Baron-Cohen, Leslie, & Frith, 1985; Leslie & Frith, 1988). Others have proposed a primary deficit in symbolic thought, which would thus implicate more basic representational processes (Hermelin & O'Connor, 1970; Menyuk & Quill, 1985; Ricks & Wing, 1975). Both of these views provide a cognitive account of autism, although the "metarepresentation-deficit" hypothesis emphasizes the social rather than the cognitive implications for development (i.e., for understanding self and others vs. understanding information generally). Both differ from the position espoused by Hobson (1989), who argues for the primacy of dysfunctional affective systems in autism (also see Kanner, 1943).

These viewpoints are not necessarily mutually exclusive. Indeed, Mundy and Sigman (1989a, 1989b) have argued that both cognitive and affective systems are impaired in autism. Their findings indicate that children with autism fail to attend jointly to others and to objects or events. Behaviors such as pointing or using eye gaze to direct another's attention are notably absent, as is evidence that the children are responsive to the attempts of others to share attention. This deficit in social cognition also appears to involve an affective component (Kasari, Sigman, Mundy, & Yirmiya, 1990; Mundy, 1995). Baron-Cohen (1993) has argued that the capacity for joint attention is a prerequisite to developing a theory of mind. Put simply, we learn about others by attending to their "minds' eyes." We do not debate this, nor do we provide an exhaustive survey of the relevant literature in this chapter (see Bishop, 1993, and Happe, 1994, for recent reviews). Rather, our purpose is to consider the evidence for impairment in basic components of attention, which may contribute to, or even account for, the higher-order cognitive and social features of autism.

To state our biases from the outset, we are not convinced that the core deficit in autism is social, although clearly this aspect of development is profoundly affected. We concur with Hobson (1989) that the emotional nonresponsivity evident early in life is even more primary. On the assumption that attentional systems regulate emotional reactivity (see, e.g.,

Bornstein & Lamb, 1992; Rothbart, Ziaie, & O'Boyle, 1992), we suggest that impairments in attention may impact on the affective as well as the cognitive and social development of children with autism. We also believe that an attentional account is capable of explaining the pervasive behavioral inflexibility, which in our opinion is central to understanding the neuropsychopathology of autism.

We begin by outlining a theoretical framework for conceptualizing attention that assumes an interrelationship between operations governed by executive (anterior) and more basic (posterior) attentional systems. We then critically evaluate current research on attention in autism, including evidence for executive dysfunction, and for impairment in basic components of attention. Interested readers are referred to earlier reviews for a historical perspective on the topic (Bryson, Wainwright-Sharp, & Smith, 1990; Courchesne, 1987; Dawson & Lewy, 1989; Fein, Humes, Kaplan, Lucci, & Waterhouse, 1984; James & Barry, 1980; Kinsbourne, 1987). In this chapter, special consideration is given to behavioral evidence on attention in autism, from which we argue for a primary deficit in basic operations, namely, those subserving visual–spatial attention. We end by emphasizing the profound implications that such a deficit would have on the development of self and other awareness, and by suggesting directions for future research on attention in autism.

EXECUTIVE FUNCTION AND COMPONENTS OF ATTENTION

Attention is conceived currently as a network of interrelated processes that include the properties of selection and control (Allport, 1990; Posner & Dehaene, 1994). These properties of attention are thought to be implemented in networks that are hierarchically organized into two distinct levels and instantiated in different neural areas. Basic attentional processes, referred to by Posner and colleagues as the posterior attentional system (Posner, 1988; Posner & Petersen, 1990), appear to be deployed quickly and automatically to modality-specific stimuli. Central here is visual–spatial attention and the components responsible for moving attention and selecting locations for further processing. Voluntary control over basic attentional processes and recruitment of related systems necessary for goal-directed actions appear, on the other hand, to be governed by higher-order executive functions, also known as the anterior or supervisory attentional system (Shallice, 1988). Conceived as such, the deployment of attention relies on the interrelationship of the two systems. The anterior system provides direction and focus for the operations subserved by the posterior system, but the goals set by the anterior system will not be achieved unless the requisite lower-order attentional operations can be executed efficiently.

The construct of executive function lacks a clear, theoretically driven operational definition. Dennis (1991) notes that advances in the field will depend further on the adoption of a cognitive-developmental perspective. In her framework for differentiating and interrelating functions associated with the frontal lobes, consideration is given to such diverse phenomena as shifting set, assuming an intentional stance, and the capacity for social discourse, problems in virtually all of which have been implicated in autism (Ozonoff, 1995). Dennis convincingly argues that frontal–executive functions all depend on the ability to disengage sufficiently from the external world to allow behavior to be guided by mental representations (e.g., goals or intentions). People with autism have been described as behaviorists; that is, their behavior appears to be determined largely by external physical events (Baron-Cohen, 1989; Menyuk & Quill, 1985). A central question is whether at base the problem is one of poor executive control (including the formation/representation of intentions in the first place) or of compromised lower-order attentional operations that respond automatically to sensory (physical) stimulation. Researchers addressing these and related issues have adopted either a neuropsychological perspective or an information-processing approach.

Adoption of a neuropsychological perspective was motivated largely by the theoretical claims of Damasio and Maurer (1978), who argued for dysfunction in the frontal limbic system in autism. Research to be described has focused on standard neuropsychological measures sensitive to frontal–executive dysfunction, and more recently on understanding the component processes contributing to executive impairment in autism. For this latter purpose, an information processing approach has been adopted. As we shall see, this approach has also been used to examine the integrity of basic, lower-order attentional operations and has contributed to the development of an alternate account of autism, namely the "cerebellar–attentional hypothesis" proposed by Courchesne (1987; Courchesne et al., 1994).

Studies of executive function and related components of attention are summarized in Tables 11.1 and 11.2, respectively. Participants with autism range in age across studies, although they are typically either adolescents or young adults. Unless otherwise specified, all have normal or near normal-measured intelligence, thus minimizing the impact of general cognitive impairment.

Executive Function

In one of the earliest attempts to examine the question of whether measures of frontal–executive function distinguish people with autism, Rumsey

TABLE 10.1. Studies of Executive Function

Author(s)	Autistic sample characteristics			Comparison groups	Tasks	Results
	n (males)	$\bar{x}$ CA (range)	Level of functioning			
Rumsey (1985)	9 (9)	27 yr (18–39)	VIQ = 82–127 PIQ = 86–126	N: 19–36 yr, matched on educational level	WCST	• Groups differed on three scores: categories completed, total errors, percentage of conceptual level responses. • High variability within group with autism. • Conceptual problem solving related to IQ but not to social adaptive functioning.
Schneider & Asarnow (1987)	15 (14)	10.7 yr (N.A.)	VIQ = 80.1 PIQ = 93.7	N: $\bar{x}$ CA = 11.0 yr S: $\bar{x}$ CA = 11.1 yr VIQ = 90.8 PIQ = 92.6	WCST	• No group differences on number correct, categories completed, or ability to maintain set. • Perseverative errors: S > N; A did not differ from either group. • Nonperseverative errors: S > N *N.B.* Four participants with autism, who perseverated on one category throughout, were excluded from the analyses.
Prior & Hoffman (1990)	12 (9)	13.9 yr (10–17)	MA = 8.7–17 yr	N: CA controls: $\bar{x}$ = 13.9 yr MA controls: $\bar{x}$ CA = 11.4 yr $\bar{x}$ MA = 9.8 yr	1) Milner Maze 2) WCST 3) Rey–Osterrieth Complex Figure	1) A group took twice as long to complete; made three times the errors. 2) A made three times the sorting errors; more total and perseverative errors. 3) A showed poorer reproduction. *N.B.* Very high variability, both within and between A participants.

Study	N	CA	IQ	Subject groups	Tasks	Results
Rumsey & Hamburger (1990)	10 (10)	26.4 yr (18–39)	VIQ = 96.4 PIQ = 95.9	N: x̄ CA = 24 yr x̄ VIQ = 108.4 x̄ PIQ = 104.6 D: CA range = 18–28 yr x̄ VIQ = 99.5 x̄ PIQ = 109.5	1) WCST 2) Binet subtests: verbal and picture absurdities; problem situations 3) Word Fluency 4) Fingertip number writing 5) Grooved Pegboard	1) For categories completed: A < D = N. 2) A < D = N. 3) A = D < (30.8 vs. 37.8 vs. 42.1). 4) A = D < N (8.2 vs. 4.0 vs. 1.6). 5) A = D < N (169.8 vs. 143.5 vs. 134.4)
Szatmari, Tuff, Finlayson, & Bartolucci (1990)	17 (17)	14 yr (8–18)	x̄ FSIQ = 82.2	Children with peer problems, ADHD, or conduct disorder: x̄ CA = 14 yr x̄ FSIQ = 101.5	1) WSCT 2) Grooved Pegboard	1) After matching on IQ, no group differences on categories completed, percentage of perseverative errors, or total errors. 2) A performed significantly worse than clinical comparison group.
Ozonoff, Pennington, & Rogers (1991)	23 (21)	12.1 yr (8–21)	VIQ = 82.9 PIQ = 98.3	Mixed group of dyslexia, ADHD, mild mental retardation: x̄ CA = 12.39 yr x̄ VIQ = 87.6 x̄ PIQ = 97.0	1) WCST 2) Tower of Hanoi	1) Three times more perseverative responses than clinical comparison group; A better at maintaining set; no group differences on categories completed or total errors. 2) A less efficient than clinical comparison group. Performance on executive function tasks highly correlated with IQ for group with autism alone.

(cont.)

237

TABLE 10.1. (*continued*)

Author(s)	Autistic sample characteristics			Comparison groups	Tasks	Results
	n (males)	$\bar{x}$ CA (range)	Level of functioning			
McEvoy, Rogers, & Pennington (1993)	17 (10)	60.6 mo (40–80)	High functioning (IQ equivalents not provided)	Developmental delay: matched on nonverbal mental age. N: matched on verbal mental age	1) Piagetian AB error 2) Delayed response 3) Spatial reversal 4) Alternation	1) No group differences (ceiling effect). 2) No group differences (ceiling effect). 3) A significantly more perseverative errors. 4) No group differences (floor effect).
Ozonoff, Strayer, McMahon, & Filloux (1994)	14 (13)	12.4 yr (8–16)	$\bar{x}$ VIQ = 95.9 $\bar{x}$ PIQ = 108.4 $\bar{x}$ FSIQ = 101.9	TS: $\bar{x}$ CA = 12.9 yr $\bar{x}$ VIQ = 100.8 $\bar{x}$ PIQ = 98.9 $\bar{x}$ FSIQ = 99.9 N: $\bar{x}$ CA = 12.2 yr $\bar{x}$ VIQ = 102.4 $\bar{x}$ PIQ = 97.9 $\bar{x}$ FSIQ = 100.4	1) Go/no-go (three conditions) a) Neural inhibition b) Prepotent inhibition c) Flexibility 2) Global/local	1) a) No RT differences across group b) RT: A > TS = N. c) RT: A > TS = N. A more false alarm than TS or N A: False-alarm RTs < Hit RTs 2) No group differences.
Ozonoff & McEvoy (1994)	Time 1: 23 (21) Time 2 17 (15)	12.1 yr (SD = 3.2) 15.5 yr (SD = 3.2)	$\bar{x}$ VIQ = 82.9 $\bar{x}$ PIQ = 98.4 $\bar{x}$ FSIQ = 89.5 $\bar{x}$ VIQ = 83.0 $\bar{x}$ PIQ = 97.6 $\bar{x}$ FSIQ = 89.1	LD: $\bar{x}$ CA = 12.4 yr $\bar{x}$ VIQ = 87.6 $\bar{x}$ PIQ = 97.0 $\bar{x}$ FSIQ = 91.3 $\bar{x}$ CA = 14.7 yr $\bar{x}$ VIQ = 91.8 $\bar{x}$ PIQ = 100.6 $\bar{x}$ FSIQ = 95.6	1) WCST 2) Tower of Hanoi Each administered twice, separated by 3 yr	1) LD > A at Time 2. • A: Time 1 = Time 2; LD: Time 2 > Time 1 • 6/17 A improved, 7/17 came within 2 SD's of age norms. 2) LD > A at Time 2. • A: Time 1 = Time 2; LD: Time 2 > Time 1. • 1/17 A improved, 0/17 came within 2 SD's of age norms.

Study	N	CA	IQ/MA (clinical)	Comparison group	Task	Findings
Hughes & Russell (1993)	40	12.8 yr (6–19)	$\bar{x}$ VMA = 6.6 yr	Mentally handicapped: $\bar{x}$ CA = 10.8 yr $\bar{x}$ MA = 6.2 yr / Normal MA: $\bar{x}$ CA = 3.8 yr	Detour Reaching Task: required learning of two different (detour) responses	• A failed to reach criterion significantly more often than clinical comparison group. • A made three types of errors significantly more often: goal-directed perseverations, response perseverations, and failure to capitalize on a correct response.
Hughes, Russell & Robbins (1994)	Exp. 1: 35 (27)	12.9 yr (7–18)	$\bar{x}$ VMA = 7.21 yr $\bar{x}$ NVMA = 8.2 yr	MLD: $\bar{x}$ CA = 13.3 yr $\bar{x}$ VMA = 7.3 yr / Normal MA: $\bar{x}$ CA = 8.1 yr	1) ID/ED: learning and transfer with increasing complexity 2) Tower of London planning task: simplified Tower of Hanoi	1) Discrimination learning, rule reversal, and set maintenance: N > MLD = A. • Set shift across dimensions (ED): A < MLD < N. 2) A performed less efficiently than clinical comparison group when planning involved (four to five moves).
	Exp. 2: 30 (24)	13.2 yr (8–19)	$\bar{x}$ VMA = 7.8 yr $\bar{x}$ NVMA = 8.7 yr	MLD: $\bar{x}$ CA = 13.6 yr $\bar{x}$ VMA = 7.4 yr / Normal MA: $\bar{x}$ CA = 8.0 yr		
Ozonoff & Strayer (in press)	13 (13)	13.9 yr	$\bar{x}$ VIQ = 98.6 $\bar{x}$ PIQ = 103.7 $\bar{x}$ FSIQ = 101	N: $\bar{x}$ CA = 13.1 yr $\bar{x}$ VIQ = 101.6 $\bar{x}$ PIQ = 98.2 $\bar{x}$ FSIQ = 101.1	1) Negative priming: response to previously inhibited stimulus/location required 2) Stop-signal: inhibition of response required	1) No group differences. 2) No group differences.

Note. A, autistic; N, normal; S, schizophrenic; D, dyslexic; LD, learning disabilities; MLD, moderate learning disabled; ADHD, attention-deficit/hyperactivity disorder; TS, Tourette syndrome; CA, chronological age; MA, mental age; VIQ, Verbal IQ; PIQ, Performance IQ; FSIQ, Full Scale IQ; VMA, verbal mental age; NVMA, nonverbal mental age; WCST, Wisconsin Card Sort Test; ID/ED, intradimensional/extradimensional shift-task; RT, response time.

TABLE 10.2. Studies of Basic Attentional Processes

Author(s)	Autistic sample characteristics			Comparison groups	Tasks	Results
	n (males)	$\bar{x}$ CA (range)	Level of functioning			
Ciesielski, Courchesne, & Elmasian (1990)	10 (10)	21.4 yr (18–31)	$\bar{x}$ VIQ = 83 $\bar{x}$ PIQ = 99	N: CA range = 7–26 yr $\bar{x}$ VIQ = 109 $\bar{x}$ PIQ = 107	Trained in divided attention (attention to both modalities); examined on performance on focused attention (attention to one of two modalities)	• Hits: A < in auditory; no difference in visual modality. • False alarms: A > N in both modalities, especially in visual. • RT: N < A in both auditory and visual.
Ciesielski, Courchesne, Akshoomoff, & Elmasian (1990)		Same as above		Same as above	Divided attention and focused attention tasks	No difference between performance on divided versus focused attention tasks, and this pattern did not differ between groups. NC component, which distinguished performance between tasks, was greatly attenuated in A.
Courchesne, Akshoomoff, & Ciesielski (1990)	12 (12)	24.9 yr (17–39)	$\bar{x}$ VIQ = 87.8 $\bar{x}$ PIQ = 93.8 $\bar{x}$ FSIQ = 90.1	N: n = 11 $\bar{x}$ CA = 19.3 $\bar{x}$ VIQ = 108.5 $\bar{x}$ PIQ = 108 $\bar{x}$ FSIQ = 109.8	1) Focused auditory and visual attention tasks 2) Shift attention tasks: alternate attended modality upon detection of rare target	1) No group differences. 2) A made fewer hits, especially at short interstimulate interval, and significantly more false alarms. P700 distinguished performance on two tasks, and was greatly attenuated in A.

240

Study	N (n)	Age / IQ (autistic)	Matched / Control group	Task	Results
Courchesne et al. (1991)	13 (11)	Children: 13.9 yr $(SD = 1.6)$ Adults: 28.8 yr $(SD = 4.1)$	$\bar{x}$ VIQ = 59 $\bar{x}$ PIQ = 89 $\bar{x}$ VIQ = 82 $\bar{x}$ PIQ = 95	N: Matched on sex, age, and performance on selected PIQ subtests of WISC-R. C: $\bar{x}$ CA = 8.6 yr $\bar{x}$ VIQ = 97 $\bar{x}$ PIQ = 96	See Courchesne, Akshoomoff, & Ciesielski (1990)	1) No accuracy differences among groups. 2) When less that 2.5 sec between targets: Hits: A = C < N False alarms: A > C = N Overall RT: C > N = A
Wainwright-Sharp & Bryson (in press)	Exp. 1&3 11 (11)	25.0 yr (18–31) $\bar{x}$ PPVT-R raw score = 124	CA normal: $\bar{x}$ CA = 23.6 yr $\bar{x}$ PPVT-R raw score = 159 MA normal: $\bar{x}$ CA = 11.9 yr $\bar{x}$ PPVT-R raw score = 122.5	1) Simple detection with lateral targets only 2) Simple detection with lateral and cetral targets 3) Go/no-go with lateral and central targets	1) For both A and CA normals, LVF < RVF; no laterality effect for MA normals. 2) CA normals: LVF < RVF < Central; MA normals and autistic: LVF = RVF = Central. 3) CA and MA normals: LVF = RVF = Central; A: Central < LVF = RVF, and no relationship with IQ.
	Exp. 2 11 (11)	20.4 yr (13–27) $\bar{x}$ PPVT-R raw score = 138.3	CA normal: $\bar{x}$ CA = 20.6 yr $\bar{x}$ PPVT-R raw score = 163.5 MA normal: $\bar{x}$ CA = 14.3 yr $\bar{x}$ PPVT-R raw score = 135.8		
Wainwright-Sharp & Bryson (1993)	11 (11)	20.4 yr (13–27) $\bar{x}$ PPVT-R = 89 $\bar{x}$ Raven's = 48.6	N: $\bar{x}$ CA = 20.6 yr $\bar{x}$ PPVT-R = 117 $\bar{x}$ Raven's = 94.9	Spatial orienting with central cues	• N overall RT advantage accounted for by IQ. • After covarying IQ, A had no validity effect at 100 msec; at 800 msec validity effect significantly larger than normal; effect of invalid cue especially detrimental in LVF.

(cont.)

TABLE 10.2. (continued)

| | Autistic sample characteristics | | | | | |
Author(s)	n (males)	$\bar{x}$ CA (range)	Level of functioning	Comparison groups	Tasks	Results
Casey, Gordon, Mannheim, & Rumsey (1993)	10 (10)	29.2 yr (19–41)	$\bar{x}$ FSIQ = 82 (65–107)	N: $\bar{x}$ CA = 29.6 yr $\bar{x}$ FSIQ = 124 (97–148)	1) CPT 2) Divided attention 3) Visual discrimination 4) Spatial orienting with peripheral cues	1) Hits: A < N in visual; A = N in auditory; False alarms: A > N in auditory; A = N in visual. 2) Hits: A < N in both modalities. False alarms: A = N in both modalities. 3) RT: A > N; accuracy: A = N. 4) RT: A > N. Larger validity effect overall for A. Longer LVF invalid RT at 100 msec for A.
Garretson, Fein, & Waterhouse (1990)	23	12.4 yr (4–19)	$\bar{x}$ PPVT = 5.8 yr $\bar{x}$ NVMA = 6.0 yr	Two groups, one matched on PPVT-R, one matched on Draw-a-Design Test scores	CPT, varying rate of presentation (slow and fast), and type of reinforcement (tangible and social)	• Hit rate was significantly reduced for groups with autism relative to comparison groups, during second block of slow presentation, and only with social (vs. tangible) reinforcements. • MA was a strong predictor of performance.
Townsend, Courchesne, & Egaas (1992)	10 (9)	APA: 26 ± 7 yr APN: 29 ± 12 yr	$\bar{x}$ VIQ = 82 $\bar{x}$ PIQ = 88 $\bar{x}$ VIQ = 98 $\bar{x}$ PIQ = 105	N: CA = 22 ± 5 yr $\bar{x}$ VIQ = 102 $\bar{x}$ PIQ = 109	Spatial orienting with peripheral cues	• Valid RT at 100 msec: APA = APN > N; no difference at 800 msec. • Validity effect (invalid RT – valid RT): APA > APN = N. • Validity effect larger at 800 than at 100 msec. for APA alone.

Study		N	Age		Task	Results
Townsend & Courchesne (1994)	See Townsend, Courchesne, & Egaas (1992)			$\bar{x}$ MA = 8.35 yr $\bar{x}$ IQ = 49.5	Focused spatial attention: five potential target locations across meridian, one of which was cued for duration of block, with 25% target probability	RT to correctly detected targets: APA < N < APN; no difference in accuracy of false alarms. Enhanced processing at cued location (APA); ungraded distribution of attention (APN).
Burack (1994)		12 (10)	20.5 yr	Organic MR: $\bar{x}$ CA = 15.3 yr $\bar{x}$ MA = 8.2 yr $\bar{x}$ IQ = 56.4 Familial MR: $\bar{x}$ CA = 12.1 yr $\bar{x}$ MA = 7.8 yr $\bar{x}$ IQ = 65.5 N: $\bar{x}$ CA = 8.2 yr $\bar{x}$ MA = 8.4 yr $\bar{x}$ IQ = 103.7	Forced choice: detect one of two potential targets in central location of screen (three conditions) a) window placed in center of screen b) distractors c) distractor either inside or outside of window	• When there were no distractors, the window most improved RTs of the A group. • A did not benefit from the presence of window when distractors were present (slower RTs than the other groups). • No RT differences between the groups in the no-window condition.

Note. C, cerebellar; MR, mental retardation; APA, autistic parietal abnormal ($n = 6$); APN, autistic parietal normal ($n = 4$); WISC-R, Wechsler Intelligence Scale for Children—Revised; PPVT-R, Peabody Picture Vocabulary Test—Revised; CFT, Continuous Performance Test; LVF, left visual field; RVF, right visual field; NC, an endogenous, frontally distributed negative component; all other abbreviations as in Table 10.1.

243

(1985) employed the widely used Wisconsin Card Sort Test (WCST) (also see the case study reported by Steel, Gorman, & Flexman, 1984). This test requires that cards be sorted according to a rule (color, form, or number) that is discovered through feedback and that changes once ten consecutive correct responses are achieved. After covarying differences in IQ, three of 10 WCST measures were found to differentiate men with autism from a matched, normal comparison group. The adults with autism sorted to fewer categories, made more errors, many of which were perseverative, and were less likely to sort according to a rule (percentage of conceptual-level responses). Considerable variability existed within the autistic group (one-third performed normally), and none of the WCST measures were related to degree of impairment in social adaptation; most were highly correlated with IQ. Rumsey argued for a conceptual problem-solving deficit, thus favoring a higher-order cognitive account of the problem in autism.

Subsequent research has generally replicated Rumsey's (1985) initial findings, although poor performance on the WCST appears to distinguish people with autism from some but not all developmentally matched clinical comparison groups (Ozonoff & McEvoy, 1994; Prior & Hoffman, 1990; Schneider & Asarnow, 1987; Szatmari, Tuff, Finlayson, & Bartolucci, 1990). The most striking finding is the preponderance of perseverative responses in autism and, if anything, superior maintenance of set, which has since been attributed to cognitive inflexibility (i.e., difficulties in shifting cognitive set; Ozonoff, Pennington, & Rogers, 1991). Other frontal–executive measures have also been shown to differentiate people with autism from both well-matched normal and (nonautistic) clinical groups. Notable among these is the Tower of Hanoi (TOH; for others, see Prior & Hoffman, 1990; Rumsey & Hamburger, 1988, 1990; and Szatmari et al., 1990). In the TOH, disks are distributed across three vertical pegs and participants are required to build towers of increasing complexity on one of the three pegs. A sequence of movements needs to be planned and executed, with the constraint that a larger disk cannot be placed on a smaller one. The relatively inefficient performance of children with autism on the TOH has been attributed to poor planning and associated working memory (Ozonoff et al., 1991; Ozonoff & McEvoy, 1994). Such complex tasks clearly depend, however, on the integrity of multiple operations, dysfunction in any number of which may be distinctive of autism.

In an early attempt to identify components of executive dysfunction in autism, Hughes and Russell (1993) explored the possibility that the problem is one of mentally disengaging from a salient stimulus (see Experiment 2). Performance of a less capable group of persons with autism (see Table 10.1) was examined on a task requiring retrieval of a marble that rested on a platform inside a box. Direct reaches were possible but were not reinforced; participants had to first learn to turn a knob that invariably released the marble (knob route), and once a criterion was achieved they were taught to release a spatially distinct switch and to reach in to get the marble (switch route). Relative to both developmentally matched mentally handicapped and normal children, the persons with autism were less likely to reach criterion with the switch route. Autistic children were significantly more likely to perseverate, either on direct reaches or on the knob route response, and a significant proportion (42.5%) actually made one correct switch–reach response — but failed to do so again. Although interpretation of the findings is complicated by the added complexity of the switch route (which required two distinct acts, and the causal link between action and retrieval was less direct than in the knob route), Hughes and Russell (1993) argued that the pattern of findings suggests something other than simple "stuck-in-set" perseveration (i.e., a failure to change behavior) or a simple "disengage-from-the-object" hypothesis. The children with autism could disengage sufficiently to learn the knob route with relative ease. Many also executed one correct switch–reach response, suggesting that they could shift set but had difficulty overriding the pull to act otherwise.

In a subsequent study, Hughes, Russell, and Robbins (1994) compared somewhat higher-functioning matched groups of persons with autims, mental retardation, and typical development on the intradimensional/extradimensional shift (ID/ED) task and the Tower of London, a simplified version of the TOH. The Tower of London requires the planning and execution of moves aimed at reordering three different colored balls to match the order presented in a model. The balls are placed such that all moves must be made from the top ball (i.e., a ball cannot be moved that is under another ball), and the moves required vary in complexity (one to five steps). The ID/ED shift task, which is comparable to the WCS, is presented in nine stages, each conditional on previous stages. The first consists of a simple discrimination between two pink forms; in the second the contingencies are reversed. From this stage on, two white line patterns are pseudorandomly paired with the two pink forms and first appear adjacent to the pink forms. The white lines are then superimposed on the pink forms, and this discrimination is reversed. In the next — ID shift — stages, transfer of learning is assessed by requiring discrimination of two new pink forms and by reversing the discrimination. In the final and most difficult — ED shift — stages, transfer involves a shift to discriminating the white lines, which previously were reinforced only randomly.

On the Tower of London, the group with autism were significantly less efficient than either comparison group on the problems involving planning (four or five steps). On the ID/ED shift task, both clinical groups had more difficulty than the normal group in the five pretransfer conditions, suggesting that the easier tasks of discrimination learning, rule reversal, and maintenance of set do not distinguish autism. The children with autism differed from the matched mentally handicapped group on both trials and errors to criterion only when the task required a shift across stimulus dimensions (i.e., discrimination of white lines vs. pink forms). These results, coupled with the failure to find a relationship between performance on the two executive tasks (also see Ozonoff & McEvoy, 1994), were taken as evidence for distinct, dissociable autism-specific deficits in planning and in attentional-set shifting (Hughes et al., 1994). Note, however, that planning depends on the ability to shift set, and the failure to find a relationship between performance on the two tasks may reflect a lack of performance variability.

In the one study of young children with autism, related issues were explored using tasks designed originally for nonhuman primates (McEvoy, Rogers, & Pennington, 1993). The first and easiest (Piagetian AB error) task required that the child find a reward hidden under one of two cups, the location of which was changed with each correct response. The second (delayed response) task was the same, with the addition of a 6-second response delay. In the third (spatial reversal) task, the reward was hidden behind a screen, which was immediately raised so the child could search; the side of hiding was reversed once a criterion of four consecutive correct responses was achieved. The fourth (alternation) task was the same as the spatial reversal task, except that the hiding place was alternated with each correct response. Relative to both well-matched developmentally disabled and normal children, the group with autism had difficulty on the spatial reversal task, performance on which was correlated with measures of joint attention and social-interactive behaviors (e.g., turn taking). Children with autism were able to establish and maintain a response set but made significantly more perseverative errors and failed to shift spatial location as required. Ceiling effects on the first two tasks and floor effects on the fourth task render the otherwise null group effects uninterpretable. Nonetheless, findings for the spatial reversal task indicate that young children with autism have difficulty shifting spatial location, even when the object/dimension to be discriminated remains constant (cf. Hughes et al., 1994). The significance of such findings is underscored by the fact that most executive function tasks require, among other things, shifts in spatial location.

Ozonoff, Strayer, McMahon, and Filloux (1994) examined components of executive dysfunction using a modified version of the classic go/no-go task. Trials were blocked in an attempt to examine responses to one of two previously neutral stimuli (neutral inhibition): the ability to inhibit a previously reinforced response (prepotent inhibition), and the ability to frequently shift responses from one to the other stimulus (cognitive flexibility). Performance of children/adolescents with autism was compared to that of a normal group and a group with Tourette syndrome, each matched for age, gender, and IQ. No group differences were found on the neutral inhibition condition, but responses of the children with autism were slower than those of the comparison groups (who did not differ) on both the prepotent inhibition and cognitive flexibility conditions. The group with autism also made more false-alarm errors when the task required alternate responses (frequent shifts between the two target stimuli). Poor performance on this latter, more difficult task was taken as evidence for a deficit in cognitive flexibility, although it remains possible that dysfunctional inhibitory (attentional) mechanisms contribute to the difficulties in shifting set (as prepotent inhibition condition also yielded group differences).

Only two studies have examined inhibition more directly. Ozonoff and Strayer (in press) compared matched groups of autistic and nonautistic adolescents on two tasks. In the first (stop–signal), participants were asked to categorize words as animals or nonanimals and an auditory signal cued them to inhibit responses on a random subset of trials. In the second (negative priming) task, participants saw a series of five-letter strings and were asked whether the second and fourth letters were the same or different. The critical manipulation was whether or not target (second and fourth) letters were the same as distractor (first, third, and fifth) letters on the immediately preceding trial, in which case the decrement in performance is attributed to inhibition associated with previously ignored (nontarget) stimuli (Tipper, 1985). A careful analysis of both the response time (RT) and accuracy data yielded null group effects on all measures. Bryson and Tipper (1997; Bryson, 1995) also failed to find group differences for negative priming, but adults with autism did have more difficulty than a matched normal group on a task requiring response inhibition (vs. inhibition associated with a previously ignored stimulus, as in negative priming). Evidence of enhanced inhibition (longer RTs) in autism obtained only when the response required was in the same spatial location as that which was previously inhibited. These preliminary findings implicate dysfunctional inhibition in the difficulties shifting set, the measurement of which typically involves shifts in spatial location. Note further that such shifts may include the space traversed either externally or internally (i.e., as required in categorical shifts, when shifting, for example, occurs across stimulus dimensions).

Summary and Comments

Studies using traditional neuropsychological tests have typically found that individuals with autism fare poorly on measures of executive–frontal lobe function. While evidence for executive impairment in autism is compelling, it bears emphasizing that several clinical groups perform poorly on executive measures (see, e.g., Chelune, Ferguson, Koon, & Dickey, 1986). Findings suggest that the components of executive dysfunction that distinguish autism from other developmental disorders are planning and shifting set. Planning clearly presupposes the ability to shift set, problems with which may vary with development. Adolescents/young adults with autism appear to be selectively impaired in shifting across (vs. within) stimulus dimensions; in young autistic children the problem is apparent even when the stimulus remains constant and only spatial shifts are required. Possible differences in findings at different age levels underscore the importance of a developmental perspective in studies of autism.

Ozonoff et al. (1991) emphasize cognitive inflexibility in understanding the shift problem in autism. In contrast, Hughes et al. (1994) favor an attentional account. The latter appears more consistent with evidence of enhanced response inhibition in autism and of superior maintenance of set. We now turn to research that has examined more basic operations, which are known to be subserved by posterior attentional systems.

Basic Components of Attention

Evidence to be reviewed below converges to suggest that in autism there is a selective deficit in rapidly and accurately shifting attention. In one set of experiments, Courchesne and colleagues examined both behavioral and electrophysiological responses in tasks designed to isolate different components of attention. Both auditory stimuli (1- and 2-kilohertz tones) and visual stimuli (red and green squares) were intermixed and presented in sequence, one at a time. One of the two stimuli in each modality occurred infrequently (25% of trials), and responses were required only to the infrequent stimuli. In one version of this task (Ciesielski, Courchesne, & Elmasian, 1990), participants were trained to respond to infrequent stimuli in both modalities (divided attention); once a criterion was reached, they were required to respond only to one modality while ignoring the other (selective attention tasks). Relative to a matched normal group, adults with autism had a significantly elevated false alarm rate, evident in both tasks, but particularly marked in the selective visual task. They erred specifically by responding to infrequent stimuli in the to-be-ignored modality. The group with autism also had significantly fewer correct detections (hits) in the selective auditory task, and their RTs tended to be longer in both selective attention tasks. Markedly attenuated event-related potentials (ERPs) in the frontal and parietal areas of the autistic adults suggested further that, despite adequate task performance, stimulus selection is abnormal both between and within modalities (for a detailed description of ERP findings, see Ciesielski, Courchesne, & Elmasian, 1990).

In a related report (Ciesielski, Courchesne, Akshoomoff, & Elmasian, 1990), performance on the selective/focused attention tasks was compared to that on the divided attention task used in the training phase described above (responses required to infrequent stimuli in both vs. one modality). Performance (percentage of target hits and RT) did not differ between tasks, and there were no significant interactions involving the group. Again, all frontal and to a lesser extent parietal ERP components were reduced in the autistic group. Among the several tested, (NC) was the only component that reliably distinguished performance in the divided and focused attention tasks, and this nonspecific modality effect was absent in the young adults with autism, again despite adequate task performance. This apparent insensitivity to the differential attentional demands across tasks was taken as evidence of all-or-none rather than selective neural responsivity in autism.

A variant of the same task was used to examine attentional shifts across modalities in matched autistic and normal groups and a group with acquired neocerebellar lesions (Courchesne, Akshoomoff, & Ciesielski, 1990; Courchesne et al., 1991; also reviewed in Courchesne et al., 1994). Presence of an infrequent target in one modality served as a cue to alternate attention and respond to the previously ignored modality. The two focused (auditory and visual) attention tasks served as controls; task requirements were the same, except that attentional shifts were not required. The main finding was the significant decrement in performance, evident in both the groups with autism and neocerebellar groups, when required to rapidly switch back and forth between the two modalities (i.e., with less than 2.5 seconds between targets). Both groups performed significantly more poorly than the normal groups in the shift task but not in the focused attention tasks (see also Akshoomoff & Courchesne, 1992, for related findings in neocerebellar vs. cortical lesion groups). A high false-alarm rate (responses to stimuli in the to-be-ignored modality) distinguished the persons with autism from both the neocerebellar and normal groups. Consistent with the behavioral evidence, a parietal ERP response peaking at about 700 milliseconds following the cue to shift attention was evident in the normal group but greatly diminished or absent in the autistic and neocerebellar groups. The pattern of findings, coupled with magnetic resonance imaging data specifically implicating cerebellar (particularly neocerebellar) abnormalities in autism (Courchesne, Yeung-Courchesne, Press, Hesselink, & Jernigan, 1988; Courchesne et al., 1994), was taken as evidence of a time-related, cerebellar-mediated deficit in shifting attention.

Subsequent research has explored related components of attention within the visual modality, using a standard visual laterality paradigm (Wainwright-Sharp & Bryson, in press). In Experiment 1, participants were asked to fixate a central point and respond to a simple stimulus (+s) projected either to the left or right of fixation. Performance of relatively high-functioning adults with autism was compared to that of two normal comparison groups, one matched for chronological age (CA) and the other for mental age (MA). The younger normal MA controls failed to show a laterality effect, and their overall RT resembled that of the group with autism, both of which RTs exceeded those of the normal CA controls. Nonetheless, the autistic group, like the CA controls, showed the well-documented left-field advantage for orienting in visual space, suggesting that their visual orienting is lateralized to the right hemisphere.

Two additional experiments were the same except that single target stimuli appeared at, as well as to the left or right of, central fixation (Wainwright-Sharp & Bryson, in press). Experiment 2 required simple detection (as above); Experiment 3 required responses to one of two simple stimuli (identification vs. detection alone). Unlike both normal groups, the adults with autism responded faster to central than to lateral stimuli, an effect that was not related to IQ and was significant only when the task required identification. Specifically, presence of the central stimuli (at fixation) served to attenuate responses to either side in the group with autism but not in the two normal groups. This difficulty in rapidly allocating visual–spatial attention is consistent with evidence of overfocused attention in autism (Rincover & Ducharme, 1987) and of deficits in attentional shifts (e.g., Ciesielski et al., 1990).

Wainwright-Sharp and Bryson (1993) pursued these findings further, using Posner's visual orienting paradigm in which participants fixate a central point and the lateral location of single stimuli is precued, either validly or invalidly. Centrally positioned arrows cued the location of target stimuli, and on 20% of trials attention was invalidly cued to the opposite side, thus requiring a shift across the visual field to the actual target location. Target detection was compared in young adults with autism and a CA-matched normal group; IQ was covaried to control for group differences in general ability level (which eliminated the overall group RT difference alone). The data for the normal group replicate those reported earlier (e.g., Posner & Petersen, 1980); validly cued targets were detected faster than invalidly cued targets (which is referred to as the "validity effect"), and the size of the effect did not vary with the delay between cue and target. In contrast, the group with autism showed no validity effect at 100-millisecond cue–target delays, suggesting that with short delays they had insufficient time to shift attention to the invalidly cued location. With delays of 800 milliseconds, the group with autism had a larger than normal validity effect, which was nonsignificantly greater for left visual field–right hemisphere (LVF-RH) stimulus presentations (attention was miscued to the right side, thus requiring a shift to the left).

Similar findings have been reported by Casey, Gordon, Mannheim, and Rumsey (1993), who examined several components of attention in savant adults with autism. Comparisons with a CA-matched normal group alone, who had considerably higher IQs than the group with autism, limit interpretation of the data. Nonetheless, the savant group with autism performed relatively well on measures of focused and sustained attention, thus replicating the earlier findings of Garretson, Fein, and Waterhouse (1990). On a task requiring discrimination of different stimulus attributes (form and color), RTs were longer for the group with autism, but the percentage of RT change did not differ between groups when the task required a shift in set (stimulus attributes were intermixed) versus a shift in target location alone (stimulus attributes were blocked). This null group effect, coupled with essentially perfect accuracy in both groups, suggested that the increased RTs of the group with autism reflected the time taken to shift spatial location and not stimulus attribute. Finally, on Posner's visual orienting task, using peripheral cues (appearing at target locations), the savant–autistic group had abnormally large validity effects at 100(vs. 800)-millisecond cue–target delays, which reached significance only for LVF-RH presentations (but see Burack & Iarocci, 1995, for a failure to replicate). Parallel asymmetries have been reported for patients with acquired visuospatial neglect (e.g., Peterson, Robinson, & Currie, 1989), which is typically, although not exclusively, associated with right parietal lesions (Posner, 1988). The findings of Casey et al. (1993) extend those of Wainwright-Sharp and Bryson (1993) by showing that in autism the disengage–shift problem is evident with peripheral as well as central cues, thus implicating more automatic (vs. controlled) shifts of attention (Jonides, 1981).

Related research has shown that subgroups with autism are deficient in the disengage and/or shift subcomponents of visual–spatial attention (Townsend, Courchesne, & Egaas, 1992). In a task similar to that just described, using peripheral cues, data were analyzed separately for visual orienting (RTs to validly cued targets) and for validity effects (RT difference for invalidly cued targets). High-functioning autistic adults, all with magnetic resonance imaging evidence of cerebellar abnormalities, were subgrouped into those with and without additional bilateral parietal abnormalities. Relative to CA-matched normals, both groups with autism took abnormally long to orient visual attention to validly cued targets at 100- but not at 800-millisecond cue–target delays. Abnormally long RTs to invalidly cued targets were found only in the subgroup with autism and parietal (plus cerebellar) abnormalities and were related to the degree of parietal involvement. Townsend et al. (1992) concluded that this subgroup is deficient in disengaging visual attention once it is focused and that deficits in rapidly orienting and shifting attention are characteristic of the entire population of persons with autism.

Townsend and Courchesne (1994) have since explored the nature of the disengage problem in autism. The question of whether attention is disproportionately allocated to attended relative to unattended locations was examined in a task requiring detection of a stimulus appearing in one of five laterally positioned boxes, which was primed. Once again, adults with autism and with and without parietal (in addition to cerebellar) abnormalities were compared to a CA-matched normal group. Overall accuracy did not distinguish the groups, but the subgroup with autism and parietal abnormalities had the fastest RTs to the primed target location. Evidence for enhanced attention to attended (vs. unattended) locations in this subgroup also came from ERP data, notably larger than normal P1 attention effects combined with shorter-latency P3b components to target stimuli. The findings were taken as evidence of a narrow "attention spotlight" and concurrent enhancement of the loci of focus in the subgroup with autism and parietal–cerebellar abnormalities (cf. earlier claims of overfocused attention or "tunnel vision" in autism; Lovaas, Schreibman, Koegel, & Rehm, 1971; Rincover & Ducharme, 1987).

Finally, Burack (1994) has provided evidence for a selective filtering deficit in autism, suggestive of a broad rather than a narrow beam of attention. In an RT task requiring differential responses to two stimuli, each presented centrally, the presence of distractor stimuli and a window (intended to focus attention) were systematically varied. Performance of lower-functioning adults with autism was compared to that of a normal group and two mentally handicapped groups (familial vs. organic), each matched on MA. The group with autism showed the most improvement in RT with the window, except when distractors were also present. In this case (vs. without the window), the group with autism had significantly longer RTs regardless of whether the distractors were within or outside the window. This differential window effect of distractors is puzzling. It also bears emphasizing that the findings have not been replicated with more capable people with autism (J. A. Burack, personal communication, June 1995), who have been shown elsewhere to perform well on visual search tasks involving competing stimuli (Brian & Bryson, 1997; Ozonoff, 1995; Ozonoff et al., 1991; Shah & Frith, 1983). Taken together, it may be that deficits in selective filtering are more characteristic of lower-functioning or less developmentally advanced individuals with autism. Note further that such deficits may coexist with problems disengaging and/or shifting attention once it is focused. In either case, attention may be unduly pulled by external physical events.

Summary and Comments

Studies of basic attentional processes in high-functioning adults with autism suggest that both focused and sustained attention are spared; deficits in selective filtering may be particularly characteristic of lower-functioning autistic individuals. Converging evidence points instead to a selective impairment in rapidly and accurately shifting attention both across and within modalities. Findings suggest further that there are dissociable subgroups with autism. The entire group, all with evidence of cerebellar abnormalities, appears deficient in both orienting and shifting visual attention; a subgroup (40–45%) with both parietal and cerebellar involvement have difficulty disengaging attention as well. This subgroup responds abnormally quickly to primed locations, suggesting that in autism the disengage problem may be one of narrowed attention with concommitant attentional enhancement at the loci of focus (Townsend & Courchesne, 1994). Preliminary evidence of enhanced inhibition (Bryson, 1995; Bryson & Tipper, 1997) is consistent with this possibility and may also be relevant to understanding the orienting and shift problems characteristic of the larger group with autism.

CONCLUDING REMARKS

In the research reviewed, considerable overlap exists between tasks used to examine frontal–executive functions (e.g., spatial reversal or ID/ED shift tasks) and those sensitive to more basic processes governed by posterior attentional systems (e.g., tasks requiring responses to one of two modality specific stimuli). Most are variants on the classic go/no-go task, originally designated a "frontal" task, but with no theoretical rationale (Dennis, 1991). There is a consensus that the regulation or control of attention is a central feature of frontal–executive functions (e.g., Shallice, 1988). Attention is also conceived as a network of interrelated, hierarchically organized component processes (Allport, 1990; Posner & Dehaene, 1994). The question for our purposes is whether deficits in lower-order, posterior-mediated attentional processes contribute to the frontal–executive dysfunction documented in autism?

To date, there is evidence that high-functioning children/adults with autism are deficient on executive tasks requiring a shift in set, most (if not all) of which require shifts in spatial location (e.g., Hughes et al., 1994; Ozonoff et al., 1994). There are also problems with the complex act of planning (e.g., Hughes et al., 1994; Ozonoff et al., 1991), which involves, among other things, the ability to shift set. People with autism tend to perseverate, frequently on a previous (primed) response, and alternate responses are executed with difficulty, if at all. Variants of the same tasks, used to examine basic components of attention, include the more sensitive measure of RT as well as accuracy. Findings from these studies implicate a selective deficit in disengaging and/or shifting and orienting attention, which is evident even when attention is engaged automatically and only simple modality-specific detection is required. This apparent dysfunction in basic, lower-order attentional operations may well account for the deficient development of related executive functions in autism.

One outstanding question is whether deficits in disengaging and/or shifting and orienting attention are specific to autism or are found in other developmentally disabled groups as well. Autism is part of a spectrum of pervasive developmental disorders (PDDs) that vary in severity, overlapping with other developmental disorders that share some but not all clinical features (e.g., Tourette syndrome and fragile X syndrome). It is possible that dysfunction in some attentional processes is common to more than one disorder and that dysfunction in others is unique and universal to autism.

As noted earlier, Dennis (1991) has provided a comprehensive framework for conceptualizing frontal lobe functions in children and adolescents. Recent theoretical work suggests how deficits in the development of posterior attentional systems might relate to the maldevelopment not only of higher-order frontal–executive functions (Posner & Dehaene, 1994) but of affective systems as well (Rothbart, Posner, & Boylan, 1990; Rothbart et al., 1992), which have also been implicated in autism (Hobson, 1989; see Bauman & Kemper, 1985, for evidence of limbic abnormalities). Dysfunctional arousal and associated brainstem structures, subjects of interest to of early theorists in the field (e.g., Hutt, Hutt, Lee, & Ounsted, 1964; Rimland, 1964), may also be central to understanding the impaired development of both motivational–affective and attentional systems in autism.

One undeniably striking feature of people with autism is their difficulty in initiating and coordinating action, and their tendency to engage in a restricted, repetitive, and inflexible set of behaviors (see Smith & Bryson, 1994, for a relevant review). We concur with Courchesne et al. (1994) in suggesting that selective deficits in lower-order attentional processes are primary to an understanding of the neuropsychopathology of autism/PDD. Specifically, the ability to rapidly and accurately orient and shift attention would appear to require undue effort. Such problems, evident early in life, apparently are not specific to the more complex and unpredictable social domain but would be expected to be more pronounced in it (Dawson & Lewy, 1989). Using the phenomenon of acquired spatial neglect as a model, we have suggested elsewhere that deficits in the development of visual–spatial attention would have a profound impact on the development of self and other awareness (Bryson, Wainwright-Sharp, & Smith, 1990). Spatial inattention in the developing organism might also go a long way toward explaining other features of autism, notably the restricted and repetitive repertoire of interests/behaviors, the saliency of external physical stimuli, and the difficulty in learning from context and generalizing across experience. Theoretically informed research on attention, conceived within a developmental framework, promises to both clarify the nature of autism and tell us much about the mechanisms governing normal development.

REFERENCES

Akshoomoff, N. A., & Courchesne, E. (1992). A new role for the cerebellum in cognitive operations. *Behavioral Neuroscience, 106,* 731–738.

Allport, A. (1990). Visual attention. In M. I. Posner (Ed.), *Foundations of cogni tive science* (pp. 631–682). Cambridge, MA: MIT Press.

American Psychiatric Association. (1994). *Diagnostic and statistical manual of mental disorders* (4th ed.). Washington, DC: Author.

Baron-Cohen, S. (1989). Are autistic children behaviorists? An examination of their mental–physical and appearance–reality distinctions. *Journal of Autism and Developmental Disorders, 19,* 579–600.

Baron-Cohen, S. (1993). From attention–goal psychology to belief–desire psychology: The development of a theory of mind, and its dysfunction. In S. Baron-Cohen, H. Tager-Flusberg, & D. J. Cohen (Eds.), *Understanding other minds: Perspectives from autism.* Oxford: Oxford University Press.

Baron-Cohen, S., Leslie, A. M., & Frith, U. (1985). Does the autistic child have a "theory of mind"? *Cognition, 21,* 37–46.

Bauman, M., & Kemper, T. L. (1985). Histoanatomic observations of the brain in early infantile autism. *Neurology, 35,* 866–874.

Bishop, D. V. M. (1993). Annotation: Autism, executive functions and theory of mind: A neuropsychological perspective. *Journal of Child Psychology and Psychiatry, 34,* 279–293.

Bornstein, M., & Lamb, M. E. (1992). *Development in infancy* (3rd ed.). New York: McGraw Hill.

Brian, J., & Bryson, S.E. (1997). *Disembedding performance and recognition memory in autism.* Manuscript in preparation.

Bryson, S. E. (1995, April). *Impaired components of attention in autism.* Paper presented at the meeting of the Society for Research in Child Development, Indianapolis, IN.

Bryson, S. E., Clark, B. S., & Smith, I. M. (1988). First report of a Canadian epidemiological study of autistic syndromes. *Journal of Child Psychology and Psychiatry, 29,* 433–445.

Bryson, S. E., & Tipper, S. P. (1997). *Inhibitory dysfunction in autism.* Manuscript in preparation.

Bryson, S. E., Wainwright-Sharp, J. A., & Smith, I. M. (1990) Autism: A developmental spatial neglect syndrome? In J. Enns (Ed.), *The development of attention: Research and theory.* Amsterdam: Elsevier.

Burack, J. (1994). Selective attention deficits in persons with autism: Preliminary evidence of an inefficient attentional lens. *Journal of Abnormal Psychology, 103,* 535–543.

Burack, J., & Iarocci, G. (1995, April). *Visual filtering and covert orienting in developmentally disordered persons with and without autism.* Paper presented at the meeting of the Society for Research in Child Development, Indianapolis, IN.

Casey, B. J., Gordon, C. T., Mannheim, G. B., & Rumsey, J. M. (1993). Dysfunctional attention in autistic savants. *Journal of Clinical and Experimental Neuropsychology, 15,* 933–946.

Chelune, G. J., Ferguson, W., Koon, R., & Dickey, T. O. (1986). Frontal lobe disinhibition in attention deficit disorder. *Child Psychiatry and Human Development, 16,* 221–234.

Ciesielski, K. T., Courchesne, E., Akshoomoff, N., & Elmasian, R. (1990). *Event-related potentials in intermodality divided-attention task in autism.* Paper presented at the meeting of the International Neuropsychological Society, Orlando, FL.

Ciesielski, K. T., Courchesne, E., & Elmasian, R. (1990). Effects of focused selective attention tasks on event-related potentials in autistic and normal individuals. *Electroencephalography and Clinical Neurophysiology, 75,* 207–220.

Courchesne, E. (1987). A neurophysiological view of autism. In E. Schopler & G. Mesibov (Eds.), *Neurobiological issues in autism* (pp. 285–324). New York: Plenum Press.

Courchesne, E., Akshoomoff, N. A., & Ciesielski, K. T. (1990). *Shifting attention abnormalities in autism: ERP and performance evidence.* Poster presented at the meeting of the International Neuropsychological Society, Orlando, FL.

Courchesne, E., Akshoomoff, N. A., Townsend, J., Yeung-Couchesne, R., Lincoln, A. J., James, H. E., Haas, R. H., Schreibman, L., & Lau, L. (1991). Impairment in shifting attention in autistic and cerebellar patients. *Behavioral Neuroscience, 108,* 848–865.

Courchesne, E., Townsend, J. P., Akshoomoff, N. A., Yeung-Courchesne, R., Press, G. A., & Murakami, J. W. (1994). A new finding: Impairment in shifting attention in autistic and cerebellar patients. In S. H. Broman & J. Grafman (Eds.), *Atypical cognitive deficits in developmental disorders: Implications for brain development* (pp. 101–137). Hillsdale, NJ: Erlbaum.

Courchesne, E., Yeung-Courchesne, R., Press, G. A., Hesselink, J. R., & Jernigan, T. L. (1988). Hypoplasia of cerebellar vermal lobules VI and VII in autism. *New England Journal of Medicine, 318,* 1349–1354.

Damasio, A. R., & Maurer, R. G. (1978). A neurological model for childhood autism. *Archives of Neurology, 35,* 777–786.

Dawson, G., & Lewy, A. (1989). Arousal, attention, and the socioemotional impairments of individuals with autism. In G. Dawson (Ed.), *Autism: Nature, diagnosis, and treatment* (pp. 49–74). New York: Guilford Press.

Dennis, M. (1991). Frontal lobe function in childhood and adolescence: A heuristic for assessing attention regulation, executive control and the intentional states important for social discourse. *Developmental Neuropsychology, 7,* 327–358.

Fein, D., Humes, M., Kaplan, E., Lucci, D., & Waterhouse, L. (1984). The question of left hemisphere dysfunction in autistic children. *Psychological Bulletin, 95,* 258–281.

Frith, C. D., & Frith, U. (1991). Elective affinities in schizophrenia and childhood autism. In P. Bebbington (Ed.), *Social psychiatry: Theory, methodology and practice*. New Brunswick, NJ: Transactions.

Garretson, H. B., Fein, D., & Waterhouse, L. (1990). Sustained attention in children with autism. *Journal of Autism and Developmental Disorders, 20*, 101–114.

Happe, F. G. E. (1994). Annotation: Current psychological theories of autism: The "theory of mind" account and rival theories. *Journal of Child Psychology and Psychiatry, 35*, 215–229.

Hermelin, B., & O'Connor, N. (1970). *Psychological experiments with autistic children*. Oxford: Pergamon Press.

Hobson, R. P. (1989). Beyond cognition: A theory of autism. In G. Dawson (Ed.), *Autism: Nature, diagnosis, and treatment* (pp. 22–48). New York: Guilford Press.

Hughes, C., & Russell, J. (1993). Autistic children's difficulty with mental disengagement from an object: Its implications for theories of autism. *Developmental Psychology, 29*, 498–510.

Hughes, C., Russell, J., & Robbins, T. N. (1994). Evidence for executive dysfunction in autism. *Neuropsychologia, 32*, 477–492.

Hutt, S. J., Hutt, C., Lee, D., & Ounsted, C. (1964). Arousal and childhood autism. *Nature, 204*, 980–909.

James, A., & Barry, R. J. (1980). Respiratory and vascular responses to simple stimuli in autistic, retardates and normals. *Psychophysiology, 17*, 541–547.

Jonides, J. (1981). Voluntary versus automatic control over the mind's eye's movement. In J. Long & A. Baddeley (Eds.), *Attention and performance IX* (pp. 187–203). Hillsdale, NJ: Erlbaum.

Kanner, L. (1943). Autistic disturbances of affective contact. *Nervous Child, 2*, 217–250.

Kasari, C., Sigman, M., Mundy, P., & Yirmiya, N. (1990). Affective sharing in the context of joint attention interactions of normal, autistic, and mentally retarded children. *Journal of Autism and Developmental Disorders, 20*, 87–100.

Kinsbourne, M. (1987). Cerebral–brainstem relations in infantile austim. In E. Schopler & G. Mesibov (Eds.), *Neurobiological issues in autism*. New York: Plenum Press.

Leslie, A. M., & Frith, U. (1988). Autistic children's understanding of seeing, knowing and believing. *British Journal of Developmental Psychology, 6*, 315–324.

Lotter, V. (1966). Epidemiology of autistic conditions in young children — I: Prevalence. *Social Psychiatry, 1*, 124–137.

Lovaas, O. I., Schreibman, L., Koegel, R., & Rehm, R. (1971). Selective responding by autistic children to multiple sensory input. *Journal of Abnormal Psychology, 77*, 211–222.

McEvoy, R. E., Rogers, S. J., & Pennington, B. F. (1993). Executive function and social communication deficits in young autistic children. *Journal of Child Psychology and Psychiatry, 34*, 563–578.

Menyuk, P., & Quill, K. (1985). Semantic problems in autism. In E. Schopler

& G. Mesibov (Eds.), *Communication problems in autism* (pp. 127–145). New York: Plenum Press.

Mundy, P. (1995). Joint attention and social-emotional approach behavior in children with autism. *Development and Psychopathology, 7,* 63–82.

Mundy, P., & Sigman, M. (1989a). Specifying the nature of the social impairment in autism. In G. Dawson (Ed.), *Autism: Nature, diagnosis, and treatment* (pp. 3–21). New York: Guilford Press.

Mundy, P., & Sigman, M. (1989b). The theoretical implications of joint-attention deficits in autism. *Development and Psychopathology, 6,* 313–330.

Ozonoff, S. (1995). Executive functions in autism. In E. Schopler & G. Mesibov (Eds.), *Learning and cognition in autism* (pp. 199–219). New York: Plenum Press.

Ozonoff, S., & McEvoy, R. E. (1994). A longitudinal study of executive function and theory of mind development in autism. *Development and Psychopathology, 6,* 415–431.

Ozonoff, S., Pennington, B. F., & Rogers, S. J. (1991). Executive function deficits in high-functioning autistic individuals: Relationship to theory of mind. *Journal of Child Psychology and Psychiatry, 32,* 1081–1105.

Ozonoff, S., & Strayer, D. L. (in press). Inhibitory function in nonretarded children with autism. *Journal of Autism and Developmental Disorders.*

Ozonoff, S., Strayer, D. L., McMahon, W. M., & Filloux, F. (1994). Executive function abilities in autism: An information processing approach. *Journal of Child Psychology and Psychiatry, 35,* 1015–1032.

Posner, M. I. (1988). Structures and functions of selective attention. In T. Boll & B. Bryant (Eds.), *Master lectures in clinical neuropsychology* (pp. 173–202). Washington, DC: American Psychological Association.

Posner, M. I., & Dehaene, S. (1994). Attentional networks. *Trends in Neuroscience, 17,* 75–79.

Posner, M. I., & Petersen, S. E. (1990). The attention system of the human brain. *Annual Review of Neuroscience, 13,* 25–42.

Prior, M. R., & Hoffman, W. (1990). Neuropsychological testing of autistic children through an exploration with frontal lobe tests. *Journal of Autism and Developmental Disorders, 20,* 581–590.

Ricks, D., & Wing, L. (1975). Language, communication and the use of symbols in normal and autistic children. *Journal of Autism and Childhood Schizophrenia, 5,* 191–221.

Rimland, B. (1964). *Infantile autism.* New York: Appleton-Century-Crofts.

Rincover, A., & Ducharme, J. M. (1987). Variables influencing stimulus overselectivity and "tunnel vision" in developmentally delayed children. *American Journal of Mental Deficiency, 91,* 422–430.

Rothbart, M. K., Posner, M. I., & Boylan, A. (1990). Regulatory mechanisms in infant temperament. In J. Enns (Ed.), *The development of attention: Research and theory* (pp. 47–66). Amsterdam: Elsevier.

Rothbart, M. K., Ziaie, H., & O'Boyle, C. G. (1992). Self-regulation and emotion in infancy. In N. Eisenberg & R. A. Fabes (Eds.), *New directions for child developmen: No. 55. Emotion and its regulation in early development.* San Fransisco: Jossey-Boss.

Rumsey, J. M. (1985). Conceptual problem-solving in highly verbal, nonretarded autistic men. *Journal of Autism and Developmental Disorders, 15*, 26–36.

Rumsey, J. M., & Hamburger, S. D. (1988). Neuropsychological findings in high functioning autistic men with autism, residual state. *Journal of Clinical and Experimental Neuropsychology, 10*, 201–221.

Rumsey, J. M., & Hamburger, S. D. (1990). Neuropsychological divergence of high-level autism and severe dyslexia. *Journal of Autism and Developmental Disorders, 20*, 155–168.

Schneider, S. G., & Asarnow, R. F. (1987). A comparison of cognitive/neuropsychological impairments of non-retarded autistic and schizophrenic children. *Journal of Abnormal Child Psychology, 15*, 29–45.

Shah, A., & Frith, U. (1983). An islet of ability in autistic children: A research note. *Journal of Child Psychology and Psychiatry, 24*, 613–620.

Shallice, T. (1988). *From neuropsychology to mental structure.* Cambridge, England: Cambridge University Press.

Sigman, M., & Ungerer, J. A. (1984). Cognitive and language skills in autistic, mentally retarded and normal children. *Developmental Psychology, 20*, 293–302.

Smith, I. M., & Bryson, S. E. (1994). Imitation and action: A critical review. *Psychological Bulletin, 116*, 259–273.

Steel, J. G., Gorman, R., & Flexman, J. E. (1984). Neuropsychiatric testing in an autistic mathematical idiot savant: Evidence for nonverbal abstract capacity. *Journal of the American Academy of Child Psychiatry, 23*, 704–707.

Szatmari, P., Tuff, L., Finlayson, A. J., & Bartolucci, G. (1990). Asperger's syndrome and autism: Neurocognitive aspects. *Journal of the American Academy of Child and Adolescent Psychiatry, 29*, 130–136.

Tipper, S. P. (1985). The negative priming effect: Inhibitory priming by ignored objects. *Quarterly Journal of Experimental Psychology: Human Experimental Psychology, 37A*, 571–590.

Townsend, J., & Courchesne, E. (1994). Parietal damage and narrow "spotlight" spatial attention. *Journal of Cognitive Neuroscience, 6*, 220–232.

Townsend, J., Courchesne, E., & Egaas, B. (1992, October). *Visual attention deficits in autistic adults with cerebellar and parietal abnormalities.* Paper presented at the annual meeting of the Society for Neuroscience,

Wainwright-Sharp, J. A., & Bryson, S. E. (1993). Visual orienting deficits in high-functioning people with autism. *Journal of Autism and Developmental Disorders, 23*, 1–13.

Wainwright-Sharp, J. A., & Bryson, S. E. (in press). Visual–spatial orienting in autism. *Journal of Autism and Developmental Disorders.*

Wing, L., & Attwood, A. (1987). Syndromes of autism and atypical development. In D. Cohen, A. Donnellan, & R. Paul (Eds.), *Handbook of autism and pervasive developmental disorders* (pp. 3–19). New York: Wiley.

Wing, L., & Gould, J. (1979). Severe impairments of social interaction and associated abnormalities in children: Epidemiology and classification. *Journal of Autism and Developmental Disorders, 9*, 11–29.

SECTION V
ADULTHOOD, ATTENTION, AND PSYCHOPATHOLOGY

Paying Attention to the Brain

THE STUDY OF SELECTIVE VISUAL ATTENTION IN COGNITIVE NEUROSCIENCE

Alan Kingstone
Marcia Grabowecky
George R. Mangun
Monica A. Valsangkar
Michael S. Gazzaniga

The goal of human cognitive neuroscience is to elucidate brain mechanisms underlying mental functions such as language, memory, and attention. This is an ambitious aim, and one that cannot be achieved by any single research approach. Hence, it is an interdisciplinary emphasis that both defines and fuels this developing field.

We present four major routes for investigating the relationship between brain mechanisms and human behavior. How these approaches have contributed to our understanding of visual selective attention is then reviewed, with special emphasis placed on human lesion studies. Finally, a paradox in the split-brain attention literature is examined in detail and a solution based on recent data is presented.

EXAMINING BRAIN AND BEHAVIOR

Animal Models

An indirect route to investigating brain mechanisms in humans is provided by animal models. The human brain is largely inaccessible to the invasive approaches allowed by animal models, including experimental brain lesions and single cell or multiple unit recording. The use of carefully controlled lesions allows the relationship between different brain regions to be specified, while recording from cells gives us important physiological information. Indeed, almost everything we currently know about the microorganization of brain structure and function is derived from the study of animal brains. A complete description of human brain structure and function may ultimately rest upon our understanding of animal neuroanatomy and neurophysiology.

However, a fundamental weakness of animal models is that a full understanding of another organism's brain operations will not lead us to a complete understanding of human brain operations. Differences across species in terms of structure and function place strong limitations on our ability to generalize from one species to another and from animal models to humans. Homologous structures can be very difficult to identify across species, and the specializations of different animals leads to large differences in their neuroanatomy and neurophysiology. For example, much of the rat brain is dedicated to olfactory input and much of the human brain is dedicated to visual input. An understanding of human psychological states of mind must ultimately require the study of the human brain at work.

Behavioral Studies

Behavioral investigations of healthy human subjects can tell us much about the structure and function of the human brain. This second approach combines our knowledge of normal sensory systems with precise stimulus presentation and response recording. However, strictly behavioral studies cannot draw a specific link between behavior and underlying brain mechanisms. For example, many experiments have shown that eye movement response time (RT) is reduced if the object at fixation is turned off shortly before the presentation of an eye movement target (Saslow, 1967; Reuter-Lorenz, Hughes, & Fendrich, 1991; Kingstone & Klein, 1993a; Kingstone, Fendrich, Wessinger, & Reuter-Lorenz, 1995). Kingstone and Klein (1993b) have hypothesized that this reduction in eye movement RT is due to the fixation offset event triggering two separate components: a warning signal component that is timed from any offset event and is observed for any response modality; and a fixation offset component that is triggered only by visual offsets at fixation and is specific to the oculomotor system. Thus, the behavioral work with healthy subjects suggests that visual offsets at fixation give rise to two isolable brain operations. However, this link can only be inferred based on the findings of other investigative approaches. For instance, Taylor, Kingstone, and Klein (1996) turned to animal models (cf. Munoz & Wurtz, 1992) when speculating that the fixation offset component is mediated by disinhibition of the rostral pole of the superior colliculus.

Brain Imaging

A third route for investigating brain–behavior relations is noninvasive neuroimaging techniques that allow researchers to study how brain areas are orchestrated and how they map onto brain function and behavior. The earliest imaging technique to be developed, computed tomography, provides detailed anatomical data that revolutionized neurology and experimental neuropsychology. Magnetic resonance imaging (MRI) provides similar images but with greater spatial resolution. Both produce high-quality "snapshots" of human brain structures and as such they are very useful for localizing brain lesions, tumors, and developmental abnormalities. However, neither provides images of brain activity; their strength is in identifying abnormal structure. In contrast, event-related potentials (ERPs) recorded from the human scalp provide measures of the time course of sensory information flow in both the ascending pathways and the cortex, as well as of response-related processes (for reviews, see Harter & Aine, 1984, and Mangun, Hillyard, & Luck, 1993). ERP studies provide important clues to the neural mechanisms that underlie cognitive processes in humans. Whereas the temporal resolution of ERPs is very high, the spatial resolution of ERP recordings is relatively low. Hence, it is often difficult to localize the specific brain regions involved in ERP effects.

Other imaging techniques such as positron emission tomography (PET) or, more recently, functional magnetic resonance imaging (fMRI) have significantly higher spatial resolution than is presently available with ERPs, while allowing brain activity to be observed. However, the improved spatial resolution of these techniques is purchased at a significant cost in temporal resolution. Clearly, what is needed is high spatial and high temporal resolution information. This may be achieved by combining the evidence from multiple imaging methodologies (i.e., ERPs, PET, and fMRI). In recent years, this convergent approach has been applied to cognitive neuroscience questions with promising results. For example, a recent study by Heinze, Mangun, and colleagues (1994) combined ERP and PET data to gain a high-resolution view in both temporal and spatial domains of visual–spatial attentional processess. As these imaging techniques develop, we can expect to see a clearer picture of the human brain operating in real time.

In spite of this optimism, these new imaging approaches have some problems. Are the physiological processes that give rise to a signal for one imaging technique generated by the same neuronal activity as that measured by a different imaging technique? Do these differing physiological processes reflect different mechanisms of the same cognitive process? Additionally, many functional imaging techniques require averaging across subjects, generally requiring some algorithm for "adjusting" each subject's brain to map one person onto another. This "smearing" for intersubject averaging in ERP, PET, and fMRI investigations, and the lack of agreed-upon standards in analyzing and interpreting neuroimage data pose a serious problem currently for PET and fMRI data—but a problem that may be addressed by new techniques allowing observations within a single subject.

Human Lesion Studies

A fourth approach capitalizes on knowledge gained by studying patients with brain lesions resulting from surgical interventions or from stroke, tumors, or other diseases. These patients include those with hemispheres disconnected through a surgical section of the corpus callosum and patients with focal lesions resulting from surgery or stroke. This "damaged brain" approach is an important source of information for two major reasons.

First, by combining behavioral measures with modern imaging techniques, a direct link can be made between behavior and brain structure. With dynamic imaging techniques such as PET or fMRI, these links can be expanded to include mapping from behavior to function. For instance, certain patients with lesions to the primary visual cortex can make accurate judgments about the location of visual stimuli they claim they cannot see. This "blindsight" has been attributed to visual pathways that bypass the primary cortex (for reviews, see Weiskrantz, 1990, and Cowey & Stoerig, 1991). It has also been argued that blindsight could be due to spared functioning in the primary cortex (Pöppel, Held, & Frost, 1973; Campion, Latto, & Smith, 1983). Using psychophysical tests and an image stabilizer that allows for extended and repetitive stimulus presentations to a very small area of the retina, Fendrich, Wessinger, and Gazzaniga (1992) discovered a small and isolated island of blindsight in a hemianopic patient. This behavioral result suggested that a region of cortex was spared within the lesioned area. MRI images confirmed that there was indeed cortical sparing, and a subsequent PET investigation revealed that the spared cortex was metabolically active. Based on this combination of behavioral and neuroimaging data, Fendrich et al. (1992) were able to conclude that blindsight can result from cortical sparing within a lesioned area (see also Gazzaniga, Fendrich, & Wessinger, 1994).

A second major benefit of the lesion method is that neurological impairments of cognitive processes, which are interesting in their own right, can also reveal important information about the normal operation of the impaired processes.

The lesion approach, like the other approaches, also has its weaknesses. One shortcoming is that lesions such as strokes and tumors vary from patient to patient, and so the location and size of a lesion will typically differ. While patient groups can be selected based upon regions where their lesions overlap, it cannot be concluded with certainty that the same functional area is affected in all patients. It is likewise difficult to generalize to a population from the study of a single case. Another weakness is that damage to one area may produce a deficit that is not in fact specific to the damaged area. For instance, blindness in a visual field can be produced by damage to any number of levels of the visual system, ranging from the subcortical optical fibers to primary visual cortex. Thus in many cases a direct link between behavior, brain function, and brain structure cannot be drawn with confidence.

Finally, surgically created lesions such as those in split-brain patients hold a special place within the lesion approach. Unlike lesions produced by strokes, tumors, and other neurologic insults, split-brain lesions are surgically created, precise, and localized to the callosal fibers that connect the left and right cerebral hemispheres. Thus the cause, size, and location of split-brain lesions can be equated across patients (with any callosal sparing detected by MRI analysis). However, callosotomies are only performed on patients who suffer from intractable epilepsy for an extended period, and so, in this regard at least, the brains of callosotomy patients may be unlike healthy human brains.

COVERT SELECTIVE ATTENTION IN VISION

At its best, cognitive neuroscience melds theory and technique from the different approaches described here. Hypotheses about brain mechanisms in animal models are developed through careful control of behavior using paradigms developed in both animals and humans. Data from human behavioral studies can be interpreted within a context provided by animal studies allowing direct observation of neural functioning at a local level. Each of these sources are used when designing and interpreting experiments using functional imaging methods or human brain lesion methods. Thus natural anomalies come together with careful experimental control to elucidate the mechanisms underlying cognition. We will now examine some examples of how these approaches have been used in the study of visual attention.

Space-Based and Object-Based Attention

The ability of human observers to attend to one or a few out of many possible stimuli that are competing for the control of behavior involves complex selection mechanisms. When we move our attention by moving our eyes to an object, the shift is overt. When the eyes are not moved, the shift is covert. Covert attentional orienting, like overt orienting, enhances the perception of objects.

The benefits of covert selective attention in vision can be easily demonstrated in terms of performance. In a typical study a subject might be asked to detect the onset of a light to the left or right of a central fixation point. When the target is detected, the subject presses a button as quickly as possible. Prior to target onset, advance knowledge about where a stimulus will occur can be provided by an arrow cue that points to the left or right of fixation. On most trials the target appears at the cued spatial location (e.g., on the left when the arrow is pointing to the left), but occasionally, the target will appear at the uncued location (e.g., on the right when the cue is pointing to the left). The standard cuing effect is that RT is faster and/or more accurate when a target appears at a cued location than an uncued location. Some investigators (e.g., Duncan, 1980; Shaw, 1984; Sperling, 1984) have suggested that these cuing effects might derive from an internal response bias, that is, a tendency to lower one's decision criterion so that less information must be gathered to detect or identify a stimulus at the probable position. However, to date, the weight of empirical evidence supports the view that cuing effects reflect localized changes in perceptual sensitivity in the visual field, suggesting the involvement of a limited capacity mechanism that can be aligned covertly (with no concomitant shift in gaze) with the cued stimulus position (e.g., Downing, 1988; Hawkins et al., 1990; Posner, Snyder, & Davidson, 1980). To adopt the traditional spotlight metaphor: focused attention to a spatial location (i.e., spatial attention) "illuminates" that locus and enhances the perceptual processing efficiency of any stimulus presented within its attentional "beam."

Duncan (1984) contrasted attention to location (space-based attention) with attention to objects (object-based attention). Holding spatial distance constant he discovered that two judgments concerning the same object can be made simultaneously without loss of accuracy whereas two judgments about different objects cannot (see also Treisman, Kahneman, & Burkell, 1983; Watt, 1988). This processing limitation in attending to two objects implicates an object-based attention system in addition to a space-based system. In line with this view Egly, Driver, and Rafal (1994) demonstrated that spatial cuing effects were greater when attention was shifted between two objects than within one object.

The idea that attention to space or objects may reflect isolable systems that can be manipulated independently was tested recently by Kingstone (1992; Kingstone & Klein, 1991). Advance knowledge about what object letter would probably occur (i.e., the letter Λ or the letter V) and/or where in visual space it would probably appear was provided on a trial-by-trial basis. RT was faster for expected target objects than for unexpected ones (an object-based attention effect) and faster for objects appearing at expected locations than for objects appearing at unexpected loci (a space-based attention effect). Most importantly, attention effects were additive when object and location information were resolved simultaneously, suggesting that space-based and object-based attention effects reflect the involvement of separate mechanisms.

Neural Systems Mediating Spatial Selective Attention

The brain mechanisms of selective attention have been studied using each of the four major approaches outlined previously, but here we will focus primarily on studies with human lesion populations. Posner and colleagues have conducted extensive studies with different lesion groups that serve as an example of this approach. They hypothesize that a neural system distributed across many cortical and subcortical areas is involved in covert shifts of visual spatial attention. This system includes parts of the posterior parietal lobe, the midbrain, and the thalamus. According to this view, each brain region has a special function in the operation of covert attention, but all function together in the healthy human brain.

This model of covert attention portrays attention as consisting of three primary operations. These are *disengage, move,* and *engage*. To explain these operations, a simple analogy may be drawn to the process of grasping an object. In order to grasp an object, one must first disengage from or let go of the object currently grasped. The next operation is a movement of the hand to the target object. Finally, the target object must be grasped or engaged.

In an investigation of the disengage operation, Posner, Walker, Friedrich, and Rafal (1984, 1987) tested patients with lesions of the parietal cortex. Their task was to maintain central fixation and press a button when the onset of a light was detected in either the left or right visual field. Prior to target onset a peripheral box was brightened in the left or right field, indicating where the target was likely to appear. A standard cuing effect was found: RT was faster when a target appeared in the cued field versus the uncued field. However, RTs were exceptionally slow if patients were cued to expect a target in the ipsilesional field (the field on the same side as their lesion and therefore projecting to the nonlesioned hemisphere) and the target appeared in the uncued contralesional field (the field opposite their lesion and therefore projecting directly to the lesioned hemisphere). Posner and colleagues concluded that parietal damage does not produce a difficulty in directing covert attention to the contralesional field per se but does produce an extreme difficulty in disengaging attention from the ipsilesional field.

In contrast, Rafal and Posner (1987) found that patients with unilateral thalamic lesions produced an ipsilesional curing effect that was very similar to that for parietal patients, and a contralesional curing effect that also was very similar to that for parietal patients. The dramatic difference between the two patient groups was that the thalamic patients had elevated RTs for all contralesional targets. In other words, the contralesional engage operation that tended to equate the contralesional and ipsilesional cued locations in parietal patients never occurred for thalamic patients, suggesting that the thalamic nuclei are crucual in engaging visual attention.

Finally, the move operation was studied in patients with progressive supranuclear palsy. These patients suffer from a degenerative disease that affects the midbrain, including the superior colliculus, causing profound difficulties in making eye movements, particularly in the vertical plane. Rafal, Posner, Friedman, Inhoff, and Bernstein (1988) discovered that these patients were also profoundly impaired at moving their attention covertly (i.e., without any concomitant shifts in gaze), especially for covert shifts of attention in the vertical plane. Patients with Parkinson's disease, who suffer from a similar degenerative condition that does *not* involve the superior colliculus, do not show a similar vertical plane–horizontal plane difference in orienting covert attention. Thus, the data implicate the superior colliculus as critical for moving covert attention.

Together these data suggest that the neural network mediating spatial orienting is distributed across different brain areas — with the posterior parietal lobes involved in the disengagement of attention from its current focus, with the midbrain superior colliculus involved in the movement or shifting of attention to a new location, and with the thalamus involved in the engagement of attention upon the new location.

Neural Systems Mediating Object-Based Attention

Lesion data also support the hypothesis that attention can be independently directed to objects. For example, patients suffering from Balint syndrome (which typically involves bilateral posterior damage including the posterior parietal and anterior occipital cortex) have great difficulty perceiving more than one object at a time. One possibility is that, due to their parietal damage, these patients have difficulty disengaging from individual objects and thus cannot make judgments involving comparisons between objects. A recent study by Humphreys and Riddoch (1993) provides an illustration. Patients with Balint syndrome judged whether 32 circles were the same color or not. Dumbells were formed by black lines connecting circles of the same color (Figure 11.1a) or different colors (Figure 11.1b), or black lines were randomly placed among the circles (Figure 11.1c). Patients performed approximately at chance in discriminating single-color from two-color displays when the circles were not connected and when circles of the same color were connected. Only when

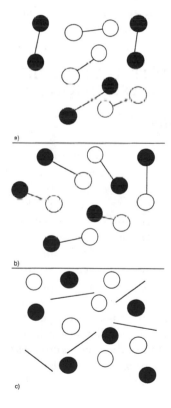

FIGURE 11.1. Examples of stimulus conditions used by Humphreys and Riddoch (1993). Dark and white circles were actually colored red and green. See the text of full details.

different colored circles were connected did patients perform well above chance, indicating that the status of the circles as parts of an object had a profound influence on the patients' decisions.

Illustrations of object-based attention also come from research on visual neglect. For example, Driver and Halligan (1991) reported that a right parietal patient neglected the left half of shapes even when these were tilted 45° so that details on the left of the shape fell to the patient's right (see also Behrmann & Moscovitch, 1994; Driver, Baylis, Goodrich, & Rafal, 1994). Data from dynamic imaging studies with healthy humans also support the distinction between space-based and object-based attention. Different timing and scalp distributions for space and object selection have been reported from ERP studies (e.g., Hillyard & Münte, 1984), and PET data have shown different extrastriate cortical regions involved in attention to space and objects (Corbetta, Miezin, Dobmeyer, Shulman, & Petersen, 1990, 1991; Corbetta, Miezin, Shulman, & Petersen, 1993). Thus while the notion that attention is space based is indisputable, there is clear evidence that attention can also be object based.

SPLIT-BRAIN STUDIES
AND AN ATTENTION PARADOX

The Split-Brain Patient

Since the commissurotomy research by Sperry and Gazzaniga began the current phase of testing callosotomy patients (Gazzaniga, Bogen, & Sperry, 1962; Sperry, Gazzaniga, & Bogen, 1969), this population has offered a powerful and interesting way to investigate the organization of perceptual and cognitive functions in the human subject. When the corpus callosum is surgically sectioned for the relief of intractable epilepsy, all major cortical connections between the two hemispheres are severed. In most patients treated recently, the anterior commisure is spared, preserving connections between the hippocampi. Subcortical structures such as the superior colliculus and the thalamus retain their interconnections, though these are much less extensive than the corpus callosum. Studies of these patients can tell us about the functions each hemisphere can carry out independent of the other. In addition, any activities that require integration between the hemispheres must rely on intact subcortical connections (see Kingstone & Gazzaniga, 1995; also Seymour, Reuter-Lorenz, & Gazzaniga, 1994, for a recent review). Traditionally studies of these patients have dealt mainly with issues of lateralization of function in processes such as speech, emotion, memory, and perceptual processing. Here we will review studies of attention in this population.

The data from callosotomy patients appear to reflect a remarkable division of processing within the split brain, with many functions lateralized, such as language, and perceptual awareness confined to a single hemisphere when stimuli are presented to one hemisphere alone. Yet these data are belied by the ease with which a split-brain patient conducts the functions of daily life. Even with specialized knowledge, experience, and testing, it may not be easy to discriminate the split-brain patient from an individual with an intact brain. The apparent ease of integration of information processed in the two disconnected hemispheres suggests that some information must be shared (albeit perhaps at a relatively low level), allowing the hemispheres to interact and maintain behavioral unity.

Most split-brain patients possess language only in the left hemisphere. The few who possess language in both hemispheres provide a unique opportunity for cognitive abilities to be compared between the hemispheres. Although language comprehension exists in both hemispheres, language production is typically restricted to the left hemisphere (i.e., the right hemisphere is mute). Visual information presented entirely in one visual field projects exclusively to the opposite, or contralateral, hemisphere. In other words, stimuli presented in the left visual field (LVF) are seen exclusively by the right hemisphere, whereas stimuli in the right visual field (RVF) project directly to the left hemisphere.

The following example will help to illustrate these main points. A split-brain patient with language comprehension in both hemispheres but language production lateralized to the left hemisphere is asked to fixate the center of a computer screen. A word is then flashed briefly to the LVF while nothing is presented to the RVF. Brief stimulus presentation is necessary to ensure that the subject does not have time to execute an eye movement to the stimulated visual field. The right hemisphere understands enough language to interpret the word, but the patient cannot articulate the word because the right hemisphere is mute. If asked what was presented the patient will respond (with his or her left, or speaking, hemisphere) that he/she does not know what was flashed on the screen. However, if asked to illustrate what was shown by drawing a picture with the left hand (which is controlled primarily by the right hemisphere), the split-brain patient can draw a picture of the stimulus.

This remarkable disconnection between the hemispheres raises the possibility that a split-brain patient might actually outperform intact subjects in situations where the information presented to the two hemispheres might normally cause confusion. Holtzman and Gazzaniga (1985) presented split-brain patient J.W. with one 3 × 3 matrix positioned in each visual field. On each trial an "X" was flashed sequentially in four of the nine cells in each matrix. The pattern in the two fields could be either the same (redundant condition) or different (mixed condition). Subsequently a probe sequence appeared in one matrix and the subject was required to respond, by pressing a key, indicating whether the probe pattern matched the stimulus pattern that had just occurred in that matrix. Comparison subjects responded correctly about 90% of the time for the redundant condition, and they were at chance in the mixed condition. In contrast, split-brain patient J.W. performed at about 75% accuracy in both conditons. Because of his disconnection the split-brain patient did not benefit from the redundant information between the visual fields and so performed worse than the controls; but he did not suffer from the conflicting information in the mixed condition, and so here he outperformed the controls. It appears as if for J.W. each hemisphere was functioning on its own, neither benefiting from corroborating information from the other hemisphere nor questioning conflicting information. At first glance, J.W. appears to have attentional resources at his disposal that are not possessed by subjects with intact brains.

A Paradox

It is unlikely that sectioning the corpus callosum in and of itself would increase the attentional capacity of the subject. However, it is possible that after the hemispheres are disconnected, each hemisphere would come to control its own attentional network. Research on this issue has produced a paradox.

To investigate the independence of attentional processing in the disconnected hemispheres, Holtzman, Volpe, and Gazzaniga (1984) tested split-brain patients in a spatial cuing experiment in which the left hemisphere was cued (by a left- or right-pointing arrow) to orient attention to the LVF or RVF; simultaneously the right hemisphere was cued (with a left- or right-pointing arrow) to direct attention to the LVF or RVF. Results showed that RTs to target stimuli were slower when the two hemispheres received different attentional instructions than when the two hemispheres received the same cues, suggesting that attentional orienting remains a unitary process in the split-brain patient (see also Holtzman & Gazzaniga, 1982; Reuter-Lorenz & Fendrich, 1990). However, Luck, Hillyard, Mangun, and Gazzaniga (1989, 1994) have recently produced data that bring this result into question. They found that split-brain patients can search through visual displays twice as fast as can healthy observers when items are divided evenly between visual fields, as though each disconnected hemisphere possessed its own attentional scanning system. This finding raises a paradox: do the disconnected hemispheres share a common attention mechanism (as suggested by Holtzman & Gazzaniga, 1982, 1985, and Reuter-Lorenz & Fendrich, 1990), or do they each orient attention independently (as suggested by Luck et al., 1989, 1994; see also Mangun et al., 1994).

A clue as to how these data can be reconciled was provided by Reuter-Lorenz and Fendrich (1990). In their experiment, split-brain patients fixated a central dot on a computer screen that displayed four empty squares. The squares were aligned in a row on the horizontal axis with two squares to the left and two squares to the right of fixation. One of the squares was brightened for 200 milliseconds (the cue) and then after a delay of 500 milliseconds an "X" was presented at the location of one of the squares. The patient's task was to push a button when the "X" was detected. The box that brightened correctly indicated where the "X" would occur on 70% of the trials, and on the remaining target trials the "X" appeared with equal probability at one of the uncued locations. The uncued location could be in the same field as the cue or in the opposite field. Results indicated that split-brain patients showed the same RT delay as did control subjects when the target appeared at an uncued location that was in the same field as the cue. However, when the target appeared at the uncued location in the opposite field, the RT delay was much greater for split-brain patients than for control subjects. These data are consistent with the notion that the two hemispheres share a common attention system (as suggested by Holtzman et al., 1984). However, in a final experiment Reuter-Lorenz and Fendrich (1990) repeated their experiment, but on this occasion the cue did not predict where the target would appear. RT was again faster when a target appeared at the cued location than when it appeared at an uncued location, but now there was little difference between whether the uncued location was in the same field as the cue or in the opposite field. Reuter-Lorenz and Fendrich (1990) speculated that each hemisphere could independently deploy attention when a target was equally likely in each visual field; in contrast, when the probability of a target was high at a cued location, the two hemispheres acted as if they were in competition for the same attentional resources.

A Solution to the Paradox?

The Reuter-Lorenz and Fendrich (1990) study draws a distinction between attending to a location because the probability is high that a target will occur there (voluntary or endogenous orienting) and attending to a location because a cue involuntarily attracts attention there (reflexive or exogenous orienting). Recent behavioral studies have suggested that endogenous and exogenous orienting may differ in the attention systems that are activated (Briand & Klein, 1987; Klein, 1994; Kingstone & Egly, 1997). Is it possible that the paradox in the split-brain literature reflects a difference between the attentional processes that have been activated, such that endogenous orienting is shared between the hemispheres, but exogenous orienting is performed independently?

To examine this question directly, Kingstone (1995) conducted the following experiment with patient J.W. (see Figure 11.2). A box was positioned 4° to the left and right of a central fixation point. On each trial one of the boxes brightened (the cue) for 100 milliseconds in the left or right field, or in both fields (a neutral cue). On 80% of all the trials a target was presented either 150 or 600 milliseconds after the cue was first presented (stimulus-onset asynchrony [SOA]). On the remaining 20% of the trials, no target appeared; these "catch trials" were included to discourage split-brain patient J.W. from responding to the onset of the cue. In the endogenous cue condition the target appeared at the cued location 80% of the time, and at the uncued location 20% of the time; in the exogenous cue condition the cue did not predict target location, so that 50% of the time the target appeared at the cued location and 50% of the time the target appeared at the uncued location. Thus endogenous and exogenous cue conditions differed only in the predictiveness of the cue. For the endogenous condition, cues reliably predicted the target location, encouraging voluntary orienting to the cue. In the exogenous cue condition, the cues were not predictive, activating reflexive orienting.

Figure 11.3 outlines three predictions for this study. If the separated

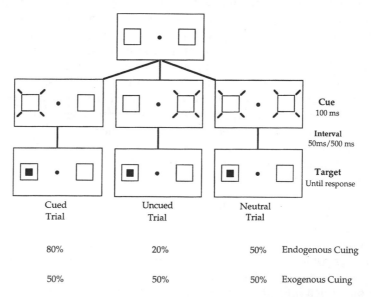

FIGURE 11.2. Example displays for cued, uncued, and neutral trials. On each trial, the cue appeared for 100 milliseconds, followed by a 50- or 500-millisecond interval (SOA = 150 or 600 milliseconds), and then the target appeared. For endogenous cues, target onset occurred at the cued location 80% of the time and at the uncued location 20% of the time. For exogenous cues and neutral cues, target onset occurred at either location 50% of the time. See the text for a complete description.

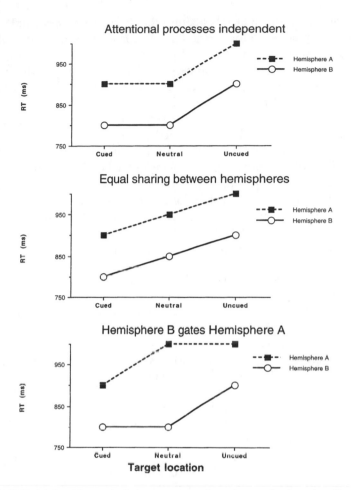

FIGURE 11.3. Theoretical data patterns based on whether the disconnected hemispheres orient attention independently, share a common attentional process, or compete for a common process with one hemisphere gating the other hemisphere.

hemispheres have independent attention systems, then response latencies on cued trials should be equivalent to neutral trials, because within each individual hemisphere the two cue types are indistiguishable. Uncued trials provide no cue information for the hemisphere detecting the target, and so the slowest latencies should occur on these trials. If, on the other hand, the two hemispheres share equally a single attentional process, then RT should be faster on cued trials than on uncued trials because the shared attentional resources will be focused on the cued location and so drawn away from the uncued location. Neutral cue trials will have RTs that fall between cued and uncued trials because the shared resources will be distributed equally between locations. Finally, consider the situation where the hemispheres compete unequally for a single attentional process, with one hemisphere gating (i.e., inhibiting) attentional access by the other. RTs for the "dominant" hemisphere on cued trials should be the same as on neutral trials and faster than on uncued trials because by definition the dominant hemisphere will orient attention to its location on cued and neutral trials. Conversely, RT for the gated, or "nondominant," hemisphere will be faster on cued trials than on neutral or uncued trials because only on cued trials will the nondominant hemisphere be able to orient attention (as on these trials the dominant hemisphere is uncued). This is roughly a winner-take-all model, with the dominant hemisphere biased to win. The nondominant hemisphere wins only when no competing signal arrives in the dominant hemisphere.

The results from this experiment are presented in Figures 11.4 and 11.5. Comparing the findings against the theoretical data patterns, we find that in the exogenous cue condition the two hemispheres orient attention independently at the short SOA, with the left hemisphere gating the right hemisphere at the long SOA. In the endogenous cue condition the the left hemisphere gates the right hemisphere at both SOA durations. These data are consistent with the view that exogenous orienting involves independent access of attentional processes between the two hemispheres at the short SOA (with endogenous orienting overiding exogenous orienting at the long SOA) and endogenous orienting involves competition for shared attentional processes between the hemispheres. In this latter situation, when the two hemispheres compete for common attentional processes, it appears that the left hemisphere is dominant and inhibits attentional orienting by the right hemisphere.

Converging evidence for this final point is provided by Kingstone, Enns, Mangun, and Gazzaniga (1995), who extended the Luck et al. (1989, 1994) standard search experiment. Luck and colleagues found that disconnected hemispheres can scan for targets independently and in parallel in a standard visual search experiment. Kingstone et al. replicated the standard search experiment and extended it by including the possibility for what is called strategic or guided visual search, that is, the selection of a small number of candidate targets and/or the rejection of a large number of distractor items based on shared feature information (cf. Egeth, Virzi, & Garbart, 1984; Wolfe, Cave, & Franzel, 1989). Figure 11.6 illustrates the difference between standard and guided search displays. Note that in Figure 11.6A the target, a black circle, is hidden among roughly an equal number of black square and gray circle distractors (this is standard search). However, in Figure 11.6B, it takes less time to find the black circle target because it can be found simply by searching among the small

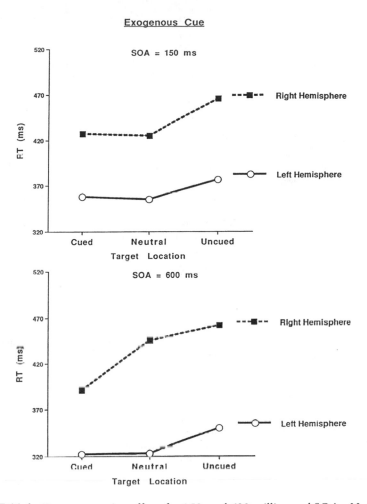

FIGURE 11.4. Exogenous cuing effects for 150- and 600-millisecond SOAs. Note that the split-brain performance pattern suggests that the two hemispheres orient attention independently at the short SOA and that the left hemisphere gates the right hemisphere at the long SOA.

set of four black square distractors. Guided search occurs when a target can be found efficiently by applying this strategic form of scanning.

In the Kingstone et al. (1995) experiment, displays consisted of 2, 4, 8, or 16 items presented in one visual field (unilateral array) or divided equally between fields (bilateral array). Subjects pressed a left-hand key for a target in the LVF and a right-hand key for a target in the RVF. In guided search trials, the division of distractors was unequal by a ratio of

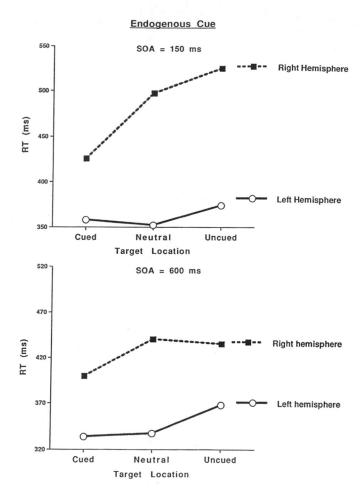

FIGURE 11.5. Endogenous cuing effects for 150- and 600-millisecond SOAs. Note that split-brain performance suggests that the left hemisphere gates the right hemisphere at both short and long SOAs.

about 5:2, with the larger number of distractors in a nontarget color or shape, a manipulation that should facilitate target detection if strategic scanning is employed. For split-brain patients but not for comparison subjects, the search rate for unilateral displays was twice that for bilateral displays, consistent with the findings of Luck et al. (1989, 1994). However, Kingstone et al. also found that the means by which each split-brain hemisphere searched its respective field differed. When provided with the opportunity to perform strategic guided search, only the left hemisphere

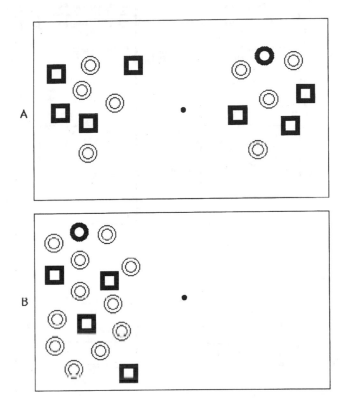

FIGURE 11.6. A bilateral search array (A) and a unilateral guided search array (B) are shown for a black circle target with display size equal to 16 (these samples are not to scale).

seized this opportunity (see Figure 11.7). One interpretation of these findings is that strategic visual–spatial control processes are lateralized to a dominant left hemisphere. An alternative interpretation, based on the cuing data reported above, is that lateralization of strategic visual search to the left hemisphere may actually reflect competition between hemispheres for a strategic (endogenous) attentional process. The right hemisphere may be capable of engaging in guided search, but it may be actively inhibited from doing so when the dominant left hemisphere is employing this strategy. This idea was tested by rerunning the guided visual search experiment with split-brain patient J.W. and eliminating the opportunity for the left hemisphere to perform guided search (no guided search displays were presented to the RVF). As predicted by the cuing data, J.W.'s right hemisphere was now found to perform strategic guided search behavior!

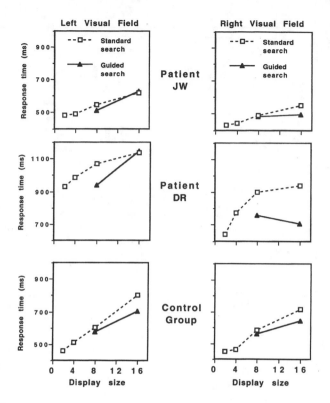

FIGURE 11.7. Standard search and guided search response times for split-brain patients and the normal control group as a function of visual field and display size. Each row represents the data from an individual patient or the control group. Left and right columns represent LVF and RVF targets, respectively. In each plot, open squares represent standard search trials and filled triangles are guided search trials. Note that the y-axes of the individual plots have different origin points but that the scales are otherwise identical.

These data provide converging evidence for the position that an interaction between the two hemispheres may reflect competition for an endogenous attention system. If the dominant left hemisphere is provided with the opportunity to use a guided search strategy, it will do so, and this will interfere with the right hemisphere's ability to perform guided search. When the guided search opportunity is not provided to the left hemisphere, the (endogenous) attentional processes required to perform guided search are available to, and accessed by, the right hemisphere.

In summary, the data suggest that the hemispheres are both independent and interdependent, with exogenous orienting reflecting independence and endogenous orienting reflecting interdependence. Whether the two hemispheres orient attention independently or not appears to be critically affected by a gating operation imposed by the dominant left hemisphere.

The neural mechanisms that underly these attentional operations are not yet identified, but several possibilities exist. Exogenous attentional orienting, the system proposed to be involuntary and independent in the two hemispheres, may be mediated by midbrain systems, including the superior colliculus. These involuntary exogenous shifts of attention could be gated by cortical regions through connections between the superior colliculus and the frontal eye fields in the dorsolateral prefrontal cortex. The mechanisms underlying the gating of endogenous or voluntary attention are even more speculative. It is possible that each hemisphere directs attention to a particular spatial location, with the dominant or more active hemisphere seizing control through thalamic gating of the other hemisphere. The thalami have massive connections with the cortex and are in turn interconnected through the massa intermedia, though this is not a massive fiber tract. Further research using the four approaches to investigate brain–behavior relations may well answer these questions in the future.

CONCLUSION

The investigations into selective attention reported here have illustrated how cognitive neuroscience as a discipline attempts to understand cognitive behavior and its underlying neural mechanisms.

This chapter has focused on studies relying on brain lesions but has shown as well how these studies benefit from converging data from other approaches. We have also presented evidence that attention has both a voluntary endogenous component and an involuntary exogenous component. Furthermore, these two types of attention appear to be subserved by different brain mechanisms. In the split-brain patient, exogenous orienting appears to function independently between left and right hemispheres whereas endogenous orienting is usually controlled by the dominant hemisphere.

These split-brain data lend strong support to the idea that exogenous and endogenous orienting draw on qualitatively different attentional processes (see, e.g., Grabowecky, Robertson, & Triesman, 1993; Kingstone & Egly, 1997; Klein, 1994). This raises the the question of whether previous findings that (endogenous) attentional effects are unsupported by a nondominant hemisphere may actually reflect inhibition generated by a dominant hemisphere. An example of this is provided by the Kingstone et al. (1995) finding that guided search is a left hemisphere processes. Our most recent data suggests that the right hemisphere can support trategic visual search, but only if access to endogenous orienting is permitted by the dominant left hemisphere. Although this conclusion must currently be considered highly speculative, it is an exciting possibilty that we will pursue vigorously in future investigations.

ACKNOWLEDGMENTS

This work was supported by grants from the Natural Sciences and Engineering Research Council, the Alberta Heritage Foundation for Medical Research, the McDonnell and Pew Foundations, the National Institute of Health, the National Institute of Mental Health, and the Human Frontier Science Program Organization.

REFERENCES

Behrmann, M., & Moscovitch, M. (1994). Object-centered neglect in patients with unilateral neglect: Effects of left–right coordinates of objects. *Journal of Cognitive Neuroscience, 6,* 1–16.

Briand, K. A., & Klein, R. M. (1987). Is Posner's "beam" the same as Treisman's "glue"?: On the relation between visual orienting and feature integration theory. *Journal of Experimental Psychology: Human Perception and Performance, 13,* 228–241.

Campion, J., Latto, R., & Smith, Y. M. (1983). Is blindsight an effect of scattered light, spared cortex, and near-threshold vision? *Behavioral and Brain Sciences, 6,* 423–486.

Corbetta, M., Miezin, F., Dobmeyer, S., Shulman, G., & Petersen, S. (1990). Attentional modulation of neural processing of shape, color and velocity in humans. *Science, 248,* 1556–1559.

Corbetta, M., Miezin, F. M. , Dobmeyer, S., Shulman, G. L., & Petersen, S. E. (1991). Selective and divided attention during visual discriminations of shape, color, and speed: Functional anatomy by positron emission tomography. *Journal of Neuroscience, 11,* 2383–2402.

Corbetta, M., Miezin, F., Shulman, G., & Petersen, S. (1993). A PET study of visuospatial attention. *Journal of Neuroscience, 13,* 1202–1226.

Cowey, A., & Stoerig, P. (1991). The neurobiology of blindsight. *Trends in Neurosciences, 14,* 140–145.

Downing, C. J. (1988). Expectancy and visual–spatial attention: Effects on perceptual quality. *Journal of Experimental Psychology: Human Perception and Performance, 14,* 188–202.

Driver, J., Baylis, G. C., Goodrich, S. J., & Rafal, R. D. (1994). Axis-based neglect of visual shapes. *Neuropsychologia, 32,* 1353–1365.

Driver, J., & Halligan, P. W. (1991). Can visual neglect operate in object-centered co-ordinates?: An affirmative single-case study. *Cognitive Neuropsychology, 8,* 475–496.

Duncan, J. (1980). The demonstration of capacity limitation. *Cognitive Psychology, 12,* 75–96.

Duncan, J. (1984). Selective attention and the organization of visual information. *Journal of Experimental Psychology: General, 113,* 501–517.

Egeth, H. E., Virzi, R. A., & Garbart, H. (1984). Searching for conjunctively defined targets. *Journal of Experimental Psychology: Human Perception and Performance, 10,* 32–39.

Egly, R., Driver, J., & Rafal, R. D. (1994). Shifting visual attention between objects and locations: Evidence from normal and parietal lesion subjects. *Journal of Experimental Psychology: General, 123,* 161–177.

Fendrich, R., Wessinger, C. M., & Gazzaniga, M. S. (1992). Residual vision in a scotoma: Implications for blindsight. *Science, 258,* 1489–1491.

Gazzaniga, M. S., Bogen, J. E., & Sperry, R. W. (1962). Some functional effects of sectioning the cerebral commissures in man. *Proceedings of the National Academy of Sciences, U.S.A., 48,* 1765–1769.

Gazzaniga, M. S., Fendrich, R., & Wessinger, C. M. (1994). Blindsight reconsidered. *Current Directions in Psychological Science, 3,* 93–96.

Grabowecky, M., Robertson, L. C., & Treisman, A. (1993). Preattentive processes guide visual search: Evidence from patients with unilateral visual neglect. *Journal of Cognitive Neuroscience, 5,* 288–302.

Harter, M. R., & Aine, C. J. (1984). Brain mechanisms of visual selective attention. In R. Parasuraman & D. R. Davies (Eds.), *Varieties of attention* (pp. 293–321). Orlando, FL: Academic Press.

Hawkins, H. L., Hillyard, S. A., Luck, S. J., Mouloua, M., Downing, C. J., & Woodward, D. P. (1990). Visual attention modulates signal detectability. *Journal of Experimental Psychology: Human Perception and Performance, 16,* 802–811.

Heinze, H. J., Mangun, G. R., Burchert, W., Hinrichs, H., Scholz, M., Münte, T. F., Gös, A., Scherg, M., Johannes, S., Hundeshagen, H., Gazzaniga, M. S., & Hillyard, S. A. (1994). Combined spatial and temporal imaging of brain activity during visual selective attention in humans. *Nature, 372,* 543–546.

Hillyard, S. A., & Münte, T. F. (1984). Selective attention to color and location: An analysis with event-related brain potentials. *Perception and Psychophysics, 36,* 185–198.

Holtzman, J. D., & Gazzaniga, M. S. (1982). Dual task interactions due exclusively to limits in processing resources. *Science, 218,* 1325–1327.

Holtzman, J. D., & Gazzaniga, M. S. (1985). Enhanced dual task performance following corpus commissurotomy in humans. *Neuropsychologia, 23,* 315–321.

Holtzman, J. D., Volpe, B. T., & Gazzaniga, M. S. (1984). Spatial orienting following commissural section. In R. Parasuraman & D. R. Davies (Eds.), *Varieties of attention* (pp. 375–394). Orlando, FL: Academic Press.

Humphreys, G. W., & Riddoch, M. J. (1993). Interactions between object and space sys tems revealed through neuropsychology. In D. E. Moyer & S. Kornblum (Eds.), *Attention and performance XIV: Synergies in experimental psychology, artificial intelligence and cognitive neuroscience* (pp. 143–162). Cambridge, MA: MIT Press.

Kingstone, A. (1992). Combining expectancies. *Quarterly Journal of Experimental Psychology, 44A,* 69–104.

Kingstone, A. (1995). Covert orienting and the cerebral hemispheres: Solution to a paradox? *Cognitive Neuroscience Society Abstracts, 2,* 21.

Kingstone, A., & Egly, R. (1997). *Space-based and object-based attention effects.* Manuscript submitted for publication.

Kingstone, A., Enns, J., Mangun, G. R., & Gazzaniga, M. S. (1995). Guided visual search is a left hemisphere process in split-brain patients. *Psychological Science, 6,* 118–121.

Kingstone, A., Fendrich, R., Wessinger, C. M., & Reuter-Lorenz, P. A. (1995). Are microsaccades responsible for the gap effect? *Perception and Psychophysics, 57,* 796–801.

Kingstone, A., & Gazzaniga, M. S. (1995). Subcortical transfer of higher-order information: More illusory than real? *Neuropsychology, 9,* 321–328.

Kingstone, A., & Klein, R. M. (1991). Combining shape and position expectancies: Hierarchical processing and selective inhibition. *Journal of Experimental Psychology: Human Perception and Performance, 17,* 512–519.

Kingstone, A., & Klein, R. M. (1993a). What are human express saccades? *Perception and Psychophysics, 54,* 260–273.

Kingstone, A., & Klein, R. M. (1993b). Visual offsets facilitate saccadic latency: Does predisengagement of visuospatial attention mediate this gap effect? *Journal of Experimental Psychology: Human Perception and Performance, 19,* 1251–1265.

Klein, R. M. (1994). Perceptual–motor expectancies interact with covert visual orienting under conditions of endogenous but not exogenous control. *Canadian Journal of Experimental Psychology, 48,* 167–181.

Luck, S., Hillyard, S. A., Mangun, G. R., & Gazzaniga, M. S. (1989). Independent hemispheric attentional systems mediate visual search in split-brain patients. *Nature, 342,* 543–545.

Luck, S., Hillyard, S. A., Mangun, G. R., & Gazzaniga, M. S. (1994). Independent attentional scanning in the separated hemispheres of split-brain patients. *Journal of Cognitive Neuroscience, 6,* 84–91.

Mangun, G. R., Hillyard, S. A., & Luck, S. J. (1993). Electrocortical substrates of visual selective attention. In D. Meyer & S. Kornblum (Eds.), *Attention and performance XIV* (pp. 219–243). Cambridge, MA: MIT Press.

Mangun, G. R., Luck, S. J., Plager, R., Loftus, W., Hillyard, S. A., Handy, T., Clark, V. P., & Gazzaniga, M. S. (1994). Monitoring the visual world: Hemispheric asymmetries and subcortical processes in attention. *Journal of Cognitive Neuroscience, 6,* 267–275.

Munoz, D. P., & Wurtz, R. H. (1992). Role of the rostral superior colliculus in active visual fixation and execution of express saccades. *Journal of Neurophysiology, 67,* 1000–1002.

Pöppel, E., Held, R., & Frost, D. (1973). Residual visual function after brain wounds involving the central visual pathways in man. *Nature, 243,* 295–296.

Posner, M. I., Snyder, C. R. R., &Davidson, B. J. (1980). Attention and the detection of signals. *Journal of Experimental Psychology: General, 109,* 160–174.

Posner, M. I., Walker, J. A., Friedrich, F. J., & Rafal, R. D. (1984). Effects of parietal injury on covert orienting of attention. *Journal of Neuroscience, 4,* 1863–1874.

Posner, M. I., Walker, J. A., Friedrich, F. J., & Rafal, R. D. (1987). How do the parietal lobes direct covert attention? *Neuropsychologia, 25,* 134–145.

Rafal, R. D., & Posner, M. I. (1987). Deficits in human visual spatial attention following thalamic lesions. *Proceedings of the National Academy of Sciences, U.S.A, 84,* 7349–7353.

Rafal, R. D., Posner, M. I., Friedman, J. H., Inhoff, A. W., & Bernstein, E. (1988) Orienting of visual attention in progressive supranuclear palsy. *Brain, 111,* 267–280.

Reuter-Lorenz, P. A., & Fendrich, R. (1990). Orienting attention across the vertical meridian: Evidence from callosotomy patients. *Journal of Cognitive Neuroscience, 2,* 232–238.

Reuter-Lorenz, P. A., Hughes, H. C., & Fendrich, R. (1991). The reduction of saccadic latency by prior offset of the fixation point: An analysis of the "gap effect." *Perception and Psychophysics, 49,* 167–175.

Saslow, M. G. (1967). Effects of components of displacement-step stimuli upon latency for saccadic eye movement. *Journal of the Optical Society of America, 57,* 1024–1029.

Seymour, S. E., Reuter-Lorenz, P. A., & Gazzaniga, M. S. (1994). The disconnection syndrome: Basic findings reaffirmed. *Brain, 117,* 105–115.

Shaw, M. L. (1984). Division of attention among spatial locations: A fundamental difference between detection of letters and detection of luminance increments. In H. Bouma & D. G. Bouwhuis (Eds.), *Attention and performance X* (pp. 109–121). Hillsdale, NJ: Erlbaum.

Sperling, G. (1984). A unified theory of attention and signal detection. In R. Parasuraman & D. R. Davies (Eds.), *Varieties of attention* (pp. 103–181). Orlando, FL: Academic Press.

Sperry, R. W., Gazzaniga, M. S., & Bogen, J. E. (1969). Interhemispheric relationships: The neocortical commissures; syndromes of hemisphere disconnection. In P. J. Vinken & G.W. Bruyn (Eds.), *Handbook of clinical neurology* (Vol. 4, pp. 273–290). Amsterdam: North-Holland.

Taylor, T. Kingstone, A., & Klein, R. (1996). *Visual offsets and oculomotor disinhibition: Endogenous and exogenous contributions to the gap effect.* Manuscript submitted for publication.

Treisman, A. M., Kahneman, D., & Burkell, J. (1983). Perceptual objects and the cost of filtering. *Perception and Psychophysics, 33,* 527–532.

Watt, R. J. (1988). *Visual processing: Computational, psychophysical and cognitive research.* Hillsdale, NJ: Erlbaum.

Weiskrantz, L. (1990). The Ferrier Lecture, 1989. Outlooks for blindsight: Explicit methodologies for implicit processes. *Proceedings of the Royal Society of London, B239,* 247–278.

Wolfe, J. M., Cave, K. R., & Franzel, S. L. (1989). Guided search: An alternative to the feature integration model for visual search. *Journal of Experimental Psychology: Human Perception and Performance, 15,* 419–433.

TWELVE

Attention in Aging and Alzheimer's Disease

BEHAVIOR AND NEURAL SYSTEMS

Pamela M. Greenwood
Raja Parasuraman

H ealthy adult aging in the absence of known disease is accompanied by a number of changes in cognitive skills. Aging also brings an increased risk of degenerative brain disease, most commonly dementia of the Alzheimer type (DAT). Because DAT is primarily a disease of old age, the two states can and often do overlap in their manifestations. Studies suggesting that there are both commonalities and divergences between normal aging and DAT in neural pathology (Kemper, 1994) and in cognitive functioning (Storandt & Hill, 1989) have fueled the long-standing debate on whether DAT represents a quantitative exaggeration of normal aging or a qualitatively different condition (Berg, 1985; Drachman, 1983). Recent cognitive and neuroanatomical studies have provided important new findings relevant to that debate by showing that the very old exhibit some characteristics of mild DAT. For example, in the domain of cognition, visual attention shows progressive changes that appear to fall along a continuum—from "young" older adults, through the very old, to mild DAT patients (Greenwood & Parasuraman, 1994; Parasuraman, Greenwood, Haxby, & Grady, 1992). In the domain of neuropathology, neuronal changes appear to develop in the same orderly manner in normal aging and in DAT (Braak & Braak, 1991). These findings also underscore the importance of understanding the functional and pathological boundaries between aging and DAT. In this chapter we consider the changes in attentional functioning wrought by age and DAT. We also discuss how the changes in age and DAT in neural systems may contribute to impairment in attentional functioning.

ATTENTION AS A MODEL SYSTEM
FOR STUDYING NORMAL AGING AND DAT

Age and DAT do not uniformly dim every aspect of information processing. The more dynamic aspects of cognition are particularly vulnerable. Age alters encoding of features of words more than retrieval of meaning (Madden, 1992). Working memory is impaired, but the organization of established memory is intact (Light, 1992). Implicit memory is spared, while explicit memory is not (Howard, 1988). Divided attention declines more than selective attention (Hartley, 1992). In DAT, focusing of selective attention to simple physical features is relatively well preserved in mildly demented DAT patients, whereas attention to multiple features or tasks is impaired (Parasuraman & Haxby, 1993). Primary memory is less affected by DAT than is secondary memory, and implicit memory performance is often normal (Nebes, 1992).

Whether this pattern of selectivity in cognitive deficits is qualitatively similar for normal aging and DAT is currently a matter of some debate. The issue has been most extensively examined for memory functions. Memory is the most profoundly affected cognitive function in aging and dementia, and progressive severe memory loss is a potentially early sign of DAT. It is not surprising, therefore, that most studies of cognitive functioning in either healthy or demented older adults have focused on memory skills. However, the effects of age and DAT are not limited to memory. DAT patients also have difficulty localizing and manipulating objects in space and exhibit spatial disorientation (for a review see Nebes, 1992). Plude and Hoyer's (1986) conclusion that age effects on visual processing tasks emerge only under conditions of spatial uncertainty may apply to DAT as well. While the ability to shift visuospatial attention to location cues is unchanged in age or DAT, the ability to shift attention away from invalid cues is slowed in normal elderly over age 75 (Greenwood & Parasuraman, 1994) and markedly slowed in patients with DAT (Parasuraman et al., 1992). Feature-based visual search is unchanged with age and in DAT (Greenwood, Parasuraman, & Alexander, 1997), but conjunction-based search is slowed (Plude & Doussard-Roosevelt, 1989), even when valid location cues are used, both in normal aging (Greenwood, Parasuraman, Panicker, & Haxby, 1992; Greenwood & Parasuraman, 1997) and in DAT (Greenwood et al., 1997). This mosaic of results, whereby effects of age and DAT are similar under some conditions but not others, may arise because (1) both the pathologies of age and DAT have selective pro-

clivities for the brain areas and associated neural networks that mediate
the affected processes, and/or (2) the pathologies of age and DAT are
themselves the same, differing only in extent.

There are several reasons for viewing attention as a particularly appropriate model system for studying cognitive changes in normal aging,
DAT, and the interrelationships between aging and DAT. First, the
memory losses of early DAT and of normal aging may be increased by
inefficient attention-based selection of sensory input for further processing. Secondly, there is increasing evidence, reviewed below, that the neural systems which appear to mediate certain types of attention are
selectively vulnerable to the pathologies of advancing age and developing
DAT. Finally, if DAT and normal aging are different conditions with
unique effects on the brain, then it is unlikely that they would exert similar effects both on a given cognitive process and on the neural system mediating that process. Therefore, examining the effects of aging and DAT
on processes whose neural bases are known can contribute to current understanding of the relation between the two conditions.

We confine our discussion to visuospatial attention and divided attention. This is not to imply that these are independent categories of attention or that other aspects are unimportant. Undoubtedly organisms
use all varieties of attention in managing the demands of a complex and
changing visual environment. Rather, much of the available literature on
attention has used tasks that can be conveniently placed into these
categories: spatial cuing and visual search tasks for visuospatial attention,
and dual tasks for divided attention. Many attempts to account for age-
and disease-related changes in attentional ability have relied on constructs
that encompass whole categories of processing such as divided or selective attention. However, a better understanding of how organisms actually monitor visual space requires a more detailed description of the
mechanisms of divided and selective attention. Recent cognitive-
neuroscience investigations have provided information about the neuroanatomy of specific component processes in attention. Based on these, Posner and Petersen (1990) have posited two distinct neural systems of
attention. The ability to marshal and focus attention to locations in extrapersonal space, termed visuospatial attention, is held to depend on the
"posterior attention system" involving the parietal cortex, the pulvinar,
and the superior colliculus. In contrast, the ability to detect targets within attended channels, or to control the direction of attention, what cognitive scientists refer to as control or executive processes of attention, depends
on the "anterior attention system" involving frontal structures. Control
processes are particularly called into play under conditions of divided attention, that is, when attention has to be allocated to two separate tasks
or channels of information. Posner and Petersen assert that the anterior

attention system interacts with the posterior attention system over known corticocortical connections (Goldman-Rakic, 1988) that are themselves vulnerable to DAT (Morrison, 1993). Recent investigations combining behavioral with physiological research methods have made progress in elucidating the component processes and neural systems mediating visuospatial attention (Corbetta, Miezin, Shulman, & Petersen, 1993) and divided attention (Corbetta, Miezin, Dobmeyer, Shulman, & Petersen, 1991). That these two types of attention have been the subjects of theoretical and empirical efforts aimed at identifying their neural bases makes them well suited as model systems for examining the relative effects of aging and of DAT. Accordingly, we will discuss how visuospatial and divided attention are influenced by adult aging and by DAT. In each case our approach will be to describe what is known of the variety of attention first from a cognitive perspective, then from an anatomical perspective, and finally in terms of possible neural mechanisms.

VISUOSPATIAL ATTENTION

Visual input is generally considered to be controlled by eye and head movements. However, visual attention can also be shifted in the absence of overt orienting movements. This form of attention, visuospatial attention, may be a mechanism for bringing various processing resources to bear on a location in space where an event is expected. Visuospatial attention has been the subject of extensive investigation in the past few years. Two tasks have been used prominently in these studies, the location cue response time (RT) method developed by Posner (1980) and the visual search paradigm used by Treisman and colleagues (e.g., Treisman & Gelade, 1980).

Location Cue Paradigm

This method manipulates the validity with which a spatial precue predicts the location of a subsequent target while the participant fixates a central spot. The latency of response to detect or discriminate a cued target is measured. In the typical cued location task, responses are faster (Posner, 1980) and more accurate (Bashinski & Bacharach, 1980) to targets appearing at validly cued spatial locations than to targets at uncued locations, presumably because the focus of spatial attention is shifted to the cued location and sensory processing of the target is facilitated (Downing, 1988; Hawkins et al., 1990). Larger event-related potentials are also seen to validly cued targets (Harter & Anllo-Vento, 1991). This is termed the "benefit" of a valid cue. Responses are slower and less accurate to invalidly cued targets than to uncued targets. This is termed the "cost" of an invalid cue.

The type of precue influences the nature of the attention shift: peripheral cues appear to summon attention reflexively, and they are most effective when the interval between the cue and the target (or stimulus-onset asynchrony [SOA]) is short; whereas central, symbolic cues appear to elicit a voluntary mode of attention shifting, and they are most effective at longer SOAs (Jonides, 1981; Muller & Rabbitt, 1989). Posner and colleagues have proposed that at least three subsystems contribute to covert shifts of visuospatial attention: focusing (or engagement) of attention at the cued location, movement, and shifting (or disengagement) of attention from a cued location (Posner, Walker, Friderich, & Rafal, 1984). As will be seen below, these subsystems are differentially affected by age and by DAT.

Effects of Normal Adult Aging

Processes of visuospatial attention appear to be affected only modestly by normal aging, at least up to about 75 years of age. When simple detection tasks are used, age does not alter either the ability to allocate or to shift visuospatial attention in response to location cues (Greenwood, Parasuraman, & Haxby, 1993; Hartley, Kieley, & Slabach, 1990; Nissen & Corkin, 1985; Robinson & Kertzman, 1990), even up to age 85 (Greenwood & Parasuraman, 1994). When discrimination tasks are used, age effects do emerge, although not uniformly. Hartley and colleagues (1990) found that effects of cue validity on RT increased with age in a character discrimination task with central cues (71% valid); but in a separate experiment with peripheral cues they found no age effects. Greenwood et al. (1993) compared the effects of central and peripheral cues in the same participants on a cued letter-discrimination task in mixed blocks (60% valid; 20% invalid; 20% neutral). When participants were grouped by age decade from the 20s to the 70s, there was a small but significant increase with age group in the total costs and benefits of cue validity on RT with central cues but not with peripheral cues.

Effects of cue validity on age are less robust when cues are 100% valid. Using only valid peripheral cues, Madden (1990) saw an age effect only in the lack of cue validity effects in the older group except for a narrow range of SOAs (150–183 milliseconds). Subsequently, Madden (1992), using both valid and invalid cues, found that the benefits of 100% valid peripheral cues on discrimination RT were greater in the old than the young only when the target duration was limited to 142 milliseconds. The cost of 100% invalid cues did not differ between groups. Folk and Hoyer (1992) also used blocked trials with either 100% valid or 100% invalid cues. Whether cues were central or peripheral, no age effects were found. Considered together, these results suggest that effects of age on cue validity are strongest when cue validity is less than 100% and valid and invalid cues are intermixed; when central cues are used; and when tasks are made more difficult by use of short target durations, distractors, or a requirement to discriminate.

In each of these studies of aging and visuospatial attention, the oldest participants tested had a mean age of 72 years or less. Greenwood and Parasuraman (1994) predicted that age effects should be magnified in "old old" versus "young old" individuals and found that cue validity effects on RT were greater in a group aged 75–85 than in a group aged 65–74 (Figure 12.1). While valid cues conferred similar RT benefits on both groups, the old old group had significantly longer RTs to invalid cues (RT costs) than did the young old group.

Effects of DAT

While effects of DAT on visuospatial attention are greater than those of normal aging, they are similarly selective. When visuospatial task requirements are relatively undemanding, as in cued detection, effects of DAT are not significant in spite of clear effects of cue validity on RT (Nissen, Corkin, & Growdon, 1981; Parasuraman et al., 1992). However, effects of DAT do emerge when discrimination tasks are employed. Parasuraman et al. (1992) found that patients in early DAT showed RT benefits of location cues that were similar to those of age-matched controls, indicating that the ability to focus spatial attention was not substantially compromised by the disease. However, the DAT patients showed increased RT costs following invalid location cues, whether central or peripheral, suggesting that both automatic and voluntary forms of attentional shifting are degraded in early DAT. The result for central cues has been replicated in mild-to-moderate DAT patients (Oken, Kishiyama, Kaye, & Howieson, 1994). Figure 12.2 shows that the effect of DAT on combined RT costs and benefits is greater than the effect of advanced age but qualitatively similar (Greenwood et al., 1993).

Finally, DAT spares some functions. The difference in results between detection and discrimination tasks shows that even in dementing illness the components of visuospatial attention are functional when task demands are low. Also, development of central cue validity occurs more slowly than peripheral cue validity in DAT patients (Parasuraman et al., 1992), as well as in normal elderly and normal young (Muller & Rabbitt, 1989; Greenwood et al., 1993), showing that the time course of visuospatial processing is unaffected either by age or by DAT.

Visual Search Paradigm

The visual search paradigm does not depend on location cues to direct spatial attention but rather requires speeded search for a target appearing

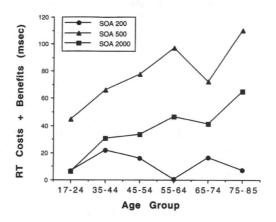

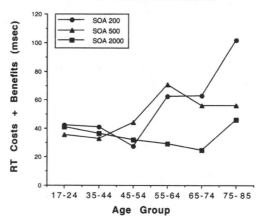

FIGURE 12.1. Total cue-validity effects (invalid − valid RT) for a cued letter-discrimination task in normal adults in six age groups from 17 to 85. Based on data reported in Greenwood and Parasuraman (1994).

unpredictably in an array of distractor stimuli. Different results are obtained at the extremes of target–distractor similarity. Where the target differs from the distractors by a unique feature, such as a pink "T" amid blue and green "N's" and "G's," the number of distractors in the array has no effect on the time to detect the target (Julesz & Bergen, 1983; Treisman, 1985). Treisman's influential feature integration theory of visual attention (Treisman & Gelade, 1980), which has guided much of the work with this paradigm, posits that visual features are encoded through pre-

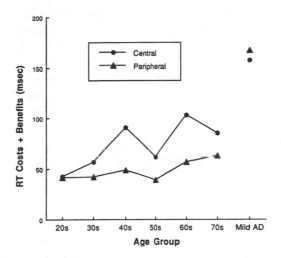

FIGURE 12.2. Total cue-validity effects (invalid RT − valid RT) for a cued letter-discimination task in normal adults in each decade from the 20s to the 70s and in patients with mild DAT. Based on data reported in Greenwood et al. (1993) and Parasuraman et al. (1992).

attentive analyses performed in parallel over the visual field, producing the phenomenon of "pop-out." The theory claims this preattentive process interprets signals from a sensory map encoding the target's unique feature. Therefore, "pop-out" is said to arise when search occurs over all items in parallel. This is termed "parallel search." In contrast, when the target differs from the distractors by a conjunction of features ("conjunction search," such as a pink "T" amid pink, blue, and green "N's" and "G's"), the time to detect the target increases linearly with the number of distractors. Treisman claims this result arises when serial deployment of visuospatial attention is required to each item. This is termed "serial search." While Treisman has partially based her theory of visual search on the independence of serial and parallel search, recent findings have tended to weaken the view that all search for conjunctions of features is necessarily serial. Wolfe and colleagues have proposed a modified version of Treisman's feature integration theory called "guided search," which attempts to account for data showing that fast, apparently parallel, conjunction search is possible (see Cave & Wolfe, 1990; Nakayama & Silverman, 1986). Rejecting the "spotlight" view of attention inherent in both Treisman's and Cave and Wolfe's accounts of visual search, Duncan and colleagues (Duncan & Humphreys, 1989; Desimone & Duncan, 1995) have postulated that attention emerges from the mechanisms that resolve the competition for visual processes that is claimed to arise between visually perceived objects.

These mechanisms are thought to be biased toward objects by spatial location or by features or conjunctions of features, so that search is always parallel. While in the present chapter we adopt the vocabulary of "spotlight" theory by using the terms of serial (conjunction) and parallel (feature) search, the phenomena might be better described as "hard" and "easy" search. From the point of view of this discussion, it is sufficient to note that these two types of search have different properties and are affected differently by age and by DAT. We will continue to discuss attention as containing both a serial and a parallel process, while acknowledging the possibility that the underlying mechanisms may be entirely parallel.

Effects of Normal Adult Aging

While age slows the ability to search through arrays of items, the effects are not uniform. Older participants are slower than young in searching for an easily discriminable target, but neither the young nor the old show an effect on RT of the number of distractors (Greenwood et al., 1992; Plude & Doussard-Roosevelt, 1989). In other words, feature search is performed similarly by young and old participants. In contrast, on conjunction search trials, the increase in RT with number of distractors was greater in the normally aged than in the young (Plude & Doussard-Roosevelt, 1989; Greenwood et al., 1992). Nevertheless, the elderly were as able as the young to selectively search through one of the relevant features of the conjunction target when the number of distractors possessing that feature was held constant, for example, in a display of pink, blue, and green letters, the number of pink distractors is held constant so that search for a pink "T" can be confined to the pink letters. According to Plude and Doussard-Roosevelt this result showed that young and old used a similar searching strategy. Greenwood et al. (1992; Greenwood & Parasuraman, 1997) reasoned that if this slowing of conjunction search with age is due to slowed shifting of visuospatial attention, then the use of precues to target location would eliminate age effects. In both young and old, RT increased with cue size; that is, as the cue enclosed more nontargets and thus became less informative, search slowed. However, when cues predicted the exact location and size of the target on conjunction trials, search in the young was speeded to the level seen on feature search trials. In the old, conjunction search was still slower than feature search even with the smallest and most precise cue size. This suggests that although location cues do produce a shift of visuospatial attention to the cued area regardless of age, only in the young does the focusing of visuospatial attention in response to the location cue eliminate the additional time needed to detect a conjunction compared to a feature target. In the old, the presence of visuospatial attention at the target location does not eliminate the slower processing of conjunction search.

Effects of DAT

The effect of parietal lesions is relevant to a discussion of the effects of DAT on visuospatial processing because the parietal lobes are the first to become hypometabolic in the early stage of DAT (Haxby, Duara, Grady, Cutler, & Rapoport, 1985; Haxby et al., 1986). Patients with unilateral neglect, regardless of visual field defects, were faster in feature search than in conjunction search, but their feature search times were slower than those of the elderly controls and, unlike those controls, increased with number of distractors (Eglin, Robertson, & Knight, 1989). The investigators concluded that the lesions underlying neglect (1) result in serial search even for feature targets, suggesting that the ability to experience "pop-out" may require intact parietal lobes, and (2) disrupt the disengagement of visuospatial attention. However, somewhat different results were obtained in patients without field defects. Carefully controlling eye movements, Arguin and colleagues studied three patients with large parieto-occipito-temporal lesions but no field defects who were slower to respond to contralesional than to ipsilesional targets following location cues (Arguin, Joanette, & Cavanagh, 1993). In a visual search task, these patients were slowed in the contralesional field in conjunction search but not in feature search.

Studying DAT itself, Saffran, Fitzpatrick-DeSalme, and Coslett (1990) observed that two patients with DAT and marked visual disturbances were able to perform feature (parallel) search with no effect of array size but were completely unable to perform serial search. In contrast, Greenwood et al. (1997) found that the pattern of parallel and serial search performance in mild DAT patients was similar to that of the normal elderly, with parallel search latency unaffected by the number of distractors whereas serial search latency increased with number of distractors. Search slopes (rate of increase in RT as a function of cue size) were smaller in DAT than in normal elderly participants, suggesting that the patients obtained less benefit from precue precision. In feature search, the effect of precue size did not alter the performance of either normal elderly or DAT patients. In conjunction search, although in normal elderly RT slowed as the size of valid precues increased, in the DAT patients valid precues had little effect on search RT, producing flatter slopes. This suggests that DAT patients may not be able to adjust the size of the attentional focus in response to changing cue size. Moreover, the overall effects of cue validity, measured by combined costs and benefits, were substantially smaller in the DAT patients than in the normal elderly. This stands in contrast to the increased effects of cue validity in DAT seen in a nonsearch directed attention task (Greenwood et al., 1993). It should be noted that Greenwood et al. (1997) found that parallel search times in DAT patients did not increase with the number of distractors as was reported for neglect patients by Eglin et al. (1989). To the extent that both neglect and DAT patients have parietal dysfunction, the two disease states should exert similar effects. An increase in search time with distractor number indicates low target–distractor discriminability, and therefore the patients of Eglin et al. may have had trouble discriminating targets and distractors.

The studies reviewed above show that while the ability to effectively deploy visuospatial attention is changed by normal aging up to 75 years, the magnitude of the effect increases beyond 75 years, becoming even greater in mild-to-moderate DAT. Specifically, while the ability to shift and engage visuospatial attention is unimpaired in normal aging, the ability to disengage visuospatial attention from invalidly cued space is vulnerable to brain changes in advanced old age, parietal injury and DAT. In addition, the ability to adjust the size of the focus of visuospatial attention, while normal in age, is altered in DAT. Finally, while parallel search is unaffected by either age or DAT, serial search is slowed in aging and even more in DAT. If, as Triesman claims, serial but not parallel search requires visuospatial attention, then the need to repeatedly shift visuospatial attention from one item to the next in visual search would necessarily involve disengagement. Therefore, slowed disengagement could underly slowed visual search. Are these selective behavioral changes a consequence of equally selective neuropathology in aging and DAT?

Functional Neuroanatomy of Visuospatial Attention

In order to determine whether brain changes common to normal aging and DAT underly the disturbances in visuospatial attention, we need to identify the mediating structures. Associating a system of attention with a certain brain region benefits from an approach that avoids broadly defined types of attention. Such an approach has arisen in recent years from neuropsychological investigations that associate components of attentional processing with neuroanatomic structures or networks of structures. Attentional processing is fractionated into components, and neural systems are postulated to mediate the components. Based on studies of unilateral neglect arising from brain damage, Mesulam (1981) proposed a network of three local cortical systems for the control of visuospatial attention: the posterior parietal area providing a sensory representation of extrapersonal space; the frontal cortex contributing a map of exploratory and orienting movements; the cingulate cortex mapping motivational values to space. Goldman-Rakic (1988) has amassed evidence from experimental lesions in monkeys that visuospatial attention is mediated by a network involving frontal and parietal areas and linked to the medial pulvinar. The most specific model was put forward by Posner and Petersen (1990), who proposed that the superior parietal lobe is involved in disengaging visuospatial attention, the midbrain in shifting the focus of attention to the target area, and the pulvinar in obtaining data from the attended location. Such models as these allow specific predictions of selective association between each processing component and brain regions or networks of regions. After considering evidence for the role of each anatomic area claimed to mediate components of visuospatial processing, we will examinine the vulnerability of these structures to pathologies of aging and DAT.

Theoretical claims have been made for a role for the pulvinar of the thalamus in visuospatial attention. However, some of the relevant evidence concerns the thalamus as a whole. Patients with unilateral hemorrhagic lesions of the thalamus have abnormally slowed responses to contralateral compared to ipsilateral targets, regardless of whether location precues are valid or invalid (Rafal & Posner, 1987). This suggests reduced ability to engage attention in the visual field contralateral to the thalamic damage. A subgroup of DAT patients with particular deficits in set shifting and visual search have decreased radiodensity in the dorsomedial thalamus (Forstl & Sahakian, 1993). Considering the pulvinar itself, LaBerge (1990) reported increased glucose metabolism in the pulvinar contralateral to a display requiring detection of a target letter flanked by distractor letters in comparison to the condition in which the target appeared alone. In contrast, Corbetta et al. (1993) did not find activation of the pulvinar during a task directing visuospatial attention with spatial cues. However, scanning occurred during a run of trials over which cues were 95% valid and therefore the components of shifting and engaging, but not disengaging, were active during the scan. Shifting and engaging are the very processing components shown to increase unit activity in the pulvinar in monkeys (Robinson & Petersen, 1992). In short, current understanding of the role of the pulvinar is limited.

The posterior parietal area was postulated by Posner and Petersen (1990) to mediate disengagement, the shifting of visuospatial attention away from invalidly cued space. Posner et al. (1984) observed that although patients with superior parietal lobe lesions were unimpaired in engaging attention following a valid cue, they were selectively slowed in disengaging attention following an invalid cue, reflected in very long RTs to invalidly cued targets. Parasuraman et al. (1992) found that patients in the early, mild stage of DAT also show an increase in RT costs of invalid cues while showing no concomitant increase in benefits of valid cues. Furthermore, combined RT costs and benefits were correlated with rates of resting glucose metabolism in the superior, but not the inferior, parietal area. Corbetta et al. (1993) found that both the superior frontal (near area 6) and the superior parietal (near area 7) cortex showed greater blood flow during a task requiring shifts of visuospatial attention but not during a detection task with the same stimuli. The importance of the parietal cortex to the process of disengagement has also been emphasized by recordings in monkey intraparietal sulcus where a subset of neurons discharged best to a target after a peripheral cue directed attention away from the target location (Robinson, Bowman, & Kertzman, 1991).

These several strands of evidence emphasize the importance of the posterior parietal area to visuospatial attention. Both pathological and imaging data agree with the view, embodied in the models put forward by Goldman-Rakic (1988) and Posner and Petersen (1990), that visuospatial attention depends on a network involving the pulvinar and both frontal and posterior parietal areas. Posterior parietal areas are linked with the disengagement of visuospatial attention from a cued location (Posner et al., 1984; Robinson et al., 1991; Parasuraman et al., 1992). Although the pulvinar seems to be involved in visuospatial attention (Rafal & Posner, 1987; LaBerge, 1990), the nature of its role is less clear. Finally, the involvement of both frontal and parietal areas in visuospatial attention argues for mediation by a corticocortical network. We are interested in the mediation of visuospatial attention in order to understand why that process is altered in age and DAT. To this point we have shown that the selective effect on processes of visuospatial attention by normal aging is magnified and extended in DAT. We have summarized the evidence implicating thalamic and posterior parietal areas in the mediation of visuospatial attention. It remains to determine whether these mediating structures (1) undergo selective alteration in age and DAT and (2) whether the alteration is similar in the two conditions.

Pathological Changes in Mediating Structures of Visuospatial Attention

What is the evidence that the two areas most strongly implicated in visuospatial attention undergo pathological changes in normal aging and in DAT? The thalamus is not usually listed as a site of major pathological change in age or DAT (Kemper, 1994). However, recent work has shown that the anterior dorsal nucleus of the thalamus as well as the entorhinal area are the first sites where age-related pathological changes are seen (Braak & Braak, 1991). Neurofibrillary tangles (NFTs), which are found as one of the pathognomonic changes of DAT, first appear in the soma and dendrites of a neuron and remain as "ghost tangles" after neuron death. In DAT there is a correlation between the number of NFTs and the severity of dementia (Berg, McKeel, Miller, Baty, & Morris, 1993) whereas no such relationship is seen for neuritic plaques. Another thalamic nucleus, the medial dorsal nucleus, develops NFTs in some normally aged brains (Grossi, Lopez, & Martinez, 1989). While reductions in overall thalamic volume are not seen in normal aging (Jernigan, Archibald, et al., 1991), such reductions are seen in mild DAT (Jernigan, Salmon, Butters, & Hesselink, 1991). Therefore, although the thalamus seems to play a role in visuospatial attention, it does not seem to be an important factor in the age-related changes seen in that process. Thalamic pathology could underly the changes in visuospatial attention in DAT. Unfortunately, much of the evidence of thalamic mediation in visuospatial attention pertains to the pulvinar of the thalamus. Although the pulvinar has not been well studied pathologically, there is a recent report of clusters of tangles in the pulvinar of DAT patients, but not of nondemented elderly (Kuljis, 1991).

The evidence is stronger for selective pathology in the posterior parietal cortex in normal aging and in DAT. In magnetic resonance imaging measurements, all cortical regions show reductions in gray matter volume in both age and DAT (Jernigan, Archibald, et al., 1991; Jernigan, Salmon, et al., 1991). Blood flow is also reduced bilaterally with age in cingulate, parahippocampal, superior temporal, medial frontal, and posterior parietal cortices (Martin, Friston, Colebatch, & Frackowiak, 1991). Even during activation tasks orbitofrontal and premotor areas are hypometabolic in old compared to young individuals. Left posterior inferior parietal areas and left posterior superior temporal areas are hypometabolic at rest in DAT and do not show increased metabolism with task-related activation (Duara, Loewenstein, & Barker, 1990). Affected cortical areas undergo mainly volumetric and metabolic changes in aging, showing frank neuropathology only at Braak and Braak's stage III (1991), which includes some individuals with DAT. The pathologies of normal aging are similar in type, although not in degree, to those seen in DAT. In mild DAT with only memory loss, parietal association areas are asymmetrically hypometabolic at rest. In moderate DAT, this hypometabolism is correlated with neuropsychological impairment (Haxby et al., 1986). Taken together, these data suggest that the declines of physiological functioning in prefrontal and posterior parietal areas in normal aging increase in DAT, becoming correlated with neuropsychological deficits.

Both age and DAT also lead to changes at the cellular level. While a body of work indicates age-related declines in cell numbers in superior frontal, superior temporal, precentral, and postcentral areas and the striatum (e.g., Ball, 1978; Ball & Lo, 1977), more recent reports find decreased cell size but minimal or no cell loss (e.g., Haug & Eggers, 1991). There is also a selective decline in synaptic parameters. In normal aging a 10% decrease in number of synapses occurs in parietal and prefrontal areas but not in motor areas (Haug & Eggers, 1991). While in normally aged brains increases in synaptic length appear to compensate for any cell loss, in mild and moderate DAT the greater cell loss is accompanied by declines in synaptic density (DeKosky & Scheff, 1990; Lippa, Hamos, Pulaski-Salo, Degennaro, & Drachman, 1992). In DAT, synaptic density in midfrontal and inferior parietal areas is correlated with cognitive impairment (Terry et al., 1991). NFTs first appear in DAT in the hippo-campal formation, subsequently develop in temporal neocortex, then in orbitofrontal, parietal, and cingulate cortices, and finally in sensorimo-tor and visual cortex (Fewster, Griffin-Brooks, MacGregor, Ojalvo-Rose, & Ball, 1991). The order and pattern of the appearance of NFTs is simi-lar in normal age and in mild DAT, although the extent is greater in DAT (Price, Davis, Morris, & White, 1991; Braak & Braak, 1991). However, the effects of age are not always linear. While dendritic extent in the den-tate gyrus increased in the 5th and 7th decades but regressed in the 8th and 9th decades of nondemented elderly (Flood, Buell, Defiore, Horwitz, & Coleman, 1985), in DAT patients dendritic extent does not increase at any age (Coleman & Flood, 1987). This finding is consistent with selec-tive slowing in disengagement of visuospatial attention in the elderly over age 75 (Greenwood & Parasuraman, 1994).

Thus, there is considerable overlap in brain regions vulnerable to effects of both age and DAT, and the course of pathological change is substantially similar in the two conditions. This review of the neuroana-tomical literature leads to the conclusion that pathological changes arise in mesial temporal, prefrontal, superior temporal, and parietal areas in both normal aging and in DAT, albeit with substantial differences in de-gree between the two. Posterior parietal cortex is subject to pathological changes in both aging and DAT. Both old age and DAT are also associat-ed with alterations in brain regions not associated with visuospatial at-tention, such as mesial and superior temporal regions. DAT eventually adds nearly all the neocortex to the list of affected regions, although in the early, mild stages in which many cognitive studies are conducted changes in regional metabolism occur selectively in parietal and temporal association areas. In fact, patients in very-early-stage DAT with no non-memory deficits have metabolic reductions largely confined to parietal as-sociation cortex (Haxby et al., 1986; Grady et al., 1988). Nevertheless, in DAT the selective degeneration of pyramidal cells giving rise to corticocor-tical connections (de Lacoste & White, 1993; Morrison, 1993) may have a particularly adverse effect on functions dependent on corticocortical com-munication, such as those proposed for visuospatial processing (Goldman-Rakic, 1988; Posner & Petersen, 1990). Although increased right/left asymmetry in frontal and parietal association areas occurs early in the course of DAT (Haxby et al., 1986), the appearance of frankly decreased frontal lobe metabolism only late in the disease (Friston & Frackowiak, 1991) may downplay its role in the behavioral effects of early DAT. Final-ly, not all regions believed to contribute to attention are altered in aging. For example, we are unaware of evidence of pathological changes in the pulvinar in aging despite its importance in several current neuropsychological models of visuospatial attention. Therefore, studies of normal elderly and mild DAT patients are to a certain extent studies of individuals with some abnormalities in mesial temporal areas (Braak & Braak, 1991) and in superior temporal and posterior parietal cortices (Martin et al., 1991), as well as with reduced corticocortical connectivity (Morrison, 1993). While the brain changes occurring in age and DAT are not global, neither are they limited to those areas believed to mediate visuospatial attention.

DIVIDED ATTENTION

The ability to perform two tasks at once is often termed "divided attention," although this term is also used to refer to single tasks in which multifeature stimuli must be attended. In this section we focus on dual-task studies, since there is a considerable literature on age-related effects in dual-task performance (Hartley, 1992). Whether dual task performance is achieved by sharing of attentional resources between the two tasks or by successive switching of attention between tasks has been debated (Hartley, 1992; Wickens, 1984). Nevertheless, many studies show that dual-task performance is poorer than performance of the component single tasks. Moreover, as will be seen below, imaging studies suggest that the ability to divide attention is dependent on frontal brain areas and, by implication, on Posner and Petersen's (1990) "anterior attention system." It is therefore of interest to enquire into the effects of age and DAT on this ability.

Age-Related Changes in Divided Attention

The appearance of a divided-attention deficit in the course of normal aging is well accepted, although there is no agreement on the source of the deficit. Divided attention has typically been studied with a dual task — two tasks performed simultaneously. However, many of the earlier studies used tasks on which the young outperformed the old on either task singly. If age differences exist on singly performed tasks, then age differences with the two tasks performed simultaneously cannot be attributed solely to a divided-attention deficit. In an effort to eliminate this problem, Salthouse and colleagues (Somberg & Salthouse, 1982; Salthouse, Rogan, & Prill, 1984) adjusted stimulus items to equate the performance of two perceptual tasks separately before presenting them together in a dual task. In these tasks, two sets of characters were presented simultaneously. Participants were induced by monetary payoffs to allocate different percentages of attention to each of the two sets, either all to one set or in intermediate stages. For example, Somberg and Salthouse (1982) used percentages of either 100/0 or 0/100 to one or the other task, and percentages of 70/30, 50/50, 30/70 to both tasks. While no age differences in divided attention were seen in the first study, the more difficult tasks used in the second study did elicit age effects (Salthouse et al. 1984). Divided-attention costs, assessed as ratios of divided-attention performance to single-task performance, were greater in the old than in the young. Subsequent work has confirmed these findings. Ponds, Brouwer, and van Wolffelaar (1988), adjusting each component task in a dual task for difficulty, found higher divided-attention costs in screened elderly compared to young and middle-aged participants in simultaneous driving and speeded dot-counting tasks. Korteling (1991) also found an older group performed more poorly when two tracking tasks, equated for average error, were performed simultaneously. Salthouse et al. (1984) argued that age differences in divided attention arise from coordination of two demanding concurrent tasks; they speculated that they found age effects whereas Somberg and Salthouse (1982) did not because the number of component mental operations was greater in the latter study. McDowd and Craik (1988) examined this suggestion that division of attention increases the complexity of a task by requiring the involvement of more mental operations. By directly plotting RT of old participants against RT of young participants from tasks varying in difficulty under dual- and single-task conditions, these investigators found that the effect of divided attention was similar to the effect of increased task complexity on single-task performance. It was concluded that although the relative costs of divided attention were higher in the old, the effects of divided attention on the elderly are equivalent to the effects of increased task complexity.

Another approach to studying the effect of age on divided attention has been to ask whether certain stages of processing are more vulnerable to divided attention in normal aging. Nestor, Parasuraman, and Haxby (1989) and Greenwood and Parasuraman (1991) used an auditory probe during a letter-match task to determine the attentional cost of various stages in the processing of letter matching, namely, the encoding and the matching/response selection stages. The primary letter-match task presented an uppercase letter followed after 1 second by a lowercase letter and required the participant to indicate whether the two letters were the same or different. It was assumed that the amount of processing ("attentional cost") demanded by one stage of this task would be reflected in the length of time taken to respond to a probe tone presented during that stage. Probes were presented either (1) before the first letter, (2) 50 milliseconds after the first letter (encoding stage), or (3) after the second letter (matching/response selection stage). In the aged, probe RT was slowed only minimally during the encoding stage but was slowed substantially during the matching/response stage (Nestor et al., 1989). The age-related slowing in probe RT during the match/response selection stage occurred similarly in both "young old'" and "old old" groups and was not mitigated by practice (Greenwood & Parasuraman, 1991). Guttentag and Madden (1987) also examined whether the age effect on divided attention occurred equally in all stages of processing. Probe tone presentation occurred either 400 millisecond before primary task presentation or up to 650 milliseconds after primary task presentation. The changes in probe tone RT over the interval between the probe tone and the primary task of visual categorization were similar for old, middle-aged, and young participants. From this Guttentag and Madden concluded that the effect of divided attention was present at all stages of the primary task. This result is consistent with Salthouse and colleagues' (1984) view (above) that age effects arise from problems in coordinating two tasks due to the increased number of task component operations when two tasks are used.

Finally, while some studies did not find effects of age on divided attention, these used individuals under the age of 65 (Baddeley, Della Sala, Logie, & Spinnler, 1986; Wickens, Braune, & Stokes, 1987). This review of the literature shows that divided-attention performance declines after age 65, but only when task demands are sufficiently great. Also, while the ability to divide attention decreases in age, the effect appears to be general with all processing stages affected similarly. The view put forward by Salthouse et al. (1984) that age effects in divided attention depend on the number of task components could be tested by comparing performance of the elderly on tasks varying in the number of objectively rated processing components. If Salthouse et al. (1984) are correct, then greater divided-attention deficits in the elderly compared to the young would be seen on tasks with larger numbers of components.

Divided Attention in DAT

The necessity of dividing attention between features of a stimulus or between two sources of stimulation seems to present an even greater problem to DAT patients than to the normally aged. Divided attention in DAT has been most commonly studied with dual-task paradigms. Baddeley et al. (1986) combined a primary task of pursuit tracking with secondary tasks of oral counting, simple auditory RT, and digit span. Single-task performance of pursuit tracking and digit span were equated for all participants. The DAT group, of mixed severity, was significantly worse on the dual-task version compared to the single-task one, while neither age-matched elderly nor young were so impaired. Progression of DAT in the same patients over 6-month testing intervals was accompanied by a greater effect of the secondary task on the primary tracking task (Baddeley, Bressi,

Della Sala, Logie, & Spinnler, 1991). Using a primary task of pursuit tracking and a secondary task of speeded discrimination, Tinklenberg, Taylor, Peabody, Redington, and Gibson (1984) also found greater effects of divided attention in moderate DAT than in mild DAT. Grober and Sliwinski (1991) required the retention of a list of digits simultaneously with performance of a letter-match task. While all participants were unimpaired in performance of each task separately, performance of the tasks together resulted in a deficit for the elderly only when the digits were required to be recalled in order. The DAT groups showed a divided attention deficit whether or not they were required to recall in order, suggesting to these investigators that the division of attention affects different processes in normal aging and DAT.

Using a different approach to study divided attention, Nebes and Brady (1989) presented letter arrays of varying sizes and required detection of a target appearing in the array on half of the trials. While normal aging did not affect performance of the tasks, DAT did cause slower target detection in mildly and moderately affected patients, particularly with the larger arrays. Filoteo et al. (1992) used the "global–local" task that divided attention between a condition requiring detection of a target number when it was formed by another number (i.e., large number "1" composed of small number "3's") and a condition in which it formed another number (i.e., a small number "1's" forming a large "3"). Consistent with the results of Nebes and Brady (1989), the mild-to-moderate DAT patients had particularly slowed RTs relative to age-matched controls, more so than on a directed-attention task in the same study.

While these studies show a divided-attention deficit in DAT, they do not provide information on the mechanisms that are vulnerable to that disease. In order to determine which stage of processing, that is, encoding of stimuli or decision making, is most affected by divided attention, Nestor, Parasuraman, and Haxby (1991) employed the probe-RT paradigm described above in which RT to a simple auditory stimulus probes the attentional demands required by each stage of processing of a letter-match task (i.e., encoding and matching/response selection). Even though mild DAT patients were able to accurately perform the letter-match and auditory RT tasks separately, they showed a dual-task deficit in the form of increased probe RT during the letter-match stage. However, probe RT was not selectively increased during either the encoding or the matching/response selection processing stages, leading the investigators to conclude that dual-task deficits in DAT can be attributed to demands of task coordination, consistent with the interpretation offered by Salthouse et al. (1984) to explain age-related deficits in divided attention.

Thus, the ability to divide attention declines in normal aging beyond age 65 or so, with an even greater decline in DAT. Divided-attention performance also appears to deteriorate as DAT progresses. Finally, in both normal aging and DAT, dividing attention affects equally the encoding and response selection stages of processing.

Functional Neuroanatomy of Divided Attention

To establish the neuroanatomic bases of divided attention, measures of regional brain function have been related to the ability to divide attention. Studying dichotic listening, Grady et al. (1989) found that the poorer dichotic performance seen in DAT patients was associated with evidence (obtained by computed-tomography scanning) of bilateral atrophy in anterior temporal regions and with reduced resting glucose metabolism in left superior temporal regions. Thus, impaired dual-task, but not single-task (monotic), performance was associated with the brain changes of DAT. Somewhat different results were obtained by Nestor, Parasuraman, Haxby, and Grady (1991), who reported that locally reduced resting metabolism in right parietal and right frontal premotor association areas in mild DAT patients was associated with slowed responding under dual-task but not under single-task conditions. In contrast, the metabolism of normal elderly individuals was not significantly associated with dual-task performance. Corbetta et al. (1991) measured regional cerebral metabolism during a task that required detection of a change in any one of three concurrent stimulus dimensions. Outside of visual areas, a metabolic increase was seen in the right prefrontal cortex and the anterior cingulate of normal young participants. This association of divided attention with increased metabolic activity in the right hemisphere is consistent with Mesulam's (1981) view of the importance of the right hemisphere in attention. The specificity of activity in the right prefrontal area to divided attention was attested to by the absence of activation in this area during selective attention. Also, during divided attention, blood flow was reduced in areas that were metabolically active during selective attention (caudate, thalamus, and premotor, insular, and lateral orbitofrontal cortices). The anterior cingulate was also selectively active during divided attention in the Corbetta et al. (1991) study. However, in light of evidence that the anterior cingulate is also active during the Stroop task (Pardo, Pardo, Janer, & Raichle, 1990) and in tasks of verbal memory (Grasby et al., 1993), cingulate activation may not be specific to divided attention. Therefore, the best indications implicate right frontal areas in divided-attention ability.

This evidence of right frontal involvement in divided attention fits with the conclusions of Moscovitch and Winocur (1992), based on neuropsychological studies, that cognitive changes in normal aging arise from modest declines in the functioning of frontal and hippocampal areas. Hartley (1993) has also argued for the importance of frontal areas in divided attention. He reasoned that since effects of age are small when visuospatial attention is required but large when divided attention is required, aging affects mainly Posner and Petersen's (1990) anterior attention system. There are two arguments against this view: First, as discussed above, the parietal lobes, which are part of the posterior attention system, do undergo age-related changes; secondly, while effects of age on the posterior attention system may not be large, they have been demonstrated (Plude & Doussard-Roosevelt, 1989; Greenwood et al., 1993; Hartley, 1993).

Pathological Changes in Mediating Structures of Divided Attention

If frontal, especially right prefrontal, areas are important for dual-task performance, what is the evidence that these areas undergo selective pathological change in normal aging and DAT? Magnetic resonance imaging studies have found that all cortical gray matter decreases in volume in aging (Jernigan, Archibald, et al., 1991). In contrast, it has been reported that the frontal lobes lose about 10% of their volume by the 80th year, while the parietal and temporal lobes undergo only insignificant losses. However, even within the frontal lobes changes are not uniform. Frontal area 6 shows neuron shrinkage beginning in the 40th year but neuron shrinkage does not occur until age 65 in frontal area 11 (Haug & Eggers, 1991). Orbitofrontal and premotor areas were selectively more hypometabolic in activation tasks in the old than in the young (Duara et al., 1990). As described above, blood flow was reduced bilaterally with age in a number of structures including two frontal areas, the cingulate and the medial frontal cortex, but unilaterally in the insula and posterior prefrontal cortex (Martin et al., 1991). In addition, correlations between blood flow and age were stronger in frontal areas (cingulate and inferior frontal) than in parietal cortices, although strong correlations were also seen for the superior temporal cortex (Martin et al., 1991). The pathology of aging and DAT overlap, with additional areas involved in DAT. The greatest losses in volume in DAT have been seen in the mesial and orbitofrontal cortex, amygdala, cingulate, and insula (Jernigan, Salmon, et al., 1991). As DAT progresses beyond the mild stage, the decline in resting frontal metabolism becomes correlated with cognitive impairment (Friston & Frackowiak, 1991). Thus, while the frontal region as a whole changes no more than any other cortical area in aging and DAT, the orbitofrontal area specifically may undergo selective pathological changes in normal aging and DAT. Such changes may underly the deficit in dual-task performance that develops in old age and increases in DAT.

CONCLUSIONS

The diverse set of cognitive, brain-imaging, and neuropathological studies we have discussed fit into the view that the effects of age and DAT emerge along a continuum of task difficulty. While healthy and demented older adults are able to attend to cued spatial locations, cue validity effects are sensitive to age and DAT only in discrimination tasks (Parasuraman et al., 1992; Greenwood et al., 1993). Also age and DAT affect search rates only when target and distractors are difficult to discriminate. Finally, divided attention in dual task performance is not affected by age unless each component task is sufficiently demanding (Salthouse et al., 1984). While task difficulty provides an organizing principle, it may be too broad a principle to be useful. Moreover, task difficulty does not act alone, since increasing age and severity of DAT heighten its effects. Dual-task deficits are not present before age 65 (Wickens et al., 1987) and increase with each stage of DAT (Baddeley et al., 1991). Cue validity effects increase with age in cued location tasks (Greenwood & Parasuraman, 1994) and search time is slowed with age in cued visual search (Greenwood et al., 1992; Greenwood & Parasuraman, 1997). Therefore, task difficulty alone cannot account for all the data.

Another approach to categorization is suggested by a proposal put forward by Duncan and Humphreys (1989) to account for parameters of visual search performance. As discussed earlier, these authors suggest that search rates arise from the competition of stimuli for processing by neural elements, with the more easily discriminable competing more successfully. This view could explain the increasing slowness of visual search with age and DAT by postulating a decline in the ability of pathologically altered neural systems to resolve competitions between stimulus elements for neural processing. Divided-attention effects could also arise from inefficiencies in mechanisms for resolving competition between events presented simultaneously for neural processing. This view is less successful in explaining the influence of age and DAT on cue validity effects. Cue validity effects cannot be governed only by bottom-up processes of neural competition. As we have discussed, neither age nor DAT change the time course of cue validity effects, suggesting that the top-down effect of task type is not vulnerable to either state. What is changed by age and DAT is the RT cost of invalid cues, the time required to disengage attention following an invalid cue (Parasuraman et al., 1992; Greenwood & Parasuraman, 1994) or in search (Greenwood et al., 1997; Greenwood & Parasuraman, 1997). These selective effects on the disengagement of visuospatial attention cannot be explained simply by appealing to inefficient neural interactions. Since a cue must be processed before knowledge of its validity is available, initial processing of valid and invalid cues must be similar. Any explanation of slowed disengagement must postulate a selective effect at the stage when attention must be redirected to the un-cued target location. Neither of the explanations discussed have sufficient precision to do this.

Does an appeal to selective pathology in mediating structures have the explanatory power to account for age- and DAT-related changes in attention? The overlap between age and DAT in functional loss of both divided and visuospatial attention indicates shared selective pathology. Some studies indicate that substantial effects of DAT on the frontal lobes appear only in the moderate stage of the disease (Friston & Frackowiak, 1991; Price et al., 1991). If so, then the apparent similarity of divided attention performance in normal aging and mild DAT together with the increase in divided-attention deficits from mild to moderate stages (Bad-deley et al., 1991) would be consistent with late-appearing frontal pathol-ogy. The best evidence of pathology in mediating structures concerns posterior parietal cortex. The specific prediction of Posner and Petersen (1990) that posterior parietal cortex mediates disengagement of visuo-spatial attention is borne out by evidence of (1) selectively slowed disen-gagement in the elderly over age 75 that increases in early DAT and (2) increases from normal aging to DAT in pathology of the posterior parie-tal cortex. Thus, selective alteration of posterior parietal areas in age and DAT can account for the slowed disengagement of visuospatial attention and hence slowed visual search. However, those areas have not been im-plicated in division of attention. Therefore, at the current level of knowledge, the neuroanatomical evidence can better account for findings on visuospatial than on divided attention.

The similarities in both behavior and pathology between normal aging and mild DAT bear on the debate concerning the relation of these two conditions. Berg (1985) concluded that aging and DAT represent the result of qualitatively different brain processes, whereas Drachman (1983) concluded that aging bears both a causal and a contributory relation to DAT. The studies we have reviewed point to changes in normal aging both in behavior and in neural integrity that are similar in type, though not in extent, to those seen in DAT. Progressive and orderly pathological changes occur with age in certain brain regions in the normal elderly and in DAT patients alike (Braak & Braak, 1991; Ohm, Kirca, Bohl, Schar-nagl, & Marz, 1994). Considered together, the behavioral and neu-ropathological findings reviewed indicate a progression of selective pathology and related functional loss that may increase nonlinearly after age 65 (Bohl, Muller, Braak, & Ohm, 1994) and, at a certain point, ac-celerate into DAT.

ACKNOWLEDGMENTS

This work was supported by an Alzheimer's Association/Ana M. Buchanan Memorial Investigator-Initiated Research Grant and National Institute on Aging Grant No. AG12387-03 to Pamela M. Greenwood, and by National Institute on Aging Grant No. AG07569 to Raja Parasuraman.

REFERENCES

Arguin, M., Joanette, Y., & Cavanagh, P. (1993). Visual search for feature and conjunction targets with an attention deficit. *Journal of Cognitive Neuroscience, 5,* 436–452.

Baddeley, A. D., Bressi, S., Della Sala, S., Logie, R., & Spinnler, H. (1991). The decline of working memory in Alzheimer's disease. *Brain, 114,* 2521–2542.

Baddeley, A. D., Della Sala, S., Logie, R., & Spinnler, H. (1986). Working memory and dementia. *Quarterly Journal of Experimental Psychology, 38A,* 603–614.

Ball, M. J. (1978). Topographic distribution of neurofibrillary tangles and granulovacuolar degeneration in hippocampal cortex of aging and demented patients: A quantitative study. *Acta Neuropathologica, 42,* 73–80.

Ball, M. J., & Lo, P. (1977). Granulovacuolar degeneration in the aging brain and in dementia. *Journal of Neuropathology and Experimental Neurology, 36,* 474–487.

Bashinski, H. S., & Bacharach, V. R. (1980). Enhancement of perceptual sensitivity as the result of selectively attending to spatial locations. *Perception and Psychophysics, 28,* 241–248.

Berg, L. (1985). Does Alzheimer's disease represent an exaggeration of normal aging? *Archives of Neurology, 42,* 737–739.

Berg, L., McKeel, D. W., Jr., Miller, J. P., Baty, J., & Morris, J. C. (1993). Neuropathological indexes of Alzheimer's disease in demented and nondemented persons aged 80 years and older. *Archives of Neurology, 50,* 349–358.

Bohl, J., Muller, H., Braak, H., & Ohm, T. G. (1994). *Analysis of staged autopsy cases uncovers pace of Alzheimer's disease-related neurofibrillary changes.* Paper presented at the annual meeting of the Society for Neuroscience, Miami, FL.

Braak, H., & Braak, E. (1991). Neuropathological stageing of Alzheimer-related changes. *Acta Neuropathologica, 82,* 239–259.

Cave, K. R., & Wolfe, J. M. (1990). Modeling the role of parallel processing in visual search. *Cognitive Psychology, 22,* 225–271.

Coleman, P. D., & Flood, D. G. (1987). Neuron numbers and dendritic extent in normal aging and Alzheimer's disease. *Neurobiology of Aging, 8,* 521–545.

Corbetta, M., Miezin, F. M., Dobmeyer, S., Shulman, G. L., & Petersen, S. E. (1991). Selective and divided attention during visual discriminations of shape, color and speed: Functional anatomy by positron emission tomography. *Journal of Neuroscience, 11,* 2383–2402.

Corbetta, M., Miezin, F. M., Shulman, G. L., & Petersen, S. E. (1993). A PET study of visuospatial attention. *Journal of Neuroscience, 13*(3), 1202–1226.

de Lacoste, M., & White, C. L. (1993). The role of cortical connectivity in Alzheimer's disease pathogenesis: A review and model system. *Neurobiology of Aging, 14,* 1–16.

DeKosky, S. T., & Scheff, S. W. (1990). Synapse loss in frontal cortex biopsies in Alzheimer's disease: Correlation with cognitive severity. *Annals of Neurology, 27,* 457–464.

Desimone, R., & Duncan, J. (1995). Neural mechanisms of selective visual attention. *Annual Review of Neuroscience, 18,* 192–222.

Downing, C. J. (1988). Expectancy and visual–spatial attention: Effects on perceptual quality. *Journal of Experimental Psychology: Human Perception and Performance, 14,* 188–202.

Drachman, D. A. (1983). How normal aging relates to dementia: A critique and a classification. In D. Samuel, S. Algeri, S. Gershon, V. E. Grimm, & G. Toffano (Eds.), *Aging of the brain* (pp. 19–30). New York: Raven Press.

Duara, R., Loewenstein, A., & Barker, W. W. (1990). Utilization of behavioral activation paradigms for positron emission tomography studies in normal young and elderly subjects and in dementia. In R. Duara (Ed.), *Positron emission tomography in dementia* (pp. 131–148). New York: Wiley-Liss.

Duncan, J., & Humphreys, G. W. (1989). Visual search and stimulus similarity. *Psychological Review, 96,* 433–458.

Eglin, M., Robertson, L. C., & Knight, R. T. (1989). Visual search performance in the neglect syndrome. *Journal of Cognitive Neuroscience, 1,* 372–385.

Fewster, P. H., Griffin-Brooks, S., MacGregor, J., Ojalvo-Rose, E., & Ball, M. J. (1991). A topographical pathway by which histopathological lesions disseminate through the brain of patients with Alzheimer's disease. *Dementia, 2,* 121–132.

Filoteo, J. V., Delis, D. C., Massman, P. J., Demadura, T., Butters, N., & Salmon, D. P. (1992). Directed and divided attention in Alzheimer's disease: Impairment in shifting of attention to global and local stimuli. *Journal of Clinical and Experimental Neuropsychology, 14,* 871–883.

Flood, D. G., Buell, S. J., Defiore, C. H., Horwitz, G. J., & Coleman, P. D. (1985). Age-related dendritic growth in dentate gyrus of human brain is followed by regression in the "oldest old." *Brain Research, 345,* 366–368.

Folk, C. L., & Hoyer, W. J. (1992). Aging and shifts of visual spatial attention. *Psychology and Aging, 7,* 453–465.

Forstl, H., & Sahakian, B. (1993). Thalamic radiodensity and cognitive performance in mild and moderate dementia of the Alzheimer type. *Journal of Psychiatric Neuroscience, 18,* 33–37.

Friston, K. J., & Frackowiak, R. S. J. (1991). Cerebral function in aging and Alzheimer's disease: The role of PET. In C. H. M. Brunia, G. Mulder, & M. N. Verbaten (Eds.), *Event-related brain research (Electroencephalography and Clinical Neurophysiology,* Suppl. 42, pp. 355–365). Amsterdam: Elsevier.

Goldman-Rakic, P. (1988). Topography of cognition: Parallel distributed networks in primate association cortex. *Annual Review of Neuroscience, 11,* 137–156.

Grady, C. L., Grimes, A. M., Patronas, N., Sunderland, T., Foster, N. L., & Rapoport, S. I. (1989). Divided attention, as measured by dichotic speech performance, in dementia of the Alzheimer type. *Archives of Neurology, 46,* 317–320.

Grady, C. L., Haxby, J. V., Horwitz, B., Sundaram, M., Berg, G., Shapiro, M., Friedland, R. P., & Rapoport, S. I. (1988). A longitudinal study of the early neuropsychological and cerebral metabolic changes in dementia of the Alzheimer type. *Journal of Clinical and Experimental Neuropsychology, 10,* 576–596.

Grasby, P. M., Frith, C. D., Friston, K. J., Bench, C., Frackowiak, R. S. J., & Dolan, R. J. (1993). Functional mapping of brain areas implicated in auditory-verbal memory function. *Brain, 116,* 1–20.

Greenwood, P. M., & Parasuraman, R. (1991). Effects of aging on the speed and attentional cost of cognitive operations. *Developmental Neuropsychology, 7,* 421–434.

Greenwood, P. M., & Parasuraman, R. (1994). Attentional disengagement deficit in nondemented elderly over 75 years of age. *Aging and Cognition, 1*(3).

Greenwood, P. M., Parasuraman, R., & Haxby, J. (1993). Changes in visuospatial attention over the adult lifespan. *Neuropsychologia, 31*(5), 471–485.

Greenwood, P. M., & Parasuraman, R. (1997). *Scale of attentional focus in visual search: Effects of adult aging.* Manuscript submitted for publication.

Greenwood, P. M., Parasuraman, R., & Alexander, G. E. (1997). Controlling the focus of spatial attention during visual search: Effects of advanced aging and Alzheimer's disease. *Neuropsychology, 11,* 3–12.

Greenwood, P. M., Parasuraman, R., Panicker, S., & Haxby, J. V. (1992). *Effects of size of attentional focus on visual search in aged adults.* Paper presented at the annual meeting of the Society for Neuroscience, Anaheim, CA.

Grober, E., & Sliwinski, M. J. (1991). Dual-task performance in demented and nondemented elderly. *Journal of Clinical and Experimental Neuropsychology, 13,* 667–676.

Grossi, D., Lopez, O. L., & Martinez, A. L. (1989). Mammillary bodies in Alzheimer's disease. *Acta Neuropathologica Scandinavica, 80,* 41–45.

Guttentag, R. E., & Madden, D. J. (1987). Adult age differences in the attentional capacity demands of letter matching. *Experimental Aging Research, 13,* 93–99.

Harter, M. R., & Anllo-Vento, L. (1991). Visual–spatial attention: Preparation and selection in children and adults. In C. H. M. Brunia, G. Mulder, & M. N. Verbaten (Eds.), *Event-related brain research (Electroencephalography and Clinical Neurophysiology* Suppl. 42, pp. 183–194). Amsterdam: Elsevier.

Hartley, A. A. (1992). Attention. In F. I. M. Craik & T. A. Salthouse (Eds.), *The handbook of aging and cognition* (pp. 3–49). Hillsdale, NJ: Erlbaum.

Hartley, A. A. (1993). Evidence for the selective preservation of spatial selective attention in old age. *Psychology and Aging, 8,* 371–379.

Hartley, A. A., Kieley, J. M., & Slabach, E. H. (1990). Age differences and similarities in the effects of cues and prompts. *Journal of Experimental Psychology: Human Perception and Performance, 16,* 523–537.

Haug, H., & Eggers, R. (1991). Morphometry of the human cortex cerebri and corpus striatum during aging. *Neurobiology of Aging, 12,* 336–338.

Hawkins, H. L., Hillyard, S. A., Luck, S. J., Mouloua, M., Downing, C. J., & Woodward, D. P. (1990). Visual attention modulates signal detectability. *Journal of Experimental Psychology, 16,* 802–811.

Haxby, J. V., Duara, R., Grady, C. L., Cutler, N. R., & Rapoport, S. I. (1985). Relations between neuropsychological and cerebral metabolic asymmetries in early Alzheimer's disease. *Journal of Cerebral Blood Flow and Metabolism, 5,* 193–200.

Haxby, J. V., Grady, C. L., Duara, R., Schlageter, N., Berg, G., & Rapoport, S. I. (1986). Neocortical metabolic abnormalities precede nonmemory cognitive impairments in early Alzheimer's-type dementia. *Archives of Neurology, 43,* 882–885.

Howard, D. V. (1988). Implicit and explicit assessment of cognitive aging. In M. L. Howe & C. J. Brainerd (Eds.), *Cognitive development in adulthood: Progress in cognitive development research* (pp. 3–37). New York: Springer-Verlag.

Jernigan, T. L., Archibald, S. L., Berhow, M. T., Sowell, E. R., Foster, D. S., & Hesselink, J. R. (1991). Cerebral structure on MRI. Part I: Localization of age-related changes. *Biological Psychiatry, 29,* 55–67.

Jernigan, T. L., Salmon, D. P., Butters, N., & Hesselink, J. R. (1991). Cerebral structure on MRI. Part II: Specific changes in Alzheimer's and Huntington's diseases. *Biological Psychiatry, 29,* 68–81.

Jonides, J. (1981). Voluntary versus automatic control over the mind's eye's movement. In J. B. Long & A. D. Baddeley (Eds.), *Attention and performance IX* (pp. 187–203). Hillsdale, NJ: Erlbaum.

Julesz, B., & Bergen, J. R. (1983). Textons, the fundamental elements in preattentive vision and perceptions of textures. *Bell Systems Technical Journal, 62,* 1619–1646.

Kemper, T. L. (1994). Neuroanatomical and neuropathological changes during aging and dementia. In M. L. Albert & J. E. Knoefel (Eds.), *Clinical neurology of aging* (pp. 3–67). New York: Oxford University Press.

Korteling, J. E. (1991). Effects of skill integration and perceptual competition on age-related differences in dual-task performance. *Human Factors, 33,* 35–44.

Kuljis, R. O. (1994). Lesions in the pulvinar in patients with Alzheimer's disease. *Journal of Neuropathology and Experimental Neurology, 53,* 202–211.

LaBerge, D. (1990). Thalamic and cortical mechanisms of attention suggested by recent positron emission tomographic experiments. *Journal of Cognitive Neuroscience, 2,* 358–372.

Light, L. L. (1992). The organization of memory in old age. In F. I. M. Craik & T. A. Salthouse (Eds.), *The handbook of aging and cognition* (pp. 111–165). Hillsdale, NJ: Erlbaum.

Lippa, C. F., Hamos, J. E., Pulaski-Salo, D., Degennaro, L. J., & Drachman, D. A. (1992). Alzheimer's disease and aging: Effects on perforant pathway perikarya and synapses. *Neurobiology of Aging, 13,* 405–411.

Madden, D. J. (1990). Adult age differences in the time course of visual attention. *Journal of Gerontology, 45,* 9–16.

Madden, D. J. (1992). Selective attention and visual search: Revision of an allocation model and application to age differences. *Journal of Experimental Psychology: Human Perception and Performance, 18,* 821–836.

Martin, A. J., Friston, K. J., Colebatch, J. G., & Frackowiak, R. S. J. (1991). Decreases in regional cerebral blood flow with normal aging. *Journal of Cerebral Blood Flow and Metabolism, 11,* 684–689.

McDowd, J. M., & Craik, F. I. M. (1988). Effects of aging and task difficulty on divided attention performance. *Journal of Experimental Psychology: Human Perception and Performance, 14,* 267–280.

Mesulam, M. M. (1981). A cortical network of directed attention and unilateral neglect. *Annals of Neurology, 19,* 309–325.

Morrison, J. H. (1993). Differential vulnerability, connectivity, and cell typology. *Neurobiology of Aging, 14,* 51–54.

Moscovitch, M., & Winocur, G. (1992). The neuropsychology of memory and aging. In F. I. M. Craik & T. A. Salthouse (Eds.), *The handbook of aging and cognition* (pp. 315–372). Hillsdale, NJ: Erlbaum.

Muller, H. J., & Rabbitt, P. M. A. (1989). Reflexive and voluntary orienting of visual attention: Time course of activation and resistance to interruption. *Journal of Experimental Psychology: Human Perception and Performance, 15,* 315–330.

Nakayama, K., & Silverman, G. H. (1986). Serial and parallel processing of visual feature conjunctions. *Nature, 320,* 264–265.

Nebes, R. D. (1989). Semantic memory in Alzheimer's disease. *Psychological Bulletin, 106,* 377–394.

Nebes, R. D. (1992). Cognitive dysfunction in Alzheimer's disease. In F. I. M. Craik & T. Salthouse (Eds.), *The handbook of aging and cognition* (pp. 373–446). Hillsdale, NJ: Erlbaum.

Nebes, R., & Brady, C. B. (1989). Focused and divided attention in Alzheimer's disease. *Cortex, 25,* 305–315.

Nestor, P. G., Parasuraman, R., & Haxby, J. V. (1989). Attentional costs of mental operations in young and old adults. *Developmental Neuropsychology, 5,* 141–158.

Nestor, P. G., Parasuraman, R., & Haxby, J. V. (1991). Speed of information processing and attention in early Alzheimer's dementia. *Developmental Neuropsychology, 7,* 243–256.

Nestor, P. G., Parasuraman, R., Haxby, J. V., & Grady, C. L. (1991). Divided attention and metabolic brain dysfunction in mild dementia of the Alzheimer's type. *Neuropsychologia, 29,* 379–387.

Nissen, M. J., & Corkin, S. (1985). Effectiveness of attentional cueing in older and younger adults. *Journal of Gerontology, 40,* 185–191.

Nissen, M. J., Corkin, S., & Growdon, J. H. (1981). *Attentional focusing in patients with Alzheimer's disease.* In paper presented at the annual conference of the American Aging Association, Chicago, IL.

Ohm, T. G., Kirca, M., Bohl, J., Scharnagl, H., & Marz, W. (1994). *APOε4 gene-dose dependent development of Alzheimer-type neurofibrillary tangles: A PCR-aided autopsy analysis.* Paper presented at the annual meeting of the Society for Neuroscience, Miami, FL.

Oken, B. S., Kishiyama, S. S., Kaye, J. A., & Howieson, D. B. (1994). Attention deficit in Alzheimer's disease is not simulated by an anticholinergic/antihistaminergic drug and is distinct from deficits in healthy aging. *Neurology, 44,* 657–662.

Parasuraman, R., Greenwood, P. M., Haxby, J. V., & Grady, C. L. (1992). Visuospatial attention in dementia of the Alzheimer type. *Brain, 115,* 711–733.

Parasuraman, R., & Haxby, J. V. (1993). Attention and brain function in Alzheimer's disease: A review. *Neuropsychology, 7,* 242–272.

Pardo, J. V., Pardo, P. J., Janer, K. W., & Raichle, M. E. (1990). The anterior cingulate cortex mediates processing selection in the Stroop attentional conflict paradigm. *Proceedings of the National Academy of Sciences, U.S.A., 87,* 256–259.

Plude, D. J. & Hoyer,W.J. (1986). Age and the selectivity of visual information processing. *Psychology and Aging, 1,* 4–10.

Plude, D. J., & Doussard-Roosevelt, J. A. (1989). Aging, selective attention and feature integration. *Psychology and Aging, 4,* 98–105.

Ponds, R. W. H. M., Brouwer, W. H., & van Wolffelaar, P. C. (1988). Age differences in divided attention in a simulated driving task. *Journal of Gerontology, 43,* P151–P156.

Posner, M. I. (1980). Orienting of attention. *Quarterly Journal of Experimental Psychology, 32,* 3–25.

Posner, M. I., & Petersen, S. E. (1990). The attention system of the human brain. *Annual Review of Neuroscience, 13,* 25–42.

Posner, M. I., Walker, J. A., Friderich, F. J., & Rafal, R. D. (1984). Effects of parietal injury on covert orienting of attention. *Journal of Neuroscience, 4,* 1863–1874.

Price, J. L., Davis, P. B., Morris, J. C., & White, D. L. (1991). The distribution of tangles, plaques and related immunohistochemical markers in healthy aging and Alzheimer's disease. *Neurobiology of Aging, 12,* 295–312.

Rafal, R. D., & Posner, M. I. (1987). Deficits in human visual spatial attention following thalamic lesions. *Proceedings of the National Academy of Sciences, U.S.A., 84,* 7349–7353.

Robinson, D. L., Bowman, E. M., & Kertzman, C. (1991). *Covert orienting of attention in macaque—II: A signal in parietal cortex to disengage attention.* Paper presented at the annual meeting of the Society for Neuroscience, New Orleans, LA.

Robinson, D. L., & Kertzman, C. (1990). Visuospatial attention: Effects of age, gender and spatial reference. *Neuropsychologia, 28,* 291–301.

Robinson, D. L., & Petersen, S. E. (1992). The pulvinar and visual salience. *Trends in Neurosciences, 15,* 127–132.

Saffran, E. M., Fitzpatrick-DeSalme, E. J., & Coslett, H. B. (1990). Visual disturbances in dementia. In M. F. Schwartz (Ed.), *Modular deficits in Alzheimer-type dementia.* Cambridge, MA: MIT Press.

Salthouse, T. A., Rogan, J. D., & Prill, K. A. (1984). Division of attention: Age differences on a visually presented memory task. *Memory and Cognition, 12,* 613–620.

Somberg, B. L., & Salthouse, T. A. (1982). Divided-attention abilities in young and old adults. *Journal of Experimental Psychology: Human Perception and Performance, 8,* 651–665.

Storandt, M., & Hill, R. D. (1989). Very mild senile dementia of the Alzheimer type — II: Psychometric test performance. *Archives of Neurology, 46,* 383–386.

Terry, R. D., Masliah, E., Salmon, D. P., Butters, N., DeTeresa, R., Hill, R., Hansen, L. A., & Katzman, R. (1991). Physical basis of cognitive alterations in Alzheimer's disease: Synapse loss is the major correlate of cognitive impairment. *Annals of Neurology, 30,* 578–580.

Tinklenberg, J. R., Taylor, J. L., Peabody, C. A., Redington, D., & Gibson, E. (1984). Dual task performance measures in geriatric studies. *Psychopharmacology Bulletin, 20,* 441–444.

Treisman, A. M. (1985). Preattentive processing in vision. *Computer Vision, Graphics and Imaging Processing, 31,* 156–177.

Treisman, A. M., & Gelade, G. (1980). A feature-integration theory of attention. *Cognitive Psychology, 12,* 97–136.

Treisman, A. M., & Gormican, S. (1988). Feature analysis in early vision: Evidence from search asymmetries. *Psychological Review, 95,* 15–48.

Wickens, C. D. (1984). Processing resources in attention. In R. Parasuraman & D. R. Davies (Eds.), *Varieties of attention.* Orlando, FL: Academic Press.

Wickens, C. D., Braune, R., & Stokes, A. (1987). Age differences in the speed and capacity of information processing: 1. A dual-task approach. *Psychology and Aging, 2,* 70–78.

Attentional Functioning in Individuals Diagnosed and at Risk for Schizophrenia

Richard A. Steffy
Jonathan M. Oakman

L isted under the Psychotic Disorders section of the latest psychiatric classification system, DSM-IV (American Psychiatric Association, 1994), schizophrenia is one of the major mental disorders. Its diagnosis is based on the presence of delusional thinking, problems of reality contact, hallucinatory experiences, along with associated difficulties in communication, emotional expression, motivation, quality of social interaction, motor coordination, and deficits in many other systems of functioning. Individuals with the disorder may manifest any portion of this range of symptoms and systemic dysfunctions. In fact, there is a remarkable diversity in the display of symptoms and deficits observed among schizophrenic patients.

As there is diversity in the symptoms of schizophrenic patients, there is also considerable variation in the life history, the course, and outcomes of the disorder. Although Kraepelin's (1913/1919) label for this disorder, "dementia praecox," suggested an origin in adolescence and a generally deteriorating outcome, onsets actually tend to occur over a wide band of early to midadulthood years, and many patients fully recover or suffer periodic bouts of disturbances interposed by at least partial remission.

With this diversity of features, it is not surprising that theories of cause and mechanism are also wide ranging. Although current trends in theorizing give heavy emphasis to the influence of hereditary and biochemical factors, one also finds the schizophrenia research literature alive with efforts to integrate those factors with malfunctions in psychological and physiological systems. This chapter tracks the voluminous and long-standing research directed toward one such system, the analysis of attentional deficits in schizophrenic populations.

As the nature of schizophrenic patients' attentional deficits has been clarified by decades of research, interest in understanding the role of attentional problems early in the lives of those who will later be afflicted with this disorder has expanded. The etiology of schizophrenia is generally held to derive from aberrant developmental processes, and so there is a strong interest in detecting early signs of its presence—both as genetic seeds and first sprouts of disturbance. Consistent with the finding of attentional deficits noted in those suffering the disorder, prospective longitudinal investigations have also found attentional system dysfunctions in children at heightened risk for the disorder. With the emergence of new assessment tools and recent models of attentional function, efforts to account for lifespan differences will continue to be an important aspect of the validation of our concepts.

CLINICAL SIGNS
OF ATTENTIONAL PROBLEMS
IN SCHIZOPHRENIC PATIENTS

Attentional problems can often be detected in casual conversations with schizophrenic individuals, who tend to be easily distracted or, alternatively, too persistent (failing to shift their attention). Conversations with some show a wandering, circumstantial quality that suggests a loss of internal focus and weak goal orientation. Others, however, show a rigid adherence to a theme, for instance, a delusional focus. Schizophrenic patients have been known to express concern (especially in early phases of the disorder) with their own attentional failings, reflecting a sense of stimulus overload, for example, "I am attending to everything at once and as a result I do not really attend to anything" (McGhie & Chapman, 1961, p. 104).

Schizophrenic patients' attention deficits are visible in their work on assigned tasks. Sluggish, disjointed, and otherwise inefficient task performances have regularly been noted (Wishner, 1955), with such observations extending from Kraepelin who, found schizophrenics unable "to keep their attention fixed for any length of time"; he observed schizophrenics to have "a kind of irresistible attraction of attention to casual external impressions" (Kraepelin, 1913/1919, pp. 6–7). Observations such as these encouraged psychological investigations of attention and collateral perceptual systems, for example, measures of perceptual constancy and size estimation (Silverman, 1964).

Although attentional deficits continue to be regarded as an important feature of the disorder, the path to understanding has been a rocky one. Observations based on diverse technologies and heterogeneous subject populations have led to many theoretical explanations of attentional problems, including deviations in persistence of perceptual traces, constricted channel capacity, inadequate transfer of information into longer-term stores, weak memory, inhibitory dysfunctions, failure to disattend, stimulus modulation problems, and others. At times, opposing models have been derived from the same technology. For example, foundation work in charting attentional deficits in schizophrenia occurred in the laboratories of David Shakow and Joseph Zubin. Both used simple reaction time tests, but procedural differences led them to derive opposite views of the nature of schizophrenics' attentional deficits. In Shakow's lab subjects were exposed to trials with long-duration preparatory interval delays (ranging from 0.5 to 25.0 seconds), and his results indicated that schizophrenic patients could not sustain a major set (thus a *too weak* focus) on a demanding task for more than a few seconds—a problem associated with severe distractibility (Shakow, 1962). Zubin (1975), however, used only short trials (approximately 1 second long) with variation in the stimulus features of the signal-to-respond and found that schizophrenics suffered *too strong* a level of attentional persistence—a failure to efficiently shift attention from the stimulus features of the previous trial (see the reviews by Nuechterlein, 1977, and Steffy & Waldman, 1993).

Theoretical conflicts of this sort continue to becloud our explanation of the attentional problems of schizophrenic patients, possibly teaching us that the concept of attention itself is too broad and vague to have been used for explanatory purposes. It is perhaps interesting to note that the term "set" that Shakow employed in his segmental set theory (as a synonym of the word "attention") was noted by Gibson (1941) to have a dozen different meanings in psychology. However, despite the imprecision in defining attentional processes and despite continued controversies over the basic nature of schizophrenics' attentional deficits, we open this chapter with a note of enthusiasm that the studies of attentional functioning have yielded research-heuristic operational definitions. Attentional measures have been useful in explicating individual differences and in generating interesting and testable views of schizophrenic performance deficits. As will be reported below, attentional deficits are linked to important external criteria such as the course and prognosis of schizophrenic disorders. They have been found to index vulnerability and to give an expanded understanding of the mechanisms and causes of this major disorder.

DEVELOPMENTAL ANTECEDENTS
TO SCHIZOPHRENIA: THE STUDY OF RISK

In recognition of the fact that direct studies of disturbed schizophrenic patients can not provide adequate information about etiology—because of confounding influences such as sick role, stigma, treatment, and incarceration—"high-risk" research designs have been devised to probe the development of schizophrenia. Free of the shortcomings of other research strategies, the prospective study of individuals with a heightened risk for the disorder (usually because one of their parents had the disorder, thus increasing the base population risk from 1% to 10%) allowed a new era of research into the developmental course of schizophrenia (Garmezy, 1974). In risk studies, vulnerable children are identified and tested periodically in their premorbid state to learn what factors in their identification—or in their periodic assessments—best account for any subsequent psychotic disturbance.

Although these studies are expensive and long drawn out, several dozen such longitudinal projects have been pursued over the last four decades. The earliest of these has reported factors associated with later breakdowns (Mednick, Parnas, & Schulsinger, 1987). Other "high-risk" projects are still awaiting adult adjustment outcome data (sometimes requiring young children to reach middle age) to determine what factors are antecedents to the disorder. In the meantime, however, there has been a fairly impressive yield from cross-sectional analyses of the differences between the high- and low-risk children. Joan R. Asarnow (1988) summarized 24 projects in which symptoms, neurointegrative dysfunctions (of attention, thinking, etc.), social maladjustment, as well as patterns of life stressors (general environment and familial) were observed to differentiate the high- from the low-risk subjects studied from birth to early adulthood years.

Illustrating this early harvest of findings, high-risk infants have shown tendencies toward abnormal motor activity and stimulus sensitivities (e.g., McNeil & Kaij, 1973). Between the 4th and 8th month of life they were noted to fall behind on Bayley Scales of Infant Development (Marcus, Auerbach, Wilkinson, & Burack, 1981) and to show attention span differences (Mednick et al., 1987). Throughout the preschool years, differences were observed on cognitive and motor coordination tests and on measures of temperament (e.g., Hanson, Gottesman, & Heston, 1976). During middle childhood and adolescent years, soft neurological signs (Hanson et al., 1976) and attention impairment (Asarnow, Steffy, MacCrimmon, & Cleghorn, 1977; Cornblatt & Erlenmeyer-Kimling, 1985) were reported along with a variety of personality difficulties (MacCrimmon, Cleghorn, Asarnow, & Steffy, 1980). Collectively these findings from prospective "high-risk" designs suggest that there are marked differences in the developmental pathways of individuals who have a genetic vunerability for the disorder and that early-occurring attentional deficits signal vulnerability to a schizophrenic disorder. Nuechterlein and Dawson (1984) also reviewed attentional deficits reported among the offspring of schizophrenic patients. They expanded the definition of populations "at risk" to include adult first-degree relatives of schizophrenic patients, individuals with schizotypic personality features, and schizophrenic patients in remission. An update on the attention tests that have best advanced understanding of schizophrenic vulnerability follows.

ATTENTIONAL MEASURES PROMISING BETTER UNDERSTANDING OF THE DEVELOPMENT OF SCHIZOPHRENIA

Several tests have especially good reliability, discriminating power, and promise as markers of vulnerability, namely, measures of the simple reaction time (SRT), and the Continuous Performance Test (CPT), and the Span of Apprehension Test. Although the testing formats of these measures vary across labs, current understanding has profited from decades of successful research with them.

Simple Reaction Time Measures

As already noted, the SRT task is one of the longest used, most studied, and effective indices of schizophrenic performance deficits, one that is reputed in the words of Cancro and colleagues to be "the closest thing to a north star in schizophrenia research" (Cancro, Sutton, Kerr, & Sugerman, 1971, p. 352). Its importance to understanding schizophrenic patients' performance deficits arose from a finding that research-cooperative, chronic schizophrenic patients were not different from nonschizophrenic subjects on various motor system tasks (including knee-jerk reflex, pursuit rotor speed, hand steadiness, and tapping speed) but were markedly impaired on SRT (Shakow, 1962). Insofar as the behavior required in the SRT task—finger press and lift—was similar in form to that required in the tapping speed measure (which yielded no schizophrenic–normal difference), Shakow concluded that the critical difference was to be found in the requirement for sustained attention during the so-called preparatory interval (PI) of each SRT trial, that is, the time between the beginning of the trial and a signal to respond. On this task, the schizophrenic patients' overall response latency was more than twice as slow as that of normal controls, and the distributions of schizophrenic and normal latency data did not overlap (Rodnick & Shakow, 1940). SRT sensitivity to pathology was documented by a very strong relationship ($r = .89$) to independent ratings of the mental health of chronically-ill schizophrenic patients (Rosenthal, Lawlor, Zahn, & Shakow, 1960).

This early SRT work had a major impact, merited by the extensive exploration of SRT task parameters conducted by Shakow's team (e.g., Zahn, Rosenthal, & Shakow, 1961, 1963), the stability of the results, and a pattern of findings that allowed a fairly precise quantitative index of schizophrenic patients' loss in attentional capacity. In particular, Shakow and his colleagues estimated that chronically disturbed schizophrenic patients could sustain a sharp attentional focus for only 4 or 5 seconds. This conclusion was based on the fact that for all subjects faster latencies were obtained from short regular-occurring (isotemporal) than from short irregular (unpredictable) trials, but schizophrenic patients lost the advantage from a regular administration of trials when PI intervals exceeded 5 seconds. In contrast, nonpatient subjects maintained the advantage of regularity for PI durations up to approximately 20 seconds (Rodnick & Shakow, 1940).

Work in our own laboratory extended Shakow's procedure (which uses lengthy blocks of regular and irregular trials) by instead embedding short, four-trial runs of regular trials within an irregular series, thus reducing the distance between regular and irregular trials and presumably reducing extraneous influences in the comparisons of these types of trials (Bellissimo & Steffy, 1972). This modification revealed that the presence of sets of long-PI regular trials embedded in a long series of irregular trials dramatically retards process schizophrenic patients' response latencies in those sets.

Use of the embedded set paradigm to probe the nature of schizophrenic attentional deficits in part confirmed Shakow's earlier observations. It also extended researchers' understanding of the impact of the regular trial manipulation in a way that challenged Shakow's segmental set theory — a position that described schizophrenics as being especially prone to distractions (Steffy & Galbraith, 1974). Shakow's position had been based on the finding that schizophrenics simply lost the attentional edge after a few seconds of a predictable (regular) SRT trial, relative to similar duration irregular trials. However, studies using the embedded set procedure consistently found that long regular trials yielded a slower reaction time than did the long-duration irregular trials, a so-called redundancy-associated deficit (Bellissimo & Steffy, 1972, 1975) — or *reaction time crossover* (RTX), as it is more generally known when referring to the interaction between the trial arrangement (regular and irregular) and trial duration (short and long trial) factors (Cromwell, 1975). This pattern was intriguing because it depicted conditions in which more information, as conferred by the regular trial arrangement, resulted in less adequate performances in schizophrenic patients.

An extensive and continuing research literature has grown out of these early SRT findings. In addition to efforts to clarify the task parameters, various investigations attempted to mine the clinical utility of this measure of attentional deficit. The RTX pattern along with general latency indices were repeatedly proven to be useful in discriminating schizophrenic and control subject performances (Steffy & Waldman, 1993), and in separating process from reactive schizophrenic subgroups (Bellissimo & Steffy, 1972, 1975).[1] Although the RTX pattern has been found in a few other groups—namely, in temporal lobe epileptic patients (Greiffenstein, Lewis, Milberg, & Rosenbaum, 1981), in Research Diagnostic Criteria (RDC)–diagnosed bipolar patients (Bohannon & Strauss, 1983), and in aging populations (Strauss, Wagman, & Quaid, 1983)—generally it discriminates process schizophrenics from most other psychiatric patients. Adding various indices of latency and RTX together, Steffy and Waldman (1993), reported that a "SRT-impairment index" showed deviant patterns in approximately 75% of process schizophrenics, 50% of reactive schizophrenics, 25% of nonschizophrenic psychiatric patients, and only 5% of nondisordered control subjects.

Other reaction time measures, including a "cross-modal shift" procedure (Spring, 1980; Mannuzza, 1980), and a probed reaction time (PRT) procedure with occasional distracting visual stimuli imposed into the RT trials (Steffy & Galbraith, 1975; Steffy, 1978) have also shown significant intergroup discriminations. In a battery of lab tests the PRT index played a major role in discriminating among DSM-III schizophrenia-spectrum disorder groups (schizophrenic, schizophreniform, schizoaffective, and schizotypic groups) and other psychiatrically disordered patient groups (Connelly, 1984).

Finally, RT technology has shown some sensitivity to populations at risk for schizophrenia. Among studies of high-risk children, there has been an uneven yield from SRT measures, with discrimination only on a latency measure that used a Shakow-based paradigm (L. M. Marcus, 1972). However, with other vulnerable populations, a cross-modal RT procedure successfully discriminated first-degree relatives of schizophrenic patients from nonschizophrenic controls (Spring, 1980). Various types of SRT procedures were found sensitive to schizotypic college students (Rosenbaum, Chapin, & Shore, 1988) and also relatives of schizophrenic patients (DeAmicis & Cromwell, 1979). Further supporting the utility of RTX as a vulnerability marker, DeAmicis and Cromwell (1979) observed that the magnitude of RTX in a schizophrenic patient group was significantly related to the magnitude of RTX in their relatives. Moreover, magnitude of patients' RTX correlated with the number of their relatives who were found disturbed (DeAmicis, Huntzinger, & Cromwell, 1981), a finding that has fostered interest in this index as a potential genetic marker (Cromwell, 1993a).

Continuous Performance Test

Emil Kraepelin, deemed to be the "parent" of modern psychiatric classifications, had observed weakness in schizophrenic capacity to apprehend briefly encountered stimuli (see the English version of Kraepelin's 1896 edition, translated and adapted by Diefendorf, 1923). As will be seen in the pages to follow, his astute observation concerning the perceptual-processing problems of schizophrenic patients has been confirmed in modern attempts to measure and understand schizophrenic deficit.

Devised by Rosvold, Mirsky, Sarason, Bransome, and Beck (1956) to measure deficits in the visual vigilance of schizophrenic patients, the CPT presents briefly flashed visual stimuli (numbers, letters, or playing card figures) throughout a lengthy series of trials, each approximately of 1-second duration. Each display is presented for approximately a half second (in some studies as little as one tenth of a second) with subjects signaling their detection of infrequently occurring target figures (typically one out of five trials) by a button press. This procedure permits several dependent variables including hit rate, latency of responding, errors of omission (defined as a failure to respond to the presence of a target), and errors of commission (a response given to a nontarget stimulus). Derived scores of sensitivity (d') and threshold for responding (β) may be calculated from signal detection formulations.[2]

Beginning in the mid-1960s, an extensive series of CPT investigations were undertaken by Maressa H. Orzack and Conan Kornetsky to examine attentional deficits in diagnosed schizophrenic patients and non-schizophrenic comparison subjects. The efforts of this team (Orzack & Kornetsky, 1966, 1971) along with those in others labs (e.g., Spohn, Lacoursiere, Thompson, & Coyne, 1977) revealed consistent differences between chronic schizophrenic patients and control groups. Nearly one in two schizophrenic patients shows CPT deficits—found to characterize acute as well as chronically ill schizophrenic patients (Bergman, Osgood, Pathak, Keefe, & Cornblatt, 1992). The CPT has shown good sensitivity as well in discriminating among RDC-diagnosed schizophrenic, schizoaffective, and affective-disordered patients (Walker, 1981). However, unlike SRT findings, differences in CPT patterns have not been identified among research-based subgroupings of schizophrenics (such as process and reactive patients).

With respect to the value of CPT scores as a vulnerability marker, Asarnow and MacCrimmon (1978) found that schizophrenic patients in clinical remission showed greater levels of CPT impairment than those with no previous psychiatric condition. Moreover, undiagnosed first-degree (blood-connected) relatives of schizophrenic patients who had exceptionally poor CPT scores were found to show significantly greater numbers of psychiatric symptoms elicited during interviews (Orzack & Kornetsky, 1971; Walker, 1981).

In attempts to assess children at risk, the use of the original Rosvold et al. (1956) procedures—using a simple "X" technique (detection of a single target figure) and an "AX" procedure (requiring a response to two consecutive letters, e.g., an "X" following an "A")—failed to find CPT-based differences between high-risk and low-risk children (Asarnow et al., 1977; Cohler, Grunebaum, Weiss, Gamer, & Gallant, 1977) unless a very young child sample was used (Grunebaum, Weiss, Gallant, & Cohler, 1974). Consequently, researchers in the last few years have further increased the processing demands of the CPT task by adding external distractors (Asarnow & MacCrimmon, 1978), by devising more complex versions (e.g., an identical pairs technique, or CPT-IP, which requires subjects to detect the occurrence of two back-to-back identical stimuli; Erlenmeyer-Kimling & Cornblatt, 1992), and by degrading the visual quality of the stimuli presented (CPT-DS). The latter technique uses stimuli flashed amid extraneous marks on the screen (Nuechterlein, 1983) and has been successful in discriminating children at risk for schizophrenia from hyperactive children.

Cornblatt and Keilp (1994) conclude their recent review of CPT research with the observation that the best CPT conditions for differentiating vulnerable populations are those that make extra-heavy demands for controlled processing. Consistent with the hope that CPT technology would become a genetic marker, the CPT has been found to have a strong heritability index (Kendler et al., 1990).

Span of Apprehension Test

Encouraged by the sensitivity of CPT measures for indexing schizophrenics' attentional deficits, researchers turned to perception/cognition laboratories for other procedures sensitive to events occurring early in the information-processing chain. For example, Sperling (1960) had created partial report strategies to estimate the amount of information that could be absorbed from a briefly presented complex visual display. His work showed that much more information is processed than can possibly be reported in open-ended full recall of a complex display. His task required subjects to report only a component of a display—with the component specified after the display had been terminated—in order to bypass the problem of output interference that occurs during subjects' attempts at full report. Extending Sperling's technique, Estes and Taylor (1964) created the Span of Apprenhension Test, which enables the number of elements processed (the span) to be calculated from performances on displays with varying signal:noise ratios. In this test, subjects are told to report which one of two possible target figures, typically letters "T" or "F" (each 50% likely), that they see in rapidly presented displays featuring the presence of a few or many irrelevant (noise) letters.

John M. Neale, working with R. L. Cromwell, first saw the advantage of using the span of apprehension technique as a measure of schizophrenic patients' selective attention deficits. A "noisy" display (featuring a target letter embedded among seven other letters) yielded a marked level of decrement for groups of schizophrenics with an average of two and a half letters recognized during a 50 millisecond display of the eight letters, in contrast to normal subjects' processing of approximately four and a half letters (Neale, McIntyre, Fox, & Cromwell, 1969). Neale (1971) followed up that initial study with the use of a wider range of displays and added psychiatric patients, penitentiary inmates, and "normal" subjects to compare to the schizophrenic patients. Despite the variations in testing procedure and diversity of the groups, Neale (1971) reported essentially the same results as noted by Neale et al. (1969). In all cases, an easy-to-detect display condition (a single target letter) showed no difference across groups, but as the signal-to-noise level was made more difficult, schizophrenic accuracy fell off more than for other groups. Subsequent work by Robert F. Asarnow (also a Cromwell student) and his colleague Duncan J. MacCrimmon (1981) found the Span of Apprehension Test capable of discriminating schizophrenics from manic-depressive patients, as well as nonpsychiatric comparison groups. This work confirmed the specificity of the technique for schizophrenia.

In recent years, span of apprehension research has followed two separate pathways, including concerns with mechanism and with individual differences. With respect to mechanism, the influence of several stimulus factors has been found unimportant to span of apprehension effects, namely, the nearness of distractor elements to targets (Neale, 1971) and target–noise similarity (Davidson & Neale, 1974), but the impact of the "partial report" response feature of the SOA task proved to be an important influence on schizophrenic performance deficits. Cash, Neale, and Cromwell (1972) found that a "full report" of letters yielded no psychopathology effect, convincing these authors that a "partial report" demand—allegedly taxing perceptual selectivity processes—is basic to the span deficit of schizophrenic patients.

This line of investigation was pursued further in an intriguing investigation by Elkins, Cromwell, and Asarnow (1992), who sought to lessen the impact of noise letters in the display by negating them with a backward masking procedure. Fifty milliseconds after a display had terminated, masking stimuli were presented in the same locations in which the noise letters (not the target loci) had originally been presented. As expected, they found accuracy under the masked-noise letter condition improved relative to the nonmasked trials in both normal and depressed patient control groups. In marked contrast, schizophrenic patients suffered a further decrement in their performances when presented masked-noise letters. Elkins and her colleagues speculated about the possible role of schizophrenic patients' hypersensitive response to "onset transients" in accounting for their increased deficit, a view comparable to other accounts of schizophrenic patients' special sensitivity to interference from signals imposed into attention-demanding tasks (Steffy, 1978).

On the other span of apprehension research frontier, the study of individual differences has been pursued most actively by Asarnow and his colleagues. For example, Marder, Asarnow, and Van Putten (1984) showed that span measures gave stable estimates of pathology over 3-month epochs despite variations in the patients' clinical condition. In a study of children at risk for schizophrenia (foster children who had schizophrenic biological mothers), high-risk subjects showed greater deficits on the Span of Apprehension Test along with other measures of selective attention and conceptual functioning (Asarnow et al., 1977). When the childrens' scores on a battery of perceptual and conceptual tasks were analyzed with clustering algorithms, a subsample of children who appeared to have an especially severe risk for the disorder on the basis of the Span of Apprehension Test and other lab tests were also found to show Minnesota Multiphasic Personality Inventory (MMPI) Schizophrenia Scale and Psychiatric Status Scale (PSS) elevations, reflecting problems in their personality organization and their social adjustment (MacCrimmon, Cleghorn, Asarnow, & Steffy, 1980). Asarnow's team then found that adults of low socioeconomic status (recruited from an employment agency) who also showed span of apprehension deficits had significant elevations on the MMPI Schizophrenia Scales and on various other indices of schizotypy (Asarnow, Nuechterlein, & Marder, 1983). Span of apprehension deficits were also observed in the first-degree relatives of schizophrenics in research conducted by Wagener, Hogarty, Goldstein, Asarnow, and Browne (1986), further confirming the value of span of appprehension as a risk-marker for schizophrenic disorders.

Taken collectively, a compelling case has been made for the value of the Span of Apprehension Test as a vulnerability marker. Reservations about this conclusion, however, were voiced by two teams, Harvey, Weintraub, and Neale (1985) and Dobson and Neufeld (1987), both of whom failed to find span deviations among children at risk for the disorder. Although these findings may educe caution as to the use of span of apprehension technology for risk work, Asarnow, Steffy, and Waldman (1985) raised the possibility that the negative results may have resulted from technical differences in the format of the tests used in the different labs. Both of the negative-finding studies used small stimulus displays (2° × 3° of visual angle) in contrast to the wider (20° × 21°) visual angle used in Asarnow's lab. Asarnow et al. (1985) argued that span might be partially affected by the size of the field required for scanning, insofar as constricted attention to peripheral stimulation in schizophrenic patients' retinal fields have been documented in perimetry investigations conducted by Cegalis, Leen, and Solomon (1977).

Other Measures of Promise

It is obvious that attention is a many-faceted construct, operationalized by quite different procedures. Tests may emphasize sustained attention, selective attention to critical features in a noisy field, shifting focus, and other subtle processes — alone or in combination. In addition to the SRT Test, CPT, and Span of Apprehension Test reviewed above as the best-explored measures of attention, other less well-researched perceptual and cognitive lab tests and various psychophysiological functions have been found sensitive to schizophrenic processes and give promise of becoming risk markers in time.

Perceptual-Cognitive Tests

Tests sensitive to schizophrenic pathology often measure the impact of irrelevant stimuli on the perception of target stimuli. As will be noted below, the presence of task-extraneous stimulation generally impairs schizophrenic functioning on attention-demanding tasks, although on some procedures task-extraneous stimulation facilitates schizophrenic performance, relative to control groups. Illustrating the exceptional variation in schizophrenic response to subtle cues are a few perceptual tasks that show special sensitivity to the disorder.

Backward-masking tasks require subjects to identify rapidly-presented displays of visual information (e.g., simple digits or letters) followed closely in time by task-extraneous stimulation superimposed on the spot vacated by the target information. Normal subjects' perceptual accuracy is seemingly unaffected by the presence of the mask when the delay is longer than one-tenth of a second, but a much longer "critical interval" (one-third to one-half of a second) is required for accurate target detection by schizophrenic patients (Saccuzzo, Hirt, & Spencer, 1974). Subjects with schizotypic personalities also have shown unusually long duration interference effects from backward masks (Saccuzzo & Schubert, 1981), indicating that individuals with less severe variants of the disorder manifest patterns of response similar to those suffering a full-blown schizophrenic disorder.

Deviations in the *prepulse inhibition of the startle reflex* has been found in subjects with schizophrenic-spectrum disorders. This effect is noted in circumstances that elicit the startle reaction (e.g., in eye-blink responses to a sudden stimulus). In nonschizophrenic subjects the amplitude of the startle reaction can be reduced by presenting a low-intensity stimulus immediately preceding the startle-inducing stimulus, but schizophrenic patients' startle reaction is not reduced by the occurrence of the early stimulus (Braff et al., 1978). This inhibition failure is also common to psychosis-prone individuals (Simons & Giardina, 1992) and to schizotypic psychiatric patients (Cadenhead & Braff, 1992).

Insensitivity to prepulse stimuli may be similar to other differences in schizophrenics or schizophrenic-prone individuals' perceptual responses to rapidly presented stimuli. In some instances schizophrenics have been found less sensitive to stimuli that elicit errors in normal control subjects, a condition that makes the patients' performances appear more accurate than those of nondisturbed subjects.[4] Several procedures have shown such a pattern. For example, in a task that simply requires *rapid counting of the number of elements* flashed onto a screen (Place & Gilmore, 1980; Wells & Leventhal, 1984), schizophrenic patients have been found less impaired than normals when the items have been arranged to approximate an organized array, a display condition that reduces the accuracy of the count among nonschizophrenic subjects. Although this advantage probably results from a difficulty in schizophrenic patients' ability to perceptually assimilate the structure of the total display, their counting accuracy is notably superior to control group subjects under such conditions (Knight, 1993).

A *negative priming effect* task also yields a better performance in schizophrenics than in nonschizophrenic subjects. On this task, subjects are trained to ignore a stimulus. When that same stimulus is later made into a target to be learned, nonpatients' efficiency in learning the target is reduced by their previous experiences with the target. In contrast, it is easier for subjects with schizotypic personalities than for comparison groups to learn the new target, presumably showing a less substantial impact from the inhibition phase of the training (Claridge, Clarke, & Beech, 1992).

Psychophysiological Measures

Some investigators have turned to the study of psychophysiological functions to explore the contribution of biological systems to attention functioning and to mine their potential as markers of schizophrenic pathology and vulnerability. These include *event-related potentials (ERPs),* which plot brain waves across short intervals. Friedman and Squires-Wheeler's (1994) recent review reports consistent evidence that late components of the waveform (N200, P300, and slow wave) tend to be reduced in schizophrenic patients; but because ERPs have not shown high levels of specificity in discriminating schizophrenic patients from patients with other major disturbances (e.g., bipolar disorders), these authors caution that the utility of ERP indices as risk markers has not been fully established. Nevertheless research of brain neurophysiology continues to be conducted with the hope that the attentional deficits associated with schizophrenia will be clarified.

Recent interest has been shown in studying brain functions when subjects are given more complex stimulus conditions than are typically used in ERP challenges. Study of the *sensory gating of the P50 ERP wave* uses a procedure similar in kind to the prepulse inhibition procedure devised to assess startle responses (described above). Freedman et al. (1993) report that the normal inhibitory effect from an initial mild stimulus — an effect that is expected to reduce the ERP to a second stimulus — is not present in schizophrenics. Like the findings in startle response studies, an early positive wave component (P50) of the evoked response (ERP) to a target signal is not reduced in schizophrenics by the presence of a previous stimulus. These findings suggest that the attentional malfunctions in schizophrenic patients extend to the earliest moments of information processing. The deficit seems to leave the schizophrenic relatively unprotected from stimulation that the normal brain automatically controls through gating functions. The fact that relatives of schizophrenic patients also have shown similar patterns of gating deficit suggests that this processing fault may be transmitted along family lines.

In addition to studies of brain physiology, considerable effort has been directed to the study of schizophrenics' autonomic nervous system functions. One of the most extensively researched areas is the *skin conductance orienting responses* (SCOR). In SCOR studies, underresponse to repeated tone stimuli is found in 40–50% of schizophrenic patients (Bernstein, 1993) and is stable over time (Spohn, Coyne, Spray, & Hayes, 1989). Although there has not been much success to date in determining the potential of SCOR deviations as a risk marker, Cannon and Mednick (1988) have found hyporesponsivity among high-risk adolescents to predict schizophrenia-spectrum disorders later in their lives. However, the picture is made cloudy by the fact that some at-risk subjects have augmented SCOR (hyperresponsivity) preceding later disturbances (Dawson, Nuechterlein, Schell &, Mintz, 1992). Given these uncertanties, Bernstein (1993) concludes his recent review of SCOR research with a caution about the place of SCOR deviations as a vulnerability marker.

The *smooth pursuit eye-tracking deviations* (ETD) procedure requires subjects to track a moving target approximating the swing of a 2-hertz pendulum; this permits researchers to study the synchrony between eye movements and the actual target velocity, and also co-occurring saccadic activity. These events may be relevant to an understanding of faults in early moments of visual attention systems. Schizophrenic patients show a choppy, dysfluent quality to their eye tracking, a finding that further confirms their difficulty in absorbing information in an efficient and effortless manner. Work with this technique has been encouraged by findings of especially good specificity and sensitivity of ETD measures in schizophrenic patients and those at risk for the disorder (see reviews by Levy, Holtzman, Matthysse, & Mendell, 1993, and Iacono, 1993).

ETD is frequently found among schizophrenic patients. For example, Holzman et al. (1974) found 84% of chronic schizophrenic patients showed ETD. Although Iacono's team reports a much lower level for various ETD indices than does Holzman's lab, even at a lower rate the test continues to have good sensitivity for schizophrenic patients (Iacono, 1993) and for schizophrenic patients in remission (Grove et al., 1991).

With respect to familial risk, Holzman et al. (1974) reported the extent of ETD to be 45% in relatives of schizophrenics, in comparison to between 8% and 11% of other psychiatric patients and nonpsychiatric subject groups. Individuals with schizotypic personality disorders also have shown ETD (Siever et al., 1990). The value of ETD as a risk marker is supported by genetic studies (Kendler et al., 1990) showing a high concordance among monozygotic twins.

Summary Impressions

The development of measures sensitive to schizophrenic patients' attentional deficits (and related psychophysiological indices) has made steady gains in the past several decades. The best and most promising measures are reliable, and they find deficits in at least one out of two schizophrenic patients, with some measures achieving excellent sensitivities. Specificity is not always as strong as sensitivity (Cornblatt & Keilp, 1994, e.g., found 90% sensitivity but only 30% specificity from the CPT measure).[4] Nevertheless, low specificity is not a cause for despair; attentional impairments may be a final common pathway for various disorders and may reflect a kinship among major pathologies. For example, reaction time deficits found in aging, temporal lobe epilepsy, and schizophrenic populations may reflect brain systems commonly affected in several disorders.

Promise for improved understanding is found in recent developments that include the charting of linkages between attentional functions and brain systems (Posner, 1994), the study of relationships between attentional deficits and individual differences in symptom patterns (Knight, 1987), and the relevance of attentional deficits for schizophrenic patients' outcomes (Cancro et al., 1971; Cornblatt & Keilp, 1994; Steffy & Waldman, 1993). For example, Steffy and Waldman (1993) reported that schizophrenic patients with excessively slow SRT latencies, in contrast to faster responders, may have longer continuing periods of hospitalization, whereas those with marked (relative to less severe) RTX patterns are more likely to have a greater number of recurrent hospitalizations.

The time may well be ripe to capitalize on the prognostic and discriminating power of these measures and establish a battery of attentional tests that can be used as clinical tools to assist in assessment of individual patients. When compared with the current diagnostic practices based on interviews, the quality of measurement in the tests reviewed here would make them good adjuncts to the currently used standard assessment techniques.

PROCESS-ORIENTED STRATEGIES: APPLICATION OF MODELS

As described above, several tests of attentional functioning yield schizophrenic performance deficits that have proven to be reliable, sensitive, and able to detect vulnerability for a schizophrenic disorder. Nevertheless, the use of single tasks in psychopathology research has been sternly criticized because group differences on such measures are prone to generalized deficit artifacts, are subject to the impact of nuisance variables (medication, hospitalization, etc.), and are unable to yield definitive and verifiable understandings of underlying mechanisms (e.g., Knight, 1993).

A new generation of research strategies promises to rectify these difficulties by employing constructs generated from models of information-processing and brain systems. Cognitive psychology models focus on events that occur in the brain during the first moments after fresh information is encountered, to make sense of perception, learning, memory, and other basic processes (e.g., Kahneman & Triesman, 1984; Schneider & Shiffrin, 1985). In recent years, models of the "brain at work" have also guided research into schizophrenic dysfunctions. As illustrated by the work of Knight and Neufeld discussed in the next two subsections, theoretical advances can be obtained by studying patterns of deficit performance across measures that are topographically dissimilar but converge on similar processes. The work of Posner broadens the neuropsychological focus to add neuroanatomical considerations. Cohen and Servan-Schreiber link schizophrenic deficits to neurochemical action through "artificial intelligence" (AI) modeling.

Knight's Cognitive Modeling

Ray Knight (1987) gives special credit in his thinking to the work of Place and Gilmore (1980), who demonstrated that schizophrenic patients organize information in rapidly-presented visual displays in ways different from nonschizophrenics. As already mentioned, Place and Gilmore asked schizophrenic patients and drug-abusing subjects to count the number of rapidly flashed elements (a random-appearing array of horizontal and vertical lines). The performances of the schizophrenic and drug-abuse patients were found essentially equivalent under a random line array condition. However, when the line elements were grouped—imposing structure into the display—the drug-abuse subjects' performance accuracy decreased. In contrast, the schizophrenic patients showed no impact from the change in the format. This finding was replicated by Wells and Leventhal (1984) and has been taken as evidence of a perceptual organization difficulty occurring in the earliest moments of schizophrenics' information processing—a time during which a global, relatively undifferentiated appreciation of the display occurs. Knight and his colleagues sought to provide a more exact account of the stage of processing and mechanism of such differences.

Adopting an information-processing model that divides the visual perceptual act into two distinct phases—an early 100-millisecond sensory store, and a second phase (extending from 100 to 600 milliseconds) during which short-term visual memory (STVM) processes occur (Phillips, 1974)—Knight's studies first explored which of these two phases are most likely to be implicated in process schizophrenic patients' deficits. To do this, Knight, Sherer, Putchat, and Carter (1978) used a technique based on Eriksen and Collins's (1967) study of iconic storage, a procedure in which pictures of common objects were segregated into components presented separately from each other. The target figure, although easily recognized when all components were displayed simultaneously, was not recognizable when either portion of the display was presented alone. Iconic memory was evaluated by examining the subjects' ability to see an intact figure as a function of a delay interval interposed between the two separate displays, with the expectation that progressively longer intervals would make it more difficult for anyone to grasp the full percept. In two labs, nonschizophrenic and process schizophrenics were found to have equivalent levels of decrement as a function of the interstimulus interval between the component presentations (Knight et al., 1978; Spaulding et al., 1980). This finding reveals comparable memory decays in the patients' and nonpatients' iconic memory systems, and it eliminates a uniquely weak iconic store as an explanation of schizophrenics' perceptual organizational difficulties.

Since the organization of a perceptual field must occur rapidly to make sense out of the complex sensory environment impinging on one's receptor organs, and since this research had eliminated the icon as a source of schizophrenics' perceptual organization problem, Knight's next research focused on phase 2, the STVM store, as a likely source of the visual-attentional problems common to process schizophrenics. That work corroborated the importance of STVM processes, by showing that backward-masking strategies impaired process schizophrenics' performances relative to good premorbid schizophrenic, nonschizophrenic patients, and non-ill subjects primarily in the phase 2 (100–600 milliseconds) time zone (Knight, Elliott, & Freedman, 1985). As we discussed earlier, the critical interval during which schizophrenics have been found impaired by a masking stimulus (following and superimposed upon the space previously occupied by a target display) extends up to 500 milliseconds, a time that falls well within the second phase.

As Knight continues to clarify the exact nature of the processes involved in STVM deficits, he is also interested in its association to individual differences, hoping to understand why his findings are mainly germane to the more severely disabled process schizophrenics. He hopes to see his work linked directly to understanding of particular symptoms as well as models of neural functioning (Knight, 1987, 1992).

Neufeld's Stochastic Modeling of Schizophrenic Information Processes

Richard (Jim) Neufeld's laboratory has studied paranoid schizophrenics' task performances. Despite the generally better level of cognitive and language functioning observed in paranoid relative to nonparanoid schizophrenic patients (Magaro, 1981), tests of attentional functioning (e.g., Span of Apprehension Test, according to Asarnow & MacCrimmon, 1978; Dobson & Neufeld, 1982) generally do not elicit paranoid–nonparanoid performance differences. To clarify paranoid schizophrenic patients' particular limitations, Neufeld and his group have turned their research focus to memory functioning where there is long-standing evidence of performance impairments that distinguish the paranoid schizophrenic patient from both nonschizophrenic patients and nonparanoid schizophrenics (Neufeld, 1991).

Complex, conceptually demanding memory task performances have been repeatedly found to be impaired in paranoid schizophrenic patients by Neufeld's research (Broga & Neufeld, 1981; Dobson & Neufeld, 1982). Illustrating his team's tests, Vollick's (1994) study used pictures containing drawings of common objects (toasters, washing machines, chairs, etc. — with the number of items varying to create different levels of memory demands). Pictures of these objects were displayed briefly for subjects to memorize the items. Afterward, a single target object (different from the memory set items) was presented and subjects were asked if the target figure is similar in "real life" size to any of the items in the memorized set. "Yes/no" answers were timed to give estimates of information-processing speed. Such a task requires subjects to transform objects into a physical (size) dimension, a task further complicated by the use of diverse stimulus-encoding operations—contrasting either verbally labeled or pictorial target stimuli.

Neufeld's team typically submits the latency and error data generated from these procedures to stochastic-modeling "goodness of fit" tests to infer mental operations that may account for subjects' pattern of response latencies. Findings from their lab suggest that paranoid schizophrenics manage these complex tasks rather well. Task demands (such as the level of memory load) on processing have the same relative degree of impact on the performance of schizophrenics as they do on other subjects. Neufeld and his colleagues interpret their findings to suggest that paranoid schizophrenics' basic attentional and memory functions do not differ from non-ill populations. However, the intercept of the performance gradients reflecting overall speed of patient and normal performances is distinguishable, and that difference is attributed through the stochastic-modeling computations to the paranoid patients' use of a more complex and unwieldy set of independent subprocesses as they transform stimuli into a usable mode (Neufeld, Vollick, & Highgate-Maynard, 1993).

The exact nature of the subprocesses Neufeld infers from his calculations has not been specified, but suggests that schizophrenics (particularly paranoids) may recruit extraneous mental operations, and may be inefficient in handling complex displays as a simple gestalt, favoring instead a focus on separate components (Neufeld & Williamson, 1996). Neufeld (1991) speculates, for example, that schizophrenic patients' well-established difficulties on the Wisconsin Card Sorting Test may result from extraneous activities that impair selective attention whenever the subjects' eyes are drawn to consider the rich stimulus array occurring on each trial (the four key stimuli, the target stimulus, along with the four discard piles). Indeed, Neufeld's concept of overly abundant subprocesses may reflect factors familiar to those working strictly within the attention domain, namely, factors akin to self-generated irrelevancies. Although Neufeld's procedures do not as yet seem ready for the investigation of individual differences or the exploration of high risk populations needed to learn the pertinence of these mechanisms for vulnerability, his group has a strong interest in the use of complex memory tasks and stochastic modeling for charting stages of the disorder.

Posner's Neuropsychological Laboratory

Michael I. Posner and his colleagues have explored visual–spatial attentional functioning in schizophrenics, in normal controls, and in subjects with known sites of focal brain damage (Posner, Early, Reiman, Pardo, & Dhawan, 1988). On the basis of others' view that schizophrenic deficits may lie predominantly in the left hemisphere (e.g., Gruzelier & Flor-Henry, 1979), they expected that schizophrenics would show greater processing delays to signals presented in the right visual field than to those in the left visual field, when a signal-detection task drew upon subjects' ability to process visuospatial information. In one of their tasks, subjects were required to press a key whenever they saw a target figure presented in either the right or left visual field. Added to this demand, a position-informative cue appeared at variable durations preceding the target to hint to the subject where the target might appear. That cue was informative on 80% of the trials but misleading in the other 20% (i.e., falsely directing attention to the wrong field). As had been expected, these investigators found that a sample of schizophrenic patients showed a lateralized asymmetry in the processing of information, much like the pattern observed in patients with known left hemisphere parietal lesions. However, because schizophrenics' left visual field responses were also more inaccurate than expected, a lateralized parietal lobe impairment did not offer a full explanation for the observed deficits. Posner, Early, et al. (1988) then noted that the deficit was strongest for those of the patients who experienced auditory hallucinations, suggesting that language-processing problems might contribute to the pattern. They reasoned that the schizophrenic subjects might have suffered distraction from internally generated language (a factor that can give rise to auditory hallucinations) in addition to the demands of the visuospatial task.

To assess this possibility, Posner, Early, et al. (1988) next tested non-schizophrenic subjects whose performance on the visuospatial task was complicated by a requirement to shadow an aurally delivered story. Insofar as these nonschizophrenic subjects' performance (impaired by an attention-sharing demand) showed a pattern similar to that of schizophrenic patients, Posner's team speculated on the concurrent roles of both anterior and posterior brain attentional systems that integrate language and visuospatial attentional systems, in accounting for schizophrenic impairment. This view gained support in a further study that required subjects to press a button indicating a left or right direction in accordance with either the words "left" or "right," or arrows pointing in either direction, a task complicated by variations in the congruency of the verbal and nonverbal cues.

Although Posner's findings are not always replicated (e.g., Nestor et al., 1992), they are widely cited as models for neuropsychological strategies. If the weight of subsequent evidence finds the lateralizing effect in schizophrenic patients, the Posner task may be found useful in vulnerability research to follow. Since schizophrenia is currently diagnosed because of thought disorder symptoms, any measures of left hemisphere functions that might reflect risk for subsequent language and thought problems would be of substantial value in charting the life history of the disorder.

Cohen and Servan-Schreiber's Neural Network Modeling

Jonathan D. Cohen and David Servan-Schreiber employ parallel distributed processing (neural) networks for computer simulations of schizophrenic deficit. Derived from work in artificial intelligence (AI) technologies, computer simulations of brain systems have been developed to approximate normal human performances on tasks, and the systems are degraded selectively so that the system's performance will approximate that found in a patient population.

Cohen and Servan-Schreiber's (1992, 1993) work was guided by Chapman and Chapman's (1973) concept of schizophrenic patients' impaired use of contextual information in conceptual tasks. Schizophrenic patients have repeatedly been shown to have a reduced ability to manage tasks that require the understanding of the context in which a target stimulus is given (e.g., the word "pen" changes its meaning if it is preceded by the word "pig" or succeeded by the word "pal"), but schizophrenics tend to be overly influenced by the most often-encountered "strong" meaning of the word. Using the Chapman's construction, this team tested computer systems that simulate diverse attentional and conceptual tasks with distinctive contextual cue features (the CPT-IP, the Stroop Color-Word Test, and a lexical decision task). The computer systems were altered (made "schizophrenic") by adjusting a "gain" parameter that reduced the sensitivity of simulated neuronal units to input activation, thus influencing the units' capacity to discriminate between lower and higher activation levels. They found that the procedure resulted in computer performances equivalent in level of error to schizophrenic patients' observed performance on these same tasks. The concept of "gain" in their research was meant to simulate dopamine systems (perhaps in mesocortical regions that project to prefrontal lobe areas) that might be sites of dysfunctional areas in some schizophrenic patients and are sites deemed especially important to attentional and cognitive tasks where contextual cues are salient task features.

Cohen and Servan-Schreiber's demonstration of a computer-simulated performance deficit, guided by an explicitly described set of neuromechanisms, is perceived as a major leap forward. Although the exact model is troubled by a concept of reduced dopamine activity that contrasts with evidence that schizophrenic patients often show increased dopamine sensitivity (Jobe, Harrow, Martin, Whitfield, & Sands, 1994), Cohen and Servan-Schreiber need merely argue that there are different dopamine dynamics in different parts of the schizophrenic brain to defend their simulation.

There are many other brain hypotheses that await AI analyses. Perhaps concepts of frontal lobe dysconnection applied by Frith (1990) to explain impairments in the "supervisory attentional systems" in schizophrenics' frontal lobe functioning is a good candidate for future brain modeling. A neural developmental construction has recently been advanced by Hoffman and Dobscha (1989) to explore schizophrenic memory loss in networks degraded by a concept of "axonal pruning." Clearly these efforts at modeling are still on the horizon, requiring experimentation, but at the moment regarded as promising leads.

CONCLUSIONS

Schizophrenic attentional deficits are many-splendored things, and their complexity defies our attempts to put forward a single explanatory position. Reports in the experimental psychopathology literature often rely, therefore, on a listing of broad task-descriptive factors such as sustained, selective or focused, encoded, and shifting attention based on the features of tasks used in attentional measurement (Mirsky, 1988; Zubin, 1975). From the work reviewed here, it is clear that a number of specific measures have played an important role in documenting schizophrenic attentional difficulties. Models of deficits that may occur in various stages of information processing offer new approaches to understanding the development of attentional problems. Although no strategies have yet resulted in a comprehensive theory, there has been commendable progress in setting the stage. Our review of some of the best single-task measures (SRT, Span of Apprehension Test, and CPT), along with other less studied measures such as backward masking, prepulse inhibition of the startle reflex, SCOR, and ETD, has shown excellent discriminating power and other measurement strengths in these tasks. Strauss et al. (1993) recently showed high internal consistencies (.88 and .97) for the Span of Apprehension Test and the CPT, respectively. These measures also have adequate levels of retest reliability.

We see an advantage in collecting a set of the best laboratory tests on the same subjects to be used in multivariate analyses. Despite the fact that weak intercorrelations across tasks are often reported (Asarnow et al., 1977; Kopfstein & Neale, 1972; Strauss, Buchanan, & Hale, 1993), low intercorrelation among predictor variables is not a disadvantage to predicting criteria, such as diagnosis or postcare adjustment. Individual attentional measures often correlate with important outcome indices (Cancro et al., 1971; Steffy, 1993; Steffy & Waldman, 1993). It is conceivable, therefore, that a collection of the best-validated single-task measures may have utility when tested in multiple regression designs using life adjustment factors (response to treatment, relapse rate) as criteria. We can also envision using the best single-task measures as part of a lab technology that will be blended with standard clinical measures for assessment purposes (Connelly, 1984; Spaulding, Hargrove, Crinean, & Martin, 1981).

We anticipate that collections of such measures will eventually yield theoretical advances as well. A recent theory by Cromwell (1993b) advances the idea that attentional measures reflect either one or both of two sources of core disturbance in schizophrenia, namely, excessive excitability (supersensitivity) or excessive inhibition. When these tendencies co-occur, Cromwell suggests that the probability of a schizophrenic episode is high. He argues that these tendencies may map onto the different symptom patterns and may have separable genetic bases. Cromwell's conception of an excessive excitatory mechanism is derived from the reliable qualities of performance impairment resulting from the use of the PRT, RTX, and Cross-Modal Reaction Time measures, as well as the "overload" noted in Span of Apprehension Test performances. On the other hand, schizophrenic patients also tend to show remarkable suppressive (inhibitory) features noted in the line-enumeration (item-counting) procedure of Place and Gilmore (1980) and other indications of schizophrenics' failure to process information (e.g., prepulse inhibition, the T50 gating phenomenon, as well as underresponse in SCOR studies). Any future "master theory" of schizophrenic attentional functioning will have to account for the remarkable variations in schizophrenic patients' sensitivity to stimulation that are documented by these measures of over- and under-responsivity.

The cognitive and brain modeling approaches offer an especially exciting promise of theoretical development based on hypothetico-deductive reasoning. However, the application of this work to understanding schizophrenia is in its infancy and suffers from a surplus of alternatives. There are many suspected brain sites (e.g., frontal, septohippocampal, thalamus, basal ganglia, and temporal lobe systems) and there are also many cognitive models that might be applied. Moreover, Knight (1987) points out that some of the cognitive models that are now viewed to be promising may lose their appeal as new work in cognitive laboratories advances. If, however, there is a breakthrough resulting from a given model, the model-relevant measures will probably be validated with the same experimental strategies used by authors of the single-task measures described in the early part of this chapter, namely, study of subtypes, performance variations across phase of the illness, and antecedents in the lives of at-risk individuals that will forecast future breakdowns.

Clearly the study of attentional dysfunctions in schizophrenic disorders has been shown to deserve the emphasis it has been given in the past six decades of investigation. The demand for basic investigations that refine attention measures and explicate the underlying processes continues to be strong. As measures of attention are developed, refined, and made theoretically cogent, they become available for use in understanding the developmental precursors of schizophrenic disorders, a vital step in elucidation of its nature and in preventing breakdown among those at risk.

NOTES

1. Steffy's team repeatedly observed the effect to be specific to the process schizophrenics (those with poor premorbid adjustment and insidious onset to their disturbance), and not found in reactive (good premorbid, sudden onset) schizophrenics.

2. Although the CPT was originally devised to index decrements in attention over time, no trial factor was significant in the original Rosvold et al. (1956) study—and deterioration in performance over trials in later studies has rarely been shown (Cornblatt & Keilp, 1994)—so trial effects are not regularly reported.

3. Demonstrations of schizophrenic superiority on a task is a relatively unusual event and presents a distinct investigative advantage in providing estimates of functioning that are not an artifact of a generalized deficit.

4. Sometimes the reverse is true; Iacono (1993) reported excellent specificity but weak sensitivity in his studies of ETD. Clearly there is a need for further work on the patterning of attentional problems among diverse psychiatric populations.

REFERENCES

American Psychiatric Association. (1994) *Diagnostic and statistical manual of mental disorders* (4th ed.). Washington, DC: Author.

Asarnow, J. R. (1988). Children at risk for schizophrenia: Converging lines of evidence. *Schizophrenia Bulletin, 14,* 613–631.

Asarnow, R. F., & MacCrimmon, D. J. (1978). Residual performance deficit in clinically remitted schizophrenics: A marker of schizophrenia? *Journal of Abnormal Psychology, 87,* 597–608.

Asarnow, R. F., & MacCrimmon, D. J. (1981). Span of apprehension deficits during postpsychotic stages of schizophrenia. *Archives of General Psychiatry, 38,* 1006–1011.

Asarnow, R. F., Nuechterlein, K. H., & Marder, S. R. (1983). Span of apprehension performance, neuropsychological functioning and indices of psychosis proneness. *Journal of Nervous and Mental Disease, 171,* 662–669.

Asarnow, R. F., Steffy, R. A., MacCrimmon, D. J., & Cleghorn, J. M. (1977). An attentional assessment of foster children at risk for schizophrenia. *Journal of Abnormal Psychology, 86,* 267–275.

Asarnow, R. F., Steffy, R. A., & Waldman, I. (1985). Comment on Harvey, Weintraub, and Neale: Span of apprehension deficits in children vulnerable to psychopathology. *Journal of Abnormal Psychology, 94,* 414–417.

Bellissimo, A., & Steffy, R. A. (1972). Redundancy-associated deficit in schizophrenic reaction time performance. *Journal of Abnormal Psychology, 80,* 299–307.

Bellissimo, A., & Steffy, R. A. (1975). Contextual influences on crossover in the reaction time performance of schizophrenics. *Journal of Abnormal Psychology, 84,* 210–110.

Bergman, A., Osgood, C., Pathak, A., Keefe, R., & Cornblatt, B. (1992). Attention and the progression of psychosis [Abstract]. *Biological Psychiatry, 31,* 115.

Bernstein, A. (1993). Missing facts and other lacunae in orienting research in schizophrenia. In R. L. Cromwell & C. R. Snyder (Eds.), *Schizophrenia: Origins, processes, treatment, and outcome* (pp. 197–219). New York: Oxford University Press.

Bohannon, W. E., & Strauss, M. E. (1983). Reaction time crossover in psychiatric outpatients. *Psychiatry Research, 9,* 17–22.

Braff, D. L., Stone, C., Callaway, E., Geyer, M., Glick, I., & Bali, L. (1978). Prestimulus effects on human startle reflex in normals and schizophrenics. *Psychophysiology, 15,* 339–343.

Broga, M. I., & Neufeld, R. W. J. (1981). Multivariate cognitive performance levels and response styles among paranoid and nonparanoid schizophrenics. *Journal of Abnormal Psychology, 90,* 495–509.

Cadenhead, K., & Braff, D. L. (1992). Which criteria select "psychosis-prone" individuals? *Biological Psychiatry, 31,* 161–162.

Cancro, R., Sutton, S. Kerr, J. B., & Sugerman, A. A. (1971). Reaction time and prognosis in acute schizophrenia. *Journal of Nervous and Mental Disease, 153,* 351–359.

Cannon, T., & Mednick, S. (1988). *Autonomic nervous system antecedents of positive and negative symptoms in schizophrenia.* Paper presented at the meeting of the Society for Psychophysiological Research, San Francisco, CA.

Cash, T. F., Neale, J. M., & Cromwell, R. L. (1972). Span of apprehension in acute schizohrenics: Full-report technique. *Journal of Abnormal Psychology, 79,* 322–326.

Cegalis, J. A., Leen, D., & Solomon, E. J. (1977) Attention in schizophrenia: An analysis of selectivity in the functional visual field. *Journal of Abnormal Psychology, 86,* 470–482.

Chapman, L. J., & Chapman, J. P. (1973). *Disordered thought in schizophrenia.* New York: Appleton-Century-Crofts.

Claridge, G. S., Clarke, K. H., & Beech, A. R. (1992). Lateralization of the "negative priming" effect: Relationships with schizotypy and with gender. *British Journal of Psychology, 83,* 13–23.

Cohen, J. D., & Servan-Schreiber, D. (1992). Context, cortex, and dopamine: A connectionist approach to behavior and biology in schizophrenia. *Psychological Review, 99*(1), 45–77.

Cohen, J. D., & Servan-Schreiber, D. (1993). A theory of dopamine function and its role in cognitive deficits in schizophrenia. *Schizophrenia Bulletin, 19,* 85–104.

Cohler, B. J., Grunebaum, H. U., Weiss, J. L., Gamer, E., & Gallant, D. H. (1977). Disturbance of attention among schizophrenic, depressed and well mothers and their young children. *Journal of Child Psychology and Psychiatry, 18,* 115–135.

Connelly, W. (1984). *DSM-III schizophrenic disorder: Comparisons with other functional psychoses and borderline conditions.* Unpublished doctoral dissertation, University of Waterloo, Ontario.

Cornblatt, B. A., & Erlenmeyer-Kimling, L. (1985). Global attentional deviance in children at risk for schizophrenia: Specificity and predictive validity. *Journal of Abnormal Psychology, 94,* 470–486.

Cornblatt, B. A., & Keilp, J. G. (1994). Impaired attention, genetics, and the pathophysiology of schizophrenia. *Schizophrenia Bulletin, 20,* 31–46.

Cromwell, R. L. (1975). Assessment of schizophrenia. *Annual Review of Psychology, 26,* 593–619.

Cromwell, R. L. (1993a). Schizophrenia research: Things to do before the geneticist arrives. In R. L. Cromwell & C. R. Snyder (Eds.), *Schizophrenia: Origins, processes, treatment and outcome* (pp. 51–61). New York: Oxford University Press.

Cromwell, R. L. (1993b). A summary review of schizophrenia. In R. L. Cromwell & C. R. Snyder (Eds.), *Schizophrenia: Origins, processes, treatment and outcome* (pp. 335–349). New York: Oxford University Press.

Davidson, G. S., & Neale, J. M. (1974). The effects of signal–noise similarity on visual information processing in schizophrenics. *Journal of Abnormal Psychology, 83,* 683–686.

Dawson, M. E., Nuechterlein, K. H., Schell, A. M., & Mintz, J. (1992). Concurrent and predictive electrodermal correlates of symptomatology in recent-onset schizophrenic patients. *Journal of Abnormal Psychology, 101,* 153–164.

DeAmicis, L. A., & Cromwell, R. L. (1979). Reaction time crossover in process schizophrenic patients, their relatives, and control subjects. *Journal of Nervous and Mental Disease, 167,* 593–600.

DeAmicis, L. A., Huntzinger, R. S., & Cromwell, R. L. (1981). Magnitude of reaction time crossover in process schizophrenic patients in relation to their first-degree relatives. *Journal of Nervous and Mental Disease, 169,* 64–65.

Diefendorf, A. R. (1923). *Clinical psychiatry: A textbook for students and physicians abstracted and adapted from the seventh German edition (1896) of Kraepelin's "Lehrbuch der Psychiatrie."* New York: Macmillan.

Dobson, D. J. G., & Neufeld, R. W. J. (1982). Paranoid–nonparanoid schizophrenic distinctions in the implementation of external conceptual constraints. *Journal of Nervous and Mental Disease, 170,* 614–621.

Dobson, D. J. G., & Neufeld, R. W. J. (1987). Span of apprehension among remitted schizophrenics using small visual angles. *Journal of Nervous and Mental Disease, 175,* 362–366.

Elkins, I. J., Cromwell, R. I., & Asarnow, R. F. (1992). Span of apprehension in schizophrenics patients as a function of distractor masking and laterality. *Journal of Abnormal Psychology, 101,* 53–60.

Eriksen, C. W., & Collins, J. F. (1967). Some temporal characteristics of visual pattern perception. *Journal of Experimental Psychology, 74,* 476–484.

Erlenmeyer-Kimling, L., & Cornblatt, B. A. (1992). A summary of attentional findings in the New York High-Risk Project. *Journal of Psychiatric Research, 26,* 405–426.

Estes, W. K., & Taylor, H. A. (1964). A detection method and probabilistic models for assessing information processing from brief visual displays. *Proceedings of the National Academy of Science, U.S.A., 52,* 446–454.

Freedman, R., Waldo, M., Adler, L. E., Nagamoto, H., Cawthra, E., Madison, A., Hoffer, L., & Bickford-Wimer, P. (1993). Schizotaxia and sensory gating. In R. L. Cromwell & C. R. Snyder (Eds.), *Schizophrenia: Origins, processes, treatment, and outcome* (pp. 98–108). New York: Oxford University Press.

Friedman, D., & Squires-Wheeler, E. (1994). Event-related potentials (ERPs) as indicators of risk for schizophrenia. *Schizophrenia Bulletin, 20,* 63–74.

Frith, C. D. (1990). *The cognitive neuropsychology of schizophrenia.* Hove, East Sussex, UK: Erlbaum.

Garmezy, N. (1974). Children at risk: The search for the antecedents of schizophrenia — Part 1. Conceptual models and research methods. *Schizophrenia Bulletin,* 14–90.

Gibson, J. J. (1941). A critical review of the concept of set in contemporary psychology. *Psychological Bulletin, 38,* 781–817.

Greiffenstein, M., Lewis, R., Milberg, W., & Rosenbaum, G. (1981). Temporal lobe epilepsy and schizophrenia: Comparison of reaction time deficits. *Journal of Abnormal Psychology, 90,* 105–112.

Grove, W. M., Lebow, B. S., Clementz, B. A., Cerri, A., Medus, C., & Iacono, W. G. (1991). Familial prevalence and coaggregation of schizotypy indicators: A multitrait family study. *Journal of Abnormal Psychology, 100,* 115–121.

Grunebaum, H., Weiss, J. L., Gallant, D., & Cohler, B. J. (1974). Attention in young children of psychotic mothers. *American Journal of Psychiatry, 131,* 887–891.

Gruzelier, J., & Flor-Henry, P. (Eds.) (1979). *Hemisphere asymmetries of function in psychopathology.* Amsterdam: Elsevier/North-Holland.

Hanson, D. R., Gottesman, I. I., & Heston, L. L. (1976). Some possible childhood indicators of adult schizophrenia inferred from children of schizophrenics. *British Journal of Psychiatry, 129,* 142–154.

Harvey, P. D., Weintraub, S., & Neale, J. M. (1985). Span of apprehension deficits in children vulnerable to psychopathology: A failure to replicate. *Journal of Abnormal Psychology, 94,* 410–413.

Hoffman, R. E., & Dobscha, S. K. (1989). Cortical pruning and the development of schizophrenia: A computer model. *Schizophrenia Bulletin, 15,* 477–490.

Holzman, P. S., Proctor, L. R., Levy, D. L., Yasillo, N. J., Maltzer, H. Y., & Hurt, S. W. (1974). Eye-tracking dysfunctions in schizophrenic patients and their relatives. *Archives of General Psychiatry, 31,* 143–151.

Iacono, W. G. (1993). Smooth pursuit oculomotor dysfunction as an index of schizophrenia. In R. L. Cromwell & C. R. Snyder (Eds.), *Schizophrenia: Origins, processes, treatment, and outcome* (pp. 76–97). New York: Oxford University Press.

Jobe, T. H., Harrow, M., Martin, E. M., Whitfield, H. J., & Sands, J. R. (1994). Schizophrenic deficits: Neuroleptics and prefrontal cortex. *Schizophrenia Bulletin, 20,* 413–416.

Kahneman, D., & Treisman, A. (1984). Changing views of attention and automaticity. In R. Parasuraman & D. R. Davies (Eds.), *Varieties of attention* (pp. 29–61), Orlando, FL: Academic Press.

Kendler, K. S., Ochs, A. L., Gorman, A. M., Hewitt, J. K., Ross, D. E., & Mirsky, A. F. (1990). The structure of schizotypy: A pilot multitrait twin study. *Psychiatry Research, 36,* 19–36.

Knight, R. A. (1987). Relating cognitive processes to symptoms: A strategy to counter methodological difficulties. In P. D. Harvey & E. F. Walker (Eds.), *Positive and negative symptoms of psychosis: Description, research, and future directions* (pp. 1–29). Hillsdale, NJ: Erlbaum.

Knight, R. A. (1992). Specifying cognitive deficits in poor premorbid schizophrenics. In E. Walker, R. Dworkin, & B. Cornblatt (Eds.), *Progress in experimental personality and psychopathology research* (Vol. 15, pp. 252–289). New York: Springer.

Knight, R. A. (1993). Comparing cognitive models of schizophrenics' input dysfunction. In R. L. Cromwell & C. R. Snyder (Eds.), *Schizophrenia: Origins, processes, treatment, and outcome* (pp. 151–175). New York: Oxford University Press.

Knight, R. A., Elliott, D. S., & Freedman, M. (1985). Short-term visual memory in schizophrenics. *Journal of Abnormal Psychology, 94,* 427–442.

Knight, R. A., Sherer, M., Putchat, C., & Carter, G. (1978). A picture integration task for measuring iconic memory in schizophrenics. *Journal of Abnormal Psychology, 87,* 314–321.

Kopfstein, J. H., & Neale, J. M. (1972). A multivariate study of attention dysfunction in schizophrenia. *Journal of Abnormal Psychology, 80,* 294–298.

Kraepelin, E. (1919). *Dementia praecox and paraphrenia* (R. M. Barclay, Trans.). Edinburgh: Livingstone. (Original work published 1913)

Levy, D. L., Holzman, P. S., Matthysse, S., & Mendell, N. R. (1993). Eye tracking dysfunction and schizophrenia: A critical perspective. *Schizophrenia Bulletin, 19,* 461–536.

MacCrimmon, D. J., Cleghorn, J. M., Asarnow, R. F., & Steffy, R. A. (1980). Children at risk for schizophrenia: Clinical and attentional characteristics. *Archives of General Psychiatry, 37,* 671–674.

Magaro, P. A. (1981). The paranoid and the schizophrenic: The case for distinct cognitive style. *Schizophrenia Bulletin, 7,* 632–661.

Mannuzza, S. (1980). Cross-modal reaction time and schizophrenic attentional deficit: A critical review. *Schizophrenia Bulletin, 6,* 654–675.

Marcus, J., Auerbach, J., Wilkinson, L., & Burack, C. (1981). Infants at risk for schizophrenia: The Jerusalem infant development study. *Archives of General Psychiatry, 38,* 703–713.

Marcus, L. M. (1972). Studies of attention in children vulnerable to psychopathology (Doctoral dissertation, University of Minnesota). *Dissertation Abstracts International, 33,* 5023-B. (University Microfilms No. 73-10,606)

Marder, S. R., Asarnow, R. F., & Van Putten, T. (1984). Information processing and neuroleptic response in acute and stabilized schizophrenic patients. *Psychiatry Research, 13,* 41–49.

McGhie, A., & Chapman, J. (1961) Disorders of attention and perception in early schizophrenia. *British Journal of Medical Psychology, 34,* 103–116.

McNeil, R., & Kaij, L. (1973). Obstetrical complications and physical size of offspring of schizophrenic, schizophrenic-like, and control mothers. *British Journal of Psychiatry, 123,* 341–348.

Mednick, S. A., Parnas, J., & Schulsinger, F. (1987). The Copenhagen High-Risk Project, 1962–86. *Schizophrenia Bulletin, 13,* 485–495.

Mirsky, A. F. (1988). Research on schizophrenia in the NIMH Laboratory of Psychology and Psychopathology, 1954–1987. *Schizophrenia Bulletin, 14,* 151–156.

Neale, J. M. (1971). Perceptual span in schizophrenia. *Journal of Abnormal Psychology, 77,* 196–204.

Neale, J. M., McIntyre, C. W., Fox, R., & Cromwell, R. L. (1969). Span of apprehension in acute schizophrenics. *Journal of Abnormal Psychology, 74,* 593–596.

Nestor, P. G., Faux, S. F., McCarley, R. W., Penhune, V., Shenton, M. E., & Pollak, S. (1992). Attentional cues in chronic schizophrenia: Abnormal disengagement of attention. *Journal of Abnormal Psychology, 101,* 682–689.

Neufeld, R. W. J. (1991). Memory deficit in paranoid schizophrenia. In P. A. Magaro (Ed.), *The cognitive bases of mental disorders: Annual review of psychopathology* (pp. 31–61). New York: Sage.

Neufeld, R. W. J., Vollick, D., & Highgate-Maynard, S. (1993). Stochastic modelling of stimulus encoding and memory search in paranoid schizophrenia: Clinical and theoretical implications. In R. L. Cromwell & R. Snyder (Eds.), *Schizophrenia: Origins, processes, treatment, and outcome* (pp. 176–191). New York: Oxford University Press.

Neufeld, R. W. J., & Williamson, P. C. (1996). Neuropsychological correlates of positive symptoms: Delusions and hallucinations. In C. Pantelis, H. E. Nelson, & T. R. E. Barnes (Eds.), *Schizophrenia: A neuropsychological perspective* (pp. 205–235). New York: Wiley.

Nuechterlein, K. H. (1977). Reaction time and attention in schizophrenia: A critical evaluation of the data and the theories. *Schizophrenia Bulletin, 3,* 373–428.

Nuechterlein, K. H. (1983). Signal detection in vigilance tasks and behavioral attributes among offspring of schizophrenic mothers and among hyperactive children. *Journal of Abnormal Psychology, 92,* 4–28.

Nuechterlein, K. H., & Dawson, M. E. (1984). Information processing and attentional functioning in the developmental course of schizophrenic disorders. *Schizophrenia Bulletin, 10,* 160–203.

Orzack, M. H., & Kornetsky, C. (1966). Attention dysfunction in chronic schizophrenia. *Archives of General Psychiatry, 14,* 323–326.

Orzack, M. H., & Kornetsky, C. (1971). Environmental and familial predictors of attention behavior in chronic schizophrenics. *Journal of Psychiatric Research, 9,* 21–29.

Phillips, W. A. (1974). On the distinction between sensory storage and short-term visual memory. *Perception and Psychophysics, 16,* 283–290.

Place, E. J. S., & Gilmore, G. C. (1980). Perceptual organization in schizophrenia. *Journal of Abnormal Psychology, 89,* 409–418.

Posner, M. I. (1994) Attention: The mechanisms of consciousness. *Proceedings of the National Academy of Sciences, U.S.A., 91,* 7398–7403.

Posner, M. I., Early, T. S., Reiman, E., Pardo, P. J., & Dhawan, M. (1988). Asymmetries in hemispheric control of attention in schizophrenia. *Archives of General Psychiatry, 45,* 814–821.

Rodnick, E., & Shakow, D. (1940). Set in the schizophrenic as measured by a composite reaction time index. *American Journal of Psychiatry, 97,* 214–225.

Rosenbaum, G., Chapin, K., & Shore, D. L. (1988). Attention deficit in schizophrenia and schizotypy: Marker versus symptom variables. *Journal of Abnormal Psychology, 97,* 41–47.

Rosenthal, D., Lawlor, W. G., Zahn, R. P., & Shakow, D. (1960). The relatonship of some aspects of mental set to degree of schizophrenic disorganization. *Journal of Personality, 28,* 26–38.

Rosvold, H. E., Mirsky, A., Sarason, I., Bransome, E. D., Jr., & Beck, L. H. (1956). A continuous performance test of brain damage. *Journal of Consulting Psychology, 20,* 343–350.

Saccuzzo, D. P., Hirt, M., & Spencer, T. J. (1974). Backward masking as a measure of attention in schizophrenia. *Journal of Abnormal Psychology, 83,* 512–522.

Saccuzzo, D. P., & Schubert, D. L. (1981). Backward masking as a measure of slow processing in schizophrenia spectrum disorders. *Journal of Abnormal Psychology, 90,* 305–312.

Schneider, W., & Shiffrin, R. (1985). Categorization (restructuring) and automatization: Two separable factors. *Psychological Review, 92,* 424–428.

Shakow, D. (1962). Segmental set: A theory of the formal psychological deficit in schizophrenia. *Archives of General Psychiatry, 6,* 1–17.

Siever, L. J., Keefe, R., Bernstein, D. P., Cocavo, E. F., Klar, H. M., Zemishlang, Z., Peterson, A. E., Davidson, M., Mahon, T., Horvath, T., & Mohr, R. (1990). Eye tracking impairment in clinically identified patients with schizotypal disorder. *American Journal of Psychiatry, 147,* 740–745.

Silverman, J. (1964). Variations in cognitive control and psychophysiological defense in the schizophrenias. *Psychosomatic Medicine, 29,* 225–251.

Simons, R. F., & Giardina, B. D. (1992). Reflex modification in psychosis-prone young adults. *Psychophysiology, 29,* 8–16.

Spaulding, W., Hargrove, D., Crinean, J., & Martin, R. (1981). A micro-computer based laboratory for psychopathology research in rural settings. *Behaviour Research Methods and Instrumentation, 13*(4), 616–623.

Spaulding, W., Rosenzweig, L., Huntzinger, R., Cromwell, R. L., Briggs, D., & Hayes, T. (1980). Visual pattern integration in psychiatric patients. *Journal of Abnormal Psychology, 89,* 635–643.

Sperling, G. (1960). The information available in brief visual presentations. *Psychological Monographs, 74*(11, Whole No. 498).

Spohn, H. E., Coyne, L., Spray, J., & Hayes, K. (1989). Skin conductance orienting response in chronic schizophrenics: The role of neuroleptics. *Journal of Abnormal Psychology, 98,* 478–486.

Spohn, H. E., Lacoursiere, R. B., Thompson, K., & Coyne, L. (1977). Phenothiazine effects on psychological and psychophysiological dysfunction in chronic schizophrenics. *Archives of General Psychiatry, 34,* 633–644.

Spring, B. J. (1980). Shift of attention in schizophrenics, siblings of schizophrenics, and depressed patients. *Journal of Nervous and Mental Disease, 168,* 133–139.

Steffy, R. A. (1978). An early cue sometimes impairs process schizophrenic performance. In L. C. Wynne, R. L. Cromwell, & S. Matthysse (Eds.), *The nature of schizophrenia: New approaches to research and treatment* (pp. 225–232). New York: Wiley.

Steffy, R. A. (1993). Cognitive deficits in schizophrenia. In P. C. Kendall & K. Dobson (Eds.), *Psychopathology and cognition* (pp. 429–472). Orlando, FL: Academic Press.

Steffy, R. A.. & Galbraith, K. (1974) A comparison of segmental set and inhibitory deficit explanations of the crossover pattern in process schizophrenic reaction time. *Journal of Abnormal Psychology, 83,* 227–233.

Steffy, R. A., & Galbraith, K. A. (1975). Time-linked impairment in schizophrenic reaction time performance. *Journal of Abnormal Psychology, 84,* 315–324.

Steffy, R. A., & Waldman, I. (1993). Schizophrenic reaction time: North star or shooting star? In R. L. Cromwell & C. R. Snyder (Eds.), *Schizophrenia: Origins, processes, treatment, and outcome* (pp. 111–134). New York: Oxford University Press.

Strauss, M. E., Buchanan, R. W., & Hale, J. (1993). Relations between attentional deficits and clinical symptoms in schizophrenic outpatients. *Psychiatry Research, 47,* 205–213.

Strauss, M. E., Wagman, A. M. I., & Quaid, K. A. (1983). Preparatory intertrial influences in reaction time of elderly adults. *Journal of Gerontology, 38,* 55–57.

Vollick, D. (1994). *Stochastic modelling of encoding-latency means and variances in paranoid and nonparanoid schizophrenia.* Unpublished doctoral dissertation, Department of Psychology, University of Western Ontario, London, Ontario.

Wagener, D. K., Hogarty, G. E., Goldstein, M. J., Asarnow, R. F., & Browne, A. (1986). Information processing and communication deviance in schizophrenic patients and their mothers. *Psychiatry Research, 18,* 365–377.

Walker, E. (1981). Attentional and neuromotor functions of schizophrenics, schizoaffectives, and patients with other affective disorders. *Archives of General Psychiatry, 38,* 1355–1358.

Wells, D. S., & Leventhal, D. (1984). Perceptual grouping in schizophrenia: Replications of Place and Gilmore. *Journal of Abnormal Psychology, 93,* 231–234.

Wishner, J. (1955). The concept of efficiency in psychological health and in psychopathology. *Psychology Review, 62,* 69–80.

Zahn, T. P., Rosenthal, D., & Shakow, D. (1961). Reaction time in schizophrenic and normal subjects in relation to the sequence of a series of regular preparatory intervals. *Journal of Abnormal and Social Psychology, 61,* 161–168.

Zahn, T. P., Rosenthal, D., & Shakow, D. (1963). Effects of irregular preparatory interval in reaction time in schizophrenia. *Journal of Abnormal and Social Psychology, 67,* 44–52.

Zubin, J. (1975). Problem of attention in schizophrenia. In M. L. Kietzman, S. Sutton, & J. Zubin (Eds.), *Experimental approaches to psychopathology* (pp. 139–166). New York: Academic Press.

Information Processing in Anxiety and Depression

A COGNITIVE-DEVELOPMENTAL PERSPECTIVE

Ian H. Gotlib
Colin MacLeod

Over the past decade, researchers have focused increasingly on the role of cognitive functioning in depression and anxiety. The impetus for this swell of interest in cognitive aspects of these two disorders has come both from theoretical formulations that implicate "faulty" cognitions in the etiology and maintenance of anxiety and depression and from methodological advances in the assessment of cognitive functioning and, in particular, of attention and memory. Although considerable progress has been made in elucidating the role of these cognitive processes in anxiety and depression, it is clear that a number of important questions remain unresolved, particularly concerning implications of the co-occurrence, or comorbidity, of these two disorders for cognitive functioning, as well as developmental aspects of cognitive dysfunction in anxiety and depression.

We have two principal goals in writing this chapter. First, we will briefly present the major theoretical formulations of the role of cognition in depression and anxiety, reviewing the results of empirical studies that have tested these formulations by examining attentional and memory functioning in individuals with these disorders. As we will see, the results of investigations in this area suggest that whereas anxiety is characterized primarily by biases in attention, depression is characterized by biases in memory functioning. Second, throughout the chapter we will focus on the possible origins of cognitive dysfunction in anxiety and depression, both by highlighting investigations that illuminate this issue and by indicating what we believe are important and fruitful directions for further theory and research in this area. We begin by describing the clinical symptoms of depression and anxiety and the prevalence of the comorbidity of these two disorders. We then describe the types of thoughts that are characteristic of both adults and children experiencing anxiety and depression. Next, we describe theoretical formulations of the role of cognitive dysfunction in anxiety and depression, and we review the results of empirical studies designed to test these formulations. Finally, we consider a number of issues involving the temporal / causal nature of the relation between cognitive dysfunction and emotional disorders, and we conclude by highlighting issues and questions that must be addressed if we are to make significant progress in this area.

SYMPTOMS, PREVALENCE, AND COMORBIDITY OF ANXIETY AND DEPRESSION

Of all the psychiatric disorders, depressive and anxiety disorders are by far the most common. During the course of a lifetime, it is estimated that between 6% and 18% of the general population will experience at least one clinically significant episode of depression (Boyd & Weissman, 1981; Karno et al., 1987) and that approximately twice as many women than men will be affected by depression (Frank, Carpenter, & Kupfer, 1988; Robins et al., 1984). Moreover, depression is a recurrent disorder: Over 80% of depressed patients have more than one depressive episode (Clayton, 1983), and over 50% of depressed patients relapse within 2 years of recovery (cf. Keller & Shapiro, 1981).

The term "depression" has a number of meanings, covering a wide range of emotional states that range in severity from normal, everyday moods of sadness to psychotic episodes with increased risk of suicide. The current diagnostic system in North America, the fourth edition of the *Diagnostic and Statistical Manual of Mental Disorders* (DSM-IV; American Psychiatric Association, 1994), requires at least a 2-week period of depressed mood or a loss of interest or pleasure in almost all daily activities, as well as a number of other symptoms, such as weight loss or gain, loss of appetite, sleep disturbance, psychomotor agitation or retardation, fatigue, feelings of guilt or worthlessness, and difficulties in thinking and concentration, for a diagnosis of major depressive disorder (MDD).

Importantly, as we will see, some of these symptoms are also characteristic of anxiety disorders. For example, DSM-IV criteria for generalized anxiety disorder (GAD) include excessive anxiety and worry about a number of events or activities for at least 6 months, more days than not, as well as a number of associated symptoms, such as restlessness, fatigue, concentration difficulties, irritability, muscle tension, and sleep disturbance. The prevalence of the anxiety disorders, when considered as an entire category, is at least as great as that of the mood disorders. For example, the Epidemiologic Catchment Area (ECA) study, conducted in the 1980s, reported 6-month prevalence rates of any anxiety disorder at 8.9% and lifetime prevalence rates at 14.6% (cf. Robins & Regier, 1991), although more recent estimates are slightly lower (Wittchen, Zhao, Kessler, & Eaton, 1994).

In recent years, considerable attention has been paid to findings that depression and anxiety commonly co-occur, at both the symptom and the syndrome levels (cf. Gotlib & Cane, 1989; Maser & Cloninger, 1990). Some investigators (e.g., Gotlib, 1984; Clark & Watson, 1991) have argued that most self-report symptom measures of anxiety and depression are tapping either a state or a trait aspect of general distress or "negative affectivity" (NA), defined as a tendency to experience general negative affective symptoms. Clark and Watson hypothesize further that anxiety and depression can be distinguished on the basis of state and trait positive affectivity (PA), which reflects a sense of energy and enthusiasm about life. More specifically, depressed but not anxious individuals are hypothesized to be low on PA, reflecting fatigue and a lack of energy or enthusiasm.

Although it is apparent that there is substantial comorbidity in the symptoms of depression and anxiety, to date there has been little empirical work conducted with comorbid patients. Thus, in terms of the focus of this chapter, it is not clear how comorbid patients might differ from their diagnostically "purer" counterparts, particularly with respect to their cognitive functioning. It is possible, for example, given the high rates of comorbidity of anxiety and depression, that these two disorders share a common pattern of dysfunctional cognitive processing. Alternatively, depression and anxiety may be characterized by different patterns of cognitive functioning, and the elevated levels of comorbidity of these two disorders may reflect shared symptoms that are unrelated to cognitive functioning. In the following sections we will review cognitive theories of depression and anxiety that are relevant to these two formulations and will present the results of studies designed to examine cognitive functioning in anxiety and depression.

THOUGHT CONTENT IN
ANXIETY AND DEPRESSION

Adult Samples

It is now clear that anxiety and depression are both associated with a preponderance of negative thoughts in adult patients (Craske & Barlow,

1991; Hollon & Shelton, 1991). Furthermore, it appears that the characteristics of such negative thoughts are somewhat different in each condition. Whereas anxiety patients tend to report negative thoughts that are future oriented and that concern themes of personal danger, depressed patients more often report negative thoughts that are past oriented and that involve themes of loss and failure (Beck & Clark, 1988; Clark, Beck, & Brown, 1989; Ingram, Kendall, Smith, Donnell, & Ronan, 1987). Some researchers have proposed that these differences in the qualities of negative thoughts should reliably distinguish anxiety from depression, a postulate that has become known as the cognitive content-specificity hypothesis (e.g., Beck, Brown, Steer, Eidelson, & Riskind, 1987).

While the association between thought content and clinical status has been well established, its causal nature remains unresolved. The predominant view, espoused explicitly by many cognitive theorists (e.g., Beck, 1967; Beck, Emery, & Greenberg, 1986) and assumed by all cognitive therapists who attempt to reduce dysphoric emotion through the modification of thought content, is that negative thoughts play a causal role in the genesis of anxiety and depression. It is possible, however, that enduring patterns of negative thinking arise as a *consequence* of long term emotional distress. That is, high-trait-anxious individuals, who have likely suffered anxiety symptoms extensively during their early development, may grow preoccupied with the possible sources of danger that could trigger their anxiety. Similarly, those individuals who are vulnerable to depression, who have likely experienced depressed affect with some frequency during their development, may become preoccupied with the possibility of loss or failure, given the capacity of such events to provoke depression. Thus, the negative thinking shown by anxious and depressed adults may be a long-term consequence of childhood episodes of anxiety or depression. Virtually all of the research conducted in this area, however, has examined the cognitive functioning of depressed and anxious adults. If it is the case that negative thinking develops gradually over time as a result of extended experience with anxiety or depression, then it would be expected that anxious and depressed children should show less evidence of negative thought content than is the case for adults. It is to this literature that we now turn our attention.

Child Samples and Developmental Considerations

Although the assessment of cognitive content in children has presented methodological challenges (cf. Kendall & Chansky, 1991; Spence, 1994), relevant findings with children closely parallel those obtained with adults. For example, Francis (1988) and Kendall (1993) reviewed considerable evidence that anxious children in fourth, fifth, and sixth grade show an elevated tendency to make self-statements that contain negative content.

Such patterns of self-statements have been reported by test-anxious children (e.g., Zatz & Chassin, 1983), trait-anxious children (e.g., Ronan, Kendall, & Rowe, 1994), and socially anxious children (e.g., Dandes, LaGreca, Wick, & Shaw, 1986). There is also some evidence of cognitive content specificity in younger populations. For example, Jolly and Dykman (1994) assessed anxiety symptoms, depression symptoms, and cognitive content in a population of 162 young inpatients (mean age = 14.6 years) at a large children's hospital. These investigators found that whereas anxiety symptoms were strongly associated with an elevated frequency of thoughts concerning imminent danger, the frequency of these thoughts was unrelated to depression symptoms. In contrast, depression symptoms were strongly associated with an elevated frequency of thoughts concerning loss or failure that were unrelated to anxiety symptoms (see also Ronan et al., 1994). It appears, therefore, that both the elevated frequency of negative thought content in anxiety and depression and the tendency for negative thoughts to involve themes of loss in depression and danger in anxiety can be observed well before adulthood.

It is noteworthy that in Jolly and Dykman's (1994) study, although thoughts concerning imminent danger predicted only anxiety and thoughts concerning loss and failure predicted only depression, a third class of thoughts predicted *both* anxiety and depression. Jolly and Dykman argue that this third group of negative thoughts represents the overlap between depressogenic and anxiogenic concerns. An inspection of these general negative thoughts reveals that they commonly embodied both past failings and future threat within the same negative self-statements (e.g., "I don't deserve to be loved," "Nothing ever works out for me anymore"). Jolly and Dyman speculate that it may be an elevation in this third class of negative thinking that most distinctly characterizes individuals suffering from comorbid anxiety and depression. Interestingly, investigators have reported that the comorbidity of depression and anxiety increases across the developmental period (King, Ollendick, & Gullone, 1991; Strauss, Last, Hersen, & Kazdin, 1988), and it is possible that this pattern of comorbidity is associated with the development of this third class of negative thinking. To address this issue requires longitudinal studies designed to examine the development of negative thought content in children at risk for depression and anxiety.

Finally, it is important to note that this content specificity provides support for the causal role of cognition in these emotional conditions. It is likely, therefore, that our understanding of individual differences in emotional vulnerability will require an understanding of individual differences in styles of thinking. Several researchers have proposed detailed information-processing models that might account for the observed association between dysphoric emotion and negative cognitive content, almost all of which involve the cognitive processes of attention and memory. A large amount of data has been generated in studies designed to assess these formulations. In the following section, we will outline two of the most prominant of these models and will then consider the evidence for the predictions that can be derived from these accounts.

INFORMATION-PROCESSING MODELS OF ANXIETY AND DEPRESSION

Schema Theory

Aaron T. Beck has been greatly influential in emphasizing the types of biased thought content that characterize depression and anxiety (e.g., Beck, 1976; Beck et al., 1986; Beck & Clark, 1988). Furthermore, Beck was one of the first theorists to propose that biases in the content of anxious and depressed patients' conscious thoughts might arise as a consequence of lower-level biases in the human information-processing system. Specifically, Beck implicates the construct of cognitive schemata in the genesis of the biased thought content reported by anxious and depressed patients. A schema can be conceptualized as a representational structure that has been developed to accommodate information pertaining to a certain class of events (Bartlett, 1932; Williams, Watts, MacLeod, & Mathews, 1988). Schemata exist for those classes of events that have been encountered frequently or that have been highly significant to an individual. The schema is essentially an organizational structure that, when activated, is used to guide the processing of information that might fit within its functional domain. Thus, for example, because most people are familiar with the class of events or behaviors commonly occurring during visits to restaurants, it is likely that many of us will possess a restaurant schema containing a prototypical representation of such visits (Schank & Abelson, 1977). When we find ourselves in a novel restaurant, this schema will become activated and will impose a structure on the new experience by guiding our attention toward elements of the environment that are central to the restaurant schema (e.g., the menu, the waiter). Our memory of the experience also will be influenced by the schema, because the recollection will be facilitated for those elements that are central to the restaurant schema.

While most of us possess a restaurant schema, many schemata are highly idiosyncratic. Beck (1976; Beck et al., 1986) proposes that certain types of negative early experiences result in the creation of idiosyncratic schemata that later serve both to guide attention selectively toward negative aspects of the environment and to facilitate the subsequent retrieval of such negative information, thereby leading to the preponderance of negative thoughts that are postulated to precipitate depression or anxiety. More specifically, Beck argues that individuals who experience highly significant loss events or threats of harm early in life develop a representational schema. In later life, this "depressogenic" or "anxiogenic" schema, when activated, will guide attention selectively toward all information concerning loss or failure, or danger or threat, and will facilitate the retrieval of such information from memory, resulting in the high frequency of thoughts that elicits a depressed or anxious mood, respectively.

Although there have been a number of extensions and refinements of Beck's schema theory (e.g., Ingram & Reed, 1986; Kendall & Ronan, 1990), two consistencies across most of these variations are worth noting. First, given that these theories implicate the influence of long-term representational structures, they are essentially trait theories. Second, while schema theorists have proposed that different *content* of idiosyncratic schemata underlie vulnerability to anxiety and to depression, the particular information-processing *biases* observed are hypothesized to be equivalent in both cases. More specifically, individuals vulnerable to either disorder should show a bias in both selective attention and memory, although the content of the bias should differ: In people vulnerable to anxiety the bias should facilitate attention to, and memory for, information concerning threat and danger, whereas in people vulnerable to depression the bias should favor the processing of information concerning loss and failure.

Network Theory

A rather different type of explanation for the preponderance of negative thought content reported by anxious and depressed patients is provided by Bower's network model of emotion and cognition (Bower, 1981, 1987, 1992). This model represents a fairly simple extension of Bower's earlier general theory of human associative memory (HAM; Anderson & Bower, 1973). Within the original HAM model, human memory is conceptualized as a collection of nodes, each containing discrete representations. Accessing any representation involves activating that node to some threshold level, and associative connections develop and strengthen between those nodes that are frequently activated simultaneously. Through this network, activation of any node will lead, through "spreading," to the partial activation (or "priming") of other nodes that share associative connections with the original node. The representations contained within these primed nodes will then be disproportionately easy to access, because less additional activation will be required to bring these nodes to the threshold level for such access to occur.

Bower (1981) extended this HAM model by introducing emotion

nodes into the memory network formulation. Each emotion node corresponds to a discrete emotional state and becomes active whenever that state is experienced. Over time, each emotion node will come to develop associative connections with those nodes that are most often activated simultaneously with that emotion node. These nodes will tend to contain representations that are affectively congruent with this emotion. Thus, because individuals will often experience depression when processing information related to loss or failure, associative connections will develop between the depression node and nodes containing this class of negative information. Similarly, because individuals will often experience anxiety when processing information related to threat and danger, associative connections will develop between the anxiety node and nodes containing information about threat and danger. Bower postulates that once such associative networks have developed, the experience of a mood state will introduce a systematic bias into the memory system. Different classes of emotionally negative representations will be made more available to the cognitive system when anxiety and when depression are elevated—threat and danger representations for anxiety, and loss and failure representations for depression.

Developmental Considerations

Much of the research reviewed in the previous two subsections has been conducted with adults; little attention has been given to the importance of developmental considerations in the study of attention and memory processes in depression and anxiety. Interestingly, in a recent review Vasey (1993) suggests that associative memory networks change across developmental levels. Moreover, because associative memory networks likely originate as simple networks involving relatively few specific events, it might be expected from Bower's model that the types and number of thoughts elicited by anxious and depressed mood should differ as a function of age. Specifically, Vasey suggests that, because of their relatively limited range of experience, young children should respond to each of these moods with a fairly restricted attentional bias, the focus of which will be related directly to those few events that have been previously experienced in that mood state. As the network grows richer, these attentional biases should become more general, although anxiety should still elicit attention primarily to general threat cues whereas depression elicits attention largely to information associated with loss and failure. Consistent with this formulation, researchers have found that whereas younger anxious children report relatively specific concerns, such as a fear of separation, older anxious children report more general concerns involving a wider range of possible dangers (Last, Hersen, Kazdin, Finkelstein, & Strauss, 1987; Miller,

Boyer, & Rodoletz, 1990). The enrichment of the associative network across development might also account for the increase in the co-occurrence of thoughts concerning both threat and loss that appears to accompany the developmental increase in the comorbidity of anxiety and depression (Strauss et al., 1988). Thus, if an individual is frequently required to process information about both loss and threat simultaneously, as may be the case if losses often are experienced while the threat of further loss remains, then associative connections may develop between nodes containing information concerning loss and nodes containing information concerning threat. For individuals possessing this memory network, initial elevations in anxiety would come to indirectly prime thoughts likely to also elevate depression, and vice versa.

The development of associative networks in anxious and depressed children remains an important issue for future research. Within the present context, however, there are two general points that should be made. First, unlike schema models, network models attribute biased thought content to the influence of current mood and therefore are primarily state-based models, construing mood state as an important mediating variable in the production of processing biases in anxiety and depression. Second, like schema models, network models propose that the processing biases observed in anxious and in depressed patients reflect the same underlying cognitive mechanisms. Therefore, although the *content* of the biases observed in anxious and depressed patients may differ, the *nature* of these biases should be equivalent. Indeed, like schema theorists, Bower (1981) has specifically predicted that both anxious patients and depressed patients should selectively attend to emotion-congruent negative information and should demonstrate an advantage in the retrieval of such information.

Clearly, it is parsimonious to attribute the information-processing characteristics of anxiety and depression to the same underlying cognitive mechanisms. Nevertheless, given that emotions have evolved to serve complex social and biological functions, it is possible that the cognitive underpinnings of different emotions may also be complex and diverse. Indeed, Oatley and Johnson-Laird (1987) have proposed that each distinct emotion serves to configure the cognitive system into a unique, highly stereotyped mode of operation that facilitates the types of information processing most likely to be adaptive for that emotion. Consistent with this position, Williams et al. (1988) have developed a model within which anxiety and depression are associated with selective processing biases in quite different classes of cognitive operations. Williams et al. draw on the distinction, introduced by Graf and Mandler (1984), between the cognitive operations of *integration* and *elaboration,* both of which operate on mental representations. Integration increases the internal cohesiveness existing *within* a representation, making it easier to activate that representation. In contrast, elaboration increases and strengthens the associative connections *between* a representation and others in memory, making that representation easier to retrieve during a memory search. Thus, whereas stimuli corresponding to a highly integrated representation will "pop out" of a stimulus array and attract attention but may not be easier to recall, stimuli corresponding to highly elaborated representations will be relatively easy to recall but will not selectively attract attention during encoding. Williams et al. argue that individuals vulnerable to anxiety will respond to dysphoric mood with increased *integrative* processing of emotionally negative stimuli whereas individuals vulnerable to depression will respond to dysphoric mood with increased *elaborative* processing of negative information. In other words, whereas anxious individuals should selectively *attend* to negative stimuli without showing a memory advantage for this information, depressed individuals should show a *memory* advantage for negative stimuli without this material selectively capturing attention during encoding.

Before we consider the evidence for this formulation, it is important to note that different cognitive biases for different emotional disorders may be adaptive from an evolutionary perspective. For example, an attentional bias in anxiety may be adaptive if it facilitates perception of those environmental elements that pose an immediate threat to the organism (thereby eliciting the anxiety). Similarly, a memory bias may be adaptive in depression if it enables the organism to better compare the circumstances surrounding the recent past negative event (which triggered the depression) against those circumstances surrounding other similar negative events, thereby facilitating recognition of rules that might prevent such events in the future. Despite this intriguing evolutionary perspective, Williams and colleagues' (1988) model is silent with respect to the issue of how such attentional and memory biases might develop across childhood. It is possible that a tendency to selectively integrate and to selectively elaborate negative representations when a person is distressed might be an inherited individual difference. Alternatively, it may be that such styles of processing are acquired as a result of experience. These alternative hypotheses can be tested only by systematic comparisons of both selective attention and selective memory across the developmental period. In the following section, we review studies that have examined directly the selective attention and memory functioning of anxious and depressed persons.

SELECTIVE INFORMATION PROCESSING IN ANXIETY AND DEPRESSION

A considerable body of research has been motivated by the hypotheses, already reviewed, that anxious and depressed patients should show patterns of processing selectivity that favor emotionally negative information.

In general, there has been reasonable support for such proposals, and biases in both attention and memory have been reported within anxious and depressed samples (cf. Gotlib & McCabe, 1992; McCabe & Gotlib, 1995; MacLeod & Mathews, 1991; Mathews & MacLeod, 1994). Furthermore, some of these findings have been rather different for these two disorders, suggesting that precise styles of selective information processing might serve to discriminate anxiety and depression. In the following two subsections we will first review studies that have examined anxious patients and then turn to experiments conducted with depressed individuals; a third subsection will consider comorbidity studies.

Anxiety

Anxiety patients presented with emotionally toned verbal stimuli under conditions that make perception difficult show an enhanced ability to detect threatening, relative to nonthreatening, items. For example, Burgess et al. (1981) presented agoraphobics, social phobics, and nonanxious comparison subjects with different lists of words, played simultaneously to each ear in a dichotic listening task, and required them to detect emotionally negative and emotionally neutral target words within each list. Both groups of anxiety patients, but not the comparison subjects, showed an enhanced ability to detect the threatening target words relative to the neutral words. Similar findings have been reported by Foa and McNally (1986) for obsessional patients. Although these enhanced detection rates for threatening words might indeed reflect an attentional bias that favors the encoding of such stimuli, it is also possible that this effect could result from a response bias. That is, anxiety patients may simply set a lower evidence criterion for deciding that a threat target word has been presented, resulting in a higher hit rate for such targets in detection tasks of this sort.

An alternative experimental approach to the examination of selective processing—an approach that is not vulnerable to this response bias account—involves the use of interference tasks. In these tasks, subjects are given a central task to perform while they attempt to ignore distractor information. The degree to which different types of distractor stimuli impair performance on the central task provides a measure of the degree to which these distractor stimuli selectively "capture," or draw, attentional resources. Across a range of tasks, investigators have found that anxiety patients show greater interference effects on the central task when they are presented with emotionally negative, as compared to emotionally neutral, distractor stimuli, indicating that anxiety patients attend selectively to negative stimuli (cf. MacLeod, 1991; Mathews & MacLeod, 1994). For example, Mathews and MacLeod (1986) utilized a dichotic listening task in which lists of either emotionally negative or neutral words were presented to the unattended ear. Instead of attempting to detect these stimuli, however, subjects were required to ignore these word lists while they performed a central reaction time task, pressing a button in response to a simple visual cue. Mathews and MacLeod found that, despite reporting no awareness of the content of the words in the unattended channel, patients with GAD took significantly longer on the reaction time task when the emotionally negative, rather than the neutral, distractor words were presented; no such difference was observed in nonanxious control subjects. This finding suggests that the negative stimuli captured attentional resources to a disproportionate degree in the anxiety patients. Furthermore, the fact that this occurred without any awareness of the distractor stimulus content suggests that this anxiety-linked attentional bias may occur quite automatically, without requiring conscious mediation.

Another interference task that has been used to assess selective attention in clinical patients is a modification of the standard Stroop color conflict task (Stroop, 1938). In this task, subjects are presented with words displayed in different ink colors and must name the ink color of each word while attempting to ignore the word's semantic content. Across many experiments, anxiety patients, compared to nonanxious control subjects, are disproportionately slower to color-name words with emotionally negative content than words with neutral content. This effect has been observed in a variety of anxiety disordered populations, including patients suffering from GAD (e.g., Mathews & MacLeod, 1985), panic disorder (e.g., McNally et al., 1994), spider phobia (e.g., Lavy, van den Hout, & Arntz, 1993), social phobia (e.g., Mattia, Heimberg, & Hope, 1993), obsessive–compulsive disorder (e.g., Lavy, van Oppen, & van den Hout, 1994) and posttraumatic stress disorder (e.g., Foa, Feske, Murdock, Kozak, & McCarthy, 1991). Clearly, this is a robust effect, and most researchers have taken it to indicate that emotionally negative word content captures selective attention in anxiety patients, slowing their color-naming responses. Furthermore, this effect seems to persist even when subjects are not consciously aware of the semantic content of subliminally presented stimuli (cf. MacLeod & Mathews, 1991; Mogg, Bradley, Williams, & Mathews, 1993), supporting the formulation that selective attention to threat is an automatic cognitive bias in anxiety patients.

Because it is possible that anxious patients' impaired color-naming response to negative stimuli is a result of cognitive *avoidance* rather than cognitive *attention* (cf. de Ruiter & Brosschot, 1994), investigators have developed more direct measures of selective attention. In several studies secondary probe tasks have been used to assess the distribution of attention in response to the presentation of emotional information. For example, MacLeod, Mathews, and Tata (1986) presented patients with GAD and nonanxious control subjects with brief (500-millisecond) exposures of pairs of words, separated vertically on a computer screen. Subjects were required to detect small dot probes that, on some trials, could appear in the vicinity of either word, and detection latency for these probes was recorded. On critical trials, one word in the pair was emotionally negative while the other was emotionally neutral, and the dot probe could appear in the vicinity of either word. As predicted, the anxiety patients were faster to detect probes when they appeared in the vicinity of the negative rather than the neutral words, suggesting that they selectively attended to the screen locations where these negative stimuli appeared. In contrast, nonanxious control subjects showed a trend in the opposite direction, tending to detect probes more slowly when they occurred in the vicinity of the negative rather than the neutral words.

Finally, recent evidence suggests that the attentional bias demonstrated by anxiety patients is most pronounced for threatening material with particular personal relevance. For example, Mogg, Mathews, and Weinman (1989) reported that when patients with GAD were subdivided according to whether they worry more about social concerns or physical concerns and were required to color-name neutral words and negative words related to each class of concern, color-naming interference was greatest for those negative words related to the patients' domains of greatest personal concern. Similar specificity has been found for phobic patients (e.g., Hope, Rapee, Heimberg, & Dombeck, 1990), panic disorder patients (e.g., Ehlers, Margraf, Davies, & Roth, 1988), and patients with posttraumatic stress disorder (e.g., Foa et al., 1991).

The finding that anxiety disordered patients show an *attentional* bias toward emotionally negative stimuli is consistent with the schema and network models presented earlier. According to both Beck's model and Bower's model, anxiety patients should also show selective *memory* for such stimuli, but there is considerably less evidence to support this second prediction. Because this volume is concerned more with attentional than with memory functioning, we will state here only that there is at best inconsistent support for a negative memory bias in individuals experience anxiety disorders (e.g., MacLeod & McLaughlin, 1995; Mathews & MacLeod, 1985; Mogg et al., 1989).

Depression

Whereas anxiety patients appear to demonstrate enhanced attention, but not facilitated memory, for emotionally negative stimuli, a different pattern of findings has emerged in studies of depressed patients. Unlike anxiety patients, depressed patients do show a robust recall bias favoring emotionally negative information (cf. Blaney, 1986). Though initially observed with autobiographical memory tasks (e.g., Clark & Teasdale, 1982), subsequent studies have shown that depressed patients' facilitated ability to recall negative information extends to verbal and nonverbal stimuli learned in a laboratory setting (e.g., Bradley & Mathews, 1983; Slife, Miura, Thompson, Shapiro, & Gallagher, 1984). Such depression-linked memory biases are found most reliably following encoding tasks that require subjects to process stimuli in a self-referent manner. The most common version of this type of encoding task involves presenting subjects with negative and positive trait adjectives and requiring them to judge whether each adjective describes either themselves or some other nominated individual. Typically, when a subsequent memory task then is unexpectedly administered, depressed patients show an enhanced ability to recall negative trait adjectives, but only for those stimuli that were presented in the self-referent, and not the other-referent, encoding condition (e.g., Bradley & Mathews, 1983).

There is less consistent evidence that clinical depression is characterized by a tendency to selectively attend to and encode emotionally negative stimulus information. For example, on a tachistoscopic task that required subjects to identify briefly presented words, Powell and Hemsley (1984) found that depressed patients demonstrated particularly high accuracy rates for negative target words. However, MacLeod, Tata, and Mathews (1987) argued that this task may primarily be assessing a depression-associated guessing bias, operating when the identity of presented words is uncertain. Indeed, using the same stimulus materials, MacLeod et al. employed a lexical decision task to assess encoding speed and found that depressed patients did not differ from nondepressed controls in the relative speed with which they could correctly decide on the lexical status of positively and negatively toned words, suggesting that depressed subjects do not show facilitated encoding of negative words.

More direct tests of attentional allocation also reveal little evidence that depressed patients show a tendency to selectively attend to emotionally negative stimuli. However, such tests do suggest the possibility that depressed patients may be characterized by the absence of a tendency to avoid negative stimuli that is commonly exhibited by nondepressed subjects. For example, in MacLeod and colleagues (1986) dot-probe study described earlier, depressed patients showed equivalent detection latencies for probes in the vicinity of threat words and in the vicinity of neutral words, suggesting no attentional response either toward or away from the negative stimuli. Given that normal control subjects in this study showed a slowing to detect probes in the vicinity of the negative words (i.e., attentional avoidance of such stimuli), it appears that the depressed patients have lost a normal tendency to avoid negative stimuli. In a variant on this probe detection task, Gotlib, MacLachan, and Katz (1988) and McCabe and Gotlib (1995) also found that depressed subjects showed no selective attentional response to negative stimuli whereas nondepressed subjects showed a tendency to selectively orient attention away from negative stimuli.

Perhaps the strongest evidence to suggest that depressed patients might actually attend selectively to negative stimuli has come from interference studies, though even here there are inconsistencies. In an initial investigation, Gotlib and McCann (1984) used an interference task to examine the color-naming latencies of mildly depressed and nondepressed subjects for depressed-, manic-, and neutral-content words. Whereas nondepressed subjects did not demonstrate differential response latencies across the three types of words, depressed subjects took longer to name the colors of the depressed- than either the neutral- or manic-content words. This difficulty in ignoring the content of depressed-content words suggests that depressed individuals differ from their nondepressed counterparts with respect to their relative accessibility of positive and negative cognitive constructs. Moreover, Gotlib and McCann found in a second study that this pattern of results was not due to transient mood differences between depressed and nondepressed subjects.

In a similar study, Williams and Nulty (1986) found depressed suicide attempters to display longer color-naming latencies for those emotionally negative words that were directly related to their suicide attempt. These subjects, however, did not show increased color-naming latencies for depression-related words that were not directly associated with their suicide attempt. Therefore, this effect may reflect attention to situationally relevant words, rather than to depression-congruent words in general. Indeed, when Mogg et al. (1993) compared clinically depressed, clinically anxious, and control subjects on a color-naming task that employed anxiety-related, depression-related, and nondysphoric words, the depressed subjects did not differ from the control subjects in their patterns of color-naming latencies (while the anxiety patients showed a relative slowing of color-naming latencies on both classes of negative words).

In a recent study, McCabe and Gotlib (1993) found that depressed patients, when attempting to ignore emotional stimulus words presented to the unattended ear during a dichotic listening task, showed a disproportionate slowing on a simultaneous simple RT task to a visual cue when these distractor words were generally negative in content, rather than neutral or positive. This represents the strongest evidence to date that clinically depressed patients show any tendency toward increased attentional capture by generally negative emotional stimuli; thus this approach seems like a promising avenue for future research.

Comorbidity

At present, it appears that whereas a selective *attentional* bias for negative stimuli is more apparent in anxious patients, a selective *memory* bias
favoring recall of negative information is more evident in depressed patients (cf. Mathews & MacLeod, 1994). These differences in the primary
information-processing biases that characterize each class of emotional
disorder may help to explain the distinctive types of thought content reported by patients experiencing these conditions. Specifically, the tendency to
selectively encode negative information might account for the future-
oriented nature of the thoughts reported by anxiety patients, who are likely
to be concerned with the imminent consequences of perceived negative elements in their immediate environment. In contrast, the tendency to selectively retrieve negative events from memory might account for the past-
oriented nature of the thoughts reported by depressed patients, who are
more likely to become preoccupied with negative events that have already
occurred. This formulation suggests the intriguing possibility that vulnerability to experience comorbid anxiety and depression might result from
the simultaneous presence of both an attentional bias toward negative information *and* a memory bias favoring the retrieval of negative information. Co-occurrence of these two processing biases might reflect either the
existence of two independent effects in attention and memory, respectively,
or alternatively may arise because of a single selective-processing bias in a
more central system, such as the executive module of the working memory
system (Baddeley, 1986), which influences both attention and memory.

Although perhaps worthy of further investigation, this speculative account of anxiety–depression comorbidity is premised on the assumption
that individual differences in the selective processing of emotional information represent a trait variable and that such patterns of selective processing
are capable of mediating emotional states. An alternative possibility, however, is that processing differences between clinical patients and control
subjects might more simply reflect the cognitive *consequences* of anxious
or depressed mood states. In the next section, we will examine developmental and temporal aspects of the relation between emotion and cognition. We will consider whether empirical findings offer support for the proposal that individual differences in selective information processing might
contribute functionally to individual differences in emotional vulnerability.

DEVELOPMENTAL AND TEMPORAL ASPECTS
OF SELECTIVE PROCESSING
IN ANXIETY AND DEPRESSION

If selective information processing does play a functional role in mediating vulnerability to anxiety and/or depression, then we should expect three

specific observations when we examine the association between selective processing and emotional disorder across time. First, given that anxiety and depressive disorders both can appear in childhood, we should expect to find evidence that selective attention to negative stimuli in anxiety, and selective memory for negative stimuli in depression, can be observed in children. Second, given that vulnerability to anxiety and/or depression remains fairly stable across time, we should expect to find that individual differences in selective information-processing biases also remain stable and that such differences are related to differences in trait emotion, rather than simply to differences in emotional state. Finally, we should find that selective information processing predicts emotional responses to subsequent stressful life events. We will consider evidence for each of these requirements in turn.

Information Processing in Children

To date, patterns of selective attention in anxious children have been the focus of surprisingly little experimental scrutiny. The results of the only published study in this area supports the presence of an attentional bias toward threat stimuli in phobic children as young as 6 years of age. Martin, Horder, and Jones (1992) studied spider phobics and control subjects within three age bands: 6–7 years, 9–10 years, and 12–13 years. All subjects were presented with a version of the color-naming interference task that contained both threat words related to the phobic fear and matched neutral control words. Martin et al. found that even the youngest phobic children showed significant slowing when they sought to color-name the phobic threat words, relative to the neutral words, while the nonanxious children showed no such effect. Furthermore, the magnitude of this anxiety-linked threat interference effect did not differ across the age ranges examined. While there is obviously a great need for additional research examining the styles of selective attention shown by anxious children, these findings are consistent with the possibility that attentional biases toward threatening stimuli contribute to the development of anxiety disorders, given that the biases seem to be fully evident at the earliest ages at which anxiety disorders can be detected in children.

Similarly, there also is evidence that the patterns of selective memory displayed by depressed adults can be observed in depressed children. For example, Hammen and Zupan (1984) examined incidental recall of emotionally toned adjectives in mildly depressed an nondepressed 7- to 12-year-old children. Whereas the nondepressed children showed a pronounced recall advantage for the positive adjectives, the depressed children showed no such effect. Similar findings have been reported by Prieto, Cole, and Tageson (1992) and by Whitman and Leitenberg (1990). Across all of these studies, as has been observed in adult depressed patients, depressed children appear to have lost the positive memory bias that characterizes nondepressed children.

Stability of Information-Processing Biases

Although selective attention and retrieval biases in anxious and depressed children, respectively, are consistent with the possibility that selective-processing biases of this sort contribute to emotional vulnerability, it is also possible that such processing biases are more simply cognitive responses to elevations in these emotional states. To examine this possibility, considerable research with adults has attempted to determine whether selective attention and memory represent correlates of state or trait emotion. The results of many of these studies indicate that these selective-processing biases are state dependent. For example, Watts, McKenna, Sharrock, and Trezise (1986) reported that their spider phobic patients, who had demonstrated slowed color-naming latencies of phobia-relevant words, ceased to show this effect following successful behavior therapy for their phobic disorder. Indeed, Lavy et al. (1993) showed that the threat interference effects can be significantly attenuated in phobic patients following even a single session of behavior therapy. Mattia et al. (1993) similarly found that social phobics show reductions in their color-naming latencies on social threat words (vs. matched control words) with improvement in their mood. The elimination of attentional bias to threat in recovered anxiety patients is not restricted to phobic disorders but has also been inferred from changes in color-naming latencies observed following the treatment of patients suffering from obsessive–compulsive disorder (Foa & McNally, 1986), panic disorder (Beck, Stanley, Averill, Baldwin, & Deagle, 1992), and GAD (Mogg, Mathews, & Eysenck, 1992).

Similar patterns have been reported in depressed patients in which improvement in depressive symptomatology is associated with a reduction in selective processing. Gotlib and Cane (1987), for example, examined the performance of diagnosed clinically depressed psychiatric patients on a color-naming task both when the patients were in episode and later when they had recovered symptomatically. Nondepressed nonpsychiatric subjects served as a time-matched control group. Gotlib and Cane found that patients took longer to color-name the depressed- than the nondepressed-content words while they were depressed. More important, however, this effect was obtained only for the hospitalization session; when the patients were no longer depressed, they did not demonstrate this differential construct accessibility. Gotlib and Cane interpreted these results as suggesting that negative schemata affect cognitive functioning only during the depressive episode and that these schemata and the depressives' negative cognitive functioning may be more parsimoniously viewed as a concomitant, rather than a cause or residual, of depression.

Other studies have yielded equivalent results. For example, the selective interference effect observed by McCabe and Gotlib (1993) when depressed persons were attempting to ignore negative-content distractor stimuli was eliminated when these depressed individuals recovered. Similarly, the relative memory advantage for negative information commonly shown by depressed patients tends to disappear when mood improves either through treatment (e.g., Slife et al., 1984) or because of diurnal fluctuations in the level of depression (Clark & Teasdale, 1982). It appears, therefore, that the patterns of selective processing demonstrated by both anxious and depressed patients are observed only when these individuals are experiencing the dysphoric mood states of anxiety or depression.

The fact that selective-processing biases are not apparent in the absence of a dysphoric mood state may seem to discount the possibility that these biases play a functional role in the mediation of emotional vulnerability. However, this is not necessarily the case. Although it is clear that selective attention to or memory for, negative information may not represent individual differences that are stable in the sense of always being present, it is nevertheless possible that individuals may show stable differences in the types of selective processing biases that are elicited by dysphoric mood and that these differences may contribute to trait vulnerability. Consistent with this possibility, it does appear that the degree to which selective processing of negative information is elicited by dysphoric mood state differs across individuals. Moreover, these individual differences are associated with personality variables thought to represent trait vulnerability to anxiety and/or depression. For example, MacLeod and Mathews (1988) used the dot-probe technique to examine patterns of selective attention in high and low trait-anxious students when their state anxiety levels were low and when these state anxiety levels were high. When state anxiety was low, the two trait groups did not differ in their probe detection latencies and neither group showed any pronounced attentional response to threat. In contrast, high state anxiety served to increase attention to stress-relevant threat stimuli in the high trait-anxious subjects but served to *decrease* attention to threat in the low trait-anxiety students (see also MacLeod & Rutherford, 1993).

There is also evidence that individuals who differ in vulnerability to depression are characterized by differences in the patterns of selective processing that are elicited by depressed mood state. Ingram, Bernet, and McGlaughlin (1994) used a dichotic listening task to assess selective attention to negative stimuli in individuals who had previously experienced a depressive episode (the high depression-vulnerable group) and in individuals who had never experienced a depressive episode (the low depression-vulnerable group). No evidence of any attentional difference between these groups was obtained when they were tested in a normal mood state. However, a negative mood induction procedure served to increase attention to emotional stimuli in the high depression-vulnerable group and to decrease attention to emotional stimuli in the low depression-vulnerable group. Thus, trait affect may interact with state affect to influence selective attention and memory processes.

Studies that have compared patterns of memory in previously depressed and never depressed subjects also have revealed different cognitive responses to induced depression across these groups. For example, Teasdale and Dent (1987) utilized a self-referent encoding task followed by an incidental memory task, with and without a mood-induction procedure intended to elicit a depressed mood state. In the absence of the mood-induction procedure, previously depressed individuals showed equivalent patterns of memory to those shown by subjects who had never suffered from depression. However, the induction of depressed mood served to increase selective recall of the negative trait words to a disproportionate degree within the previously depressed group.

The general finding that trait differences in emotional vulnerability are associated with stable differences in the patterns of selective information processing elicited by dysphoric mood state strengthens the possibility that individual differences in selective processing might contribute to emotional vulnerability. Suppose, for example, that an individual tends to respond to elevations in state anxiety by selectively attending to threatening stimuli. If we assume that the selective encoding of threatening environmental elements is likely to further increase state anxiety, thereby also increasing the selective attentional bias, it is likely that minor stress may escalate into more severe anxiety as a direct result of this pattern of selective processing. Or let us consider the individual who responds to sadness with an enhanced tendency to selectively recall past failures. Again, if we assume that recollection of past failures will tend to increase sadness, thus exaggerating the memory bias, episodes of mild dysphoria are likely to spiral into more severe depression. Thus, the style of information processing elicited by dysphoric mood state might serve as the cognitive mechanism that functionally mediates emotional vulnerability.

Predictive Utility of Information-Processing Biases

Though largely speculative, this account of emotionally vulnerability does serve to generate some clear predictions. In particular, it leads to the prediction that initial measures of the patterns of selective processing elicited by dysphoria should serve to predict later emotional reactions to subsequent stressful life events. Already, some encouraging support has been obtained for this prediction. MacLeod and Hagan (1992) used a color-naming interference task to assess individual differences in selective attention to threat stimuli within a population of state-anxious women about to undergo a cervical examination. The group of women who subsequently received a diagnosis of cervical pathology were followed up, and their emotional reactions to this later stressful life event were assessed by questionnaire. Individual differences in the subsequent emotional reactions were not significantly predicted by initial questionnaire measures of trait or state anxiety but were powerfully predicted by initial measures of selective attention to threat stimuli obtained from the color-naming task: those subjects who showed the greatest evidence of automatic attentional capture by threat at the initial test session reported the greatest subsequent elevation of dysphoria in response to the later diagnosis of pathology.

In a conceptually similar study, Bellew and Hill (1991) assessed pregnant women with the Beck Depression Inventory (BDI) and with a measure of recall bias, in which subjects were given an incidental recall task with positive, negative, and self-esteem threatening (SET) words. Subjects who recalled more SET than positive words were considered to be susceptible to depression, and those who recalled more positive than SET words were considered nonvulnerable to depression. The two groups did not differ antenatally with respect to BDI scores. When subjects were assessed 3 months following delivery, susceptible individuals who had experienced negative life events showed a significant increase in depression levels; all other groups showed a decrease in depression. Thus, the recall bias for SET events was a significant and useful predictor of depression in subjects who had experienced negative life events.

In summary, therefore, it seems entirely plausible that individual differences in the selective processing of emotional information might precede, and functionally contribute to the development of, anxiety and depression. Consistent with this possibility, selective attentional biases and memory biases favoring negative information are apparent at the earliest ages that anxiety and depression, respectively, appear as disorders. Moreover, individual differences in the patterns of selective processing elicted by dysphoria are closely associated with measures of trait vulnerability for anxiety and depression. Finally, initial measures of selective attentional and memory biases can powerfully predict subsequent levels of emotional distress in response to stressful life events.

CONCLUSIONS

In this chapter we have examined a number of theoretical formulations concerning the role of cognitive functioning in depression and anxiety and have reviewed the results of studies designed to test hypotheses derived from these theories. The findings we reviewed converge to suggest that anxiety disorders are associated with biases in attentional functioning whereas depressive disorders are characterized by biases in memory functioning. More specifically, individuals suffering from anxiety, but not depressed persons, have consistently been found to demonstrate heightened attention to negative stimuli in their environment. In contrast, depressed individuals, but not anxious persons, exhibit enhanced recall for negative experiences or stimuli. Certainly, not all studies have reported results consistent with this general pattern of cognitive functioning in anxiety and depression, and it will be important in future research to delineate the parameters underlying this pattern of functioning.

In this context, researchers will have to attend closely to the precise nature of their subject sample. In particular, investigators working in the area of depression are demonstrating a growing awareness of differences between individuals experiencing clinical versus subclinical, or dysphoric, levels of depression. Moreover, it is now apparent that the differences are more complex than would be expected if these two groups of individuals differed simply in the severity of their depression. Addressing this issue, Depue and Monroe (1978) concluded that mild depressive states lack the overt behaviors, somaticized anxiety, and physical complaints that are associated with more severe levels of depression. Indeed, Gotlib (1984) found that elevated scores on self-report measures of depression appear to reflect diffuse psychological distress, as opposed to depression per se. It may be, therefore, that inconsistencies across some the studies reviewed earlier may be due in part to the use of mildly depressed subjects in some studies and clinically depressed subjects in others. In fact, Kuiper, Olinger, and MacDonald (1988) have postulated explicitly that whereas clinical depression is characterized by efficient processing of negative stimuli, mild depression is typified by inefficient processing of both positive and negative stimuli (but see also Vredenburg, Flett, & Krames, 1993). In any case, there has been even less attention paid to differences between mild and clinical levels of anxiety, and it is clear that an important task for researchers in the future involves the more explicit delineation of parameters of attentional and memory functioning in mildly and clinically anxious and depressed individuals.

Another critical issue in this area involves the *nature* of the relation between cognitive functioning and the emotional disorders. For example, a major postulate of Beck's model of anxiety and depression is that negative schemata are stable constructs that predispose individuals to these disorders and thereby play a causal role in the onset of episodes of anxiety and depression. As we noted above, the results of the majority of relevant longitudinal studies suggest that cognitive dysfunction is a concomitant, rather than an antecedent, of depression and/or anxiety. Recently, theorists have suggested that negative schematic functioning is more easily "primed" by negative mood in individuals who have experienced episodes of anxiety or depression in the past (cf. Miranda, Persons, & Byers, 1990; Teasdale, 1988), a position that is also consistent with network models of emotion. The few studies that have examined this formulation have yielded promising results, but much more work remains to be done, particularly with respect to the onset of anxiety. Similarly, the results of a small number of recent studies suggest that cognitive biases may predict subsequent levels of depression and anxiety, and this, too, is an area of research that warrants sustained effort.

Finally, throughout this chapter we have touched on evolutionary and developmental considerations in understanding cognitive functioning in the anxiety and depressive disorders. Clearly, discussions of evolutionary aspects of cognitive biases in the emotional disorders are, by necessity, speculative. Moreover, the study of information-processing biases at different developmental levels is a very recent endeavor, and we similarly have relatively little knowledge in this area. Two recent studies have examined the prevalence of negative thinking and worry at different ages in young children (Ronan et al., 1994; Vasey, Crnic, & Carter, 1994), and the results of these investigations are promising in helping to elucidate developmental aspects of the relation between cognition and anxiety and depression. Nevertheless, these investigations represent only a preliminary attempt to adopt a developmental framework in the study of cognitive functioning and the emotional disorders, and it is critical that researchers devote much more energy to the study of developmental aspects of anxiety, depression, and information processing.

In closing, we would like to raise three additional issues. First, we have spent most of this chapter discussing studies examining information-processing biases in individuals experiencing anxiety and in individuals experiencing depression. As we noted at the beginning of this chapter, however, these two disorders are characterized by a high level of comorbidity, and significant progress in this area will be made only if we begin to examine cognitive functioning in samples of individuals characterized by comorbid anxiety and depression. Second, we have focused here on studies of information-processing biases for valenced stimuli. There are large bodies of literature examining the effects of depression and anxiety on attention and memory for nonvalenced, or neutral, material (cf. Gotlib, Roberts, & Gilboa, 1996), and it will be important to consider these studies to obtain a more complete picture of the cognitive functioning of depressed and anxious individuals. Finally, there is no doubt that a comprehensive theory of depression and anxiety will go beyond an exclusive focus on information processing and will encompass social and biological factors as well. Indeed, recently proposed integrative theories of depression (e.g., Gotlib & Hammen, 1992; Lewinsohn, Hoberman, Teri, & Hautzinger, 1985) emphasize the importance of both cognitive and interpersonal factors. Thus, the overarching goal of future research in the areas of anxiety and depression will be not simply to elucidate the role of cognitive functioning of these disorders but to integrate knowledge of the information-processing biases of anxious and depressed persons with an understanding and appreciation of their interpersonal world.

REFERENCES

American Psychiatric Association. (1994). *Diagnostic and statistical manual of mental disorders* (4th ed.). Washington, DC: Author.

Anderson, J., & Bower, G. H. (1973). *Human associative memory.* Washington, DC: Winston.

Baddeley, A. D. (1986). *Working memory.* Oxford: Clarendon Press.

Bartlett, F. C. (1932). *Remembering.* Cambridge, UK: Cambridge University Press.

Beck, A. T. (1967). *Depression.* New York: Hoeber Medical.

Beck, A. T. (1976). *Cognitive therapy and the emotional disorders.* New York: International Universities Press.

Beck, A. T., Brown, G., Steer, R. A., Eidelson, J. I., & Riskind, J. H. (1987). Differentiating anxiety and depression utilising the Cognitions Checklist. *Journal of Abnormal Psychology, 96,* 179–186.

Beck, A. T., & Clark, D. M. (1988). Anxiety and depression: An information processing perspective. *Anxiety Research, 1,* 23–36.

Beck, A. T., Emery, G., & Greenberg, R. C. (1986). *Anxiety disorders and phobias: A cognitive perspective.* New York: Basic Books.

Beck, J. G., Stanley, M. A., Averill, P. M., Baldwin, L. E., & Deagle, E. A. (1992). Attention and memory for threat in panic disorder. *Behaviour Research and Therapy, 30,* 619–629.

Bellew, M., & Hill, B. (1991). Schematic processing and the prediction of depression following childbirth. *Personality and Individual Differences, 12,* 943–949.

Blaney, P. H. (1986). Affect and memory: A review. *Psychological Bulletin, 99,* 229–246.

Bower, G. H. (1981). Mood and memory. *American Psychologist, 36,* 129–148.

Bower, G. H. (1987). Commentary on mood and memory. *Behaviour Research and Therapy, 25,* 443–456.

Bower, G. H. (1992). How might emotions affect learning? In S. A. Christianson (Ed.), *Handbook of emotion and memory* (pp. 3–31). Hillsdale, NJ: Erlbaum.

Boyd, J. H., & Weissman, M. M. (1981). Epidemiology of affective disorders. *Archives of General Psychiatry, 38,* 1039–1046.

Bradley, B. P., & Mathews, A. (1983). Negative self-schemata in clinical depression. *British Journal of Clinical Psychology, 22,* 173–182.

Burgess, I. S., Jones, L. N., Robertson, S. A., Radcliffe, W. N., Emerson, E.,

Lawler, P., & Crow, T. J. (1981). The degree of control exerted by phobic and non-phobic verbal stimuli over the recognition behaviour of phobic and non-phobic subjects. *Behaviour Research and Therapy, 19,* 223–234.

Clark, D. A., Beck, A. T., & Brown, G. (1989). Cognitive mediation in general psychiatric outpatients: A test of the content specificity hypothesis. *Journal of Personality and Social Psychology, 56,* 958–964.

Clark, D. A., & Teasdale, J. D. (1982). Diurnal variations in clinical depression and accessibility of memories of positive and negative experiences. *Journal of Abnormal Psychology, 91,* 97–105.

Clark, L. A., & Watson, D. (1991). Theoretical and empirical issues in differentiating depression from anxiety. In J. Becker & A. Kleinman (Eds.), *Psychosocial aspects of depresssion* (pp. 39–65). Hillsdale, NJ: Erlbaum.

Clayton, P. J. (1983). The prevalence and course of the affective disorders. In J. M. Davis & J. W. Maas (Eds.), *The affective disorders.* Washington, DC: American Psychiatric Press.

Craske, M., & Barlow, D. H. (1991). Contributions of cognitive psychology to assessment and treatment of anxiety. In P. R. Martin (Ed.), *Handbook of behaviour therapy and psychological science: An integrative approach.* Oxford: Pergamon Press.

Dandes, S. K., LaGreca, A. M., Wick, P. L., & Shaw, K. (1986, March). *The development of the Social Anxiety Scale for Children (SASC): Part II. Relationship to peer and teacher ratings.* Paper presented at the meeting of the Southeastern Psychological Association.

Depue, R. A., & Monroe, S. M. (1978). Learned helplessness in the perspective of the depressives disorders. *Journal of Abnormal Psychology, 87,* 3–21.

de Ruiter, C., & Brosschot, J. F. (1994). The emotional Stroop interference effect in anxiety: Attentional bias or cognitive avoidance? *Behaviour Research and Therapy, 32,* 315–319.

Ehlers, A., Margraf, J., Davies, S., & Roth, W. T. (1988). Selective processing of threat cues in subjects with panic attacks. *Cognition and Emotion, 2,* 201–220.

Foa, E. B., Feske, U., Murdock, T. B., Kozak, M. J., & McCarthy, P. R. (1991). Processing of threat-related information in rape victims. *Journal of Abnormal Psychology, 100,* 156–162.

Foa, E. B., & McNally, R. J. (1986). Sensitivity to feared stimuli in obsessive compulsive disorder: A dichotic listening analysis. *Cognitive Therapy and Research, 10,* 477–486.

Francis, G. (1988). Assessing cognition in anxious children. *Behavior Modification, 12,* 267–280.

Frank, E., Carpenter, L. L., & Kupfer, D. J. (1988). Sex differences in recurrent depression: Are there any that are significant? *American Journal of Psychiatry, 145,* 41–45.

Gotlib, I. H. (1984). Depression and general psychopathology in university students. *Journal of Abnormal Psychology, 93,* 19–30.

Gotlib, I. H., & Cane, D. B. (1987). Construct accessibility and clinical depression: A longitudinal approach. *Journal of Abnormal Psychology, 96,* 199–204.

Gotlib, I. H., & Cane, D. B. (1989). Self-report assessment of depression and anxiety. In P. C. Kendall & D. Watson (Eds.), *Anxiety and depression: Distinctive and overlapping features* (pp. 131–169). Orlando, FL: Academic Press.

Gotlib, I. H., & Hammen, C. L. (1992). *Psychological aspects of depression: Toward a cognitive–interpersonal integration.* Chichester, UK: Wiley.

Gotlib, I. H., MacLachan, A. L., & Katz, A. N. (1988). Biases in visual attention in depressed and non-depressed individuals. *Cognition and Emotion, 2,* 185–200.

Gotlib, I. H., & McCabe, S. B. (1992). An information-processing approach to the study of cognitive functioning in depression. In E. F. Walker, B. A. Cornblatt, & R. H. Dworkin (Eds.), *Progress in experimental personality and psychopathology research* (Vol. 15, pp. 131–161). New York: Springer.

Gotlib, I. H., & McCann, C. D. (1984). Construct accessibility and depression: An examination of cognitive and affective factors. *Journal of Personality and Social Psychology, 47,* 427–439.

Gotlib, I. H., Roberts, J. E., & Gilboa, E. (1996). Cognitive interference in depression. In I. Sarason, B. Sarason, & G. Pierce (Eds.), *Cognitive interference: Theories, methods, and findings* (pp. 347–377). Hillsdale, NJ: Erlbaum.

Graf, P., & Mandler, G. (1984). Activation makes words more accessible, but not necessarily more retrievable. *Journal of Verbal Learning and Verbal Behavior, 23,* 553–568.

Hammen, C., & Zupan, B. A. (1984). Self schemas, depression, and the processing of personal information in children. *Journal of Child Psychology, 37,* 598–604.

Hollon, S., & Shelton, M. (1991). Contributions of cognitive psychology to assessment and treatment of depression. In P. R. Martin (Ed.), *Handbook of behaviour therapy and psychological science: An integrative approach.* Oxford: Pergamon Press.

Hope, D. A., Rapee, R. M., Heimberg, R. G., & Dombeck, M. J. (1990). Representations of the self in social phobia: Vulnerability to social threat. *Cognitive Therapy and Research, 14,* 177–189.

Ingram, R. E., Bernet, C. Z., & McGlaughlin, S. C. (1994). Attentional allocation in individuals at risk for depression. *Cognitive Therapy and Research, 8,* 317–332.

Ingram, R. E., Kendall, P. C., Smith, T. W., Donnell, C., & Ronan, K. (1987). Cognitive specificity in emotional distress. *Journal of Personality and Social Psychology, 53,* 52–59.

Ingram, R., & Reed, M. (1986). Information encoding and retrieval processes in depression: Findings, issues, and future directions. In R. Ingram (Ed.), *Information processing approaches to clinical psychology.* Orlando, FL: Academic Press.

Jolly, J. B., & Dykman, R. A. (1994). Using self-report data to differentiate anxious and depressed symptoms in adolescents: Cognitive content specificity and global distress? *Cognitive Therapy and Research, 18,* 25–37.

Karno, M., Hough, R. L., Burnam, A., Escobar, J. I., Timbers, D. M., Santana, F., & Boyd, J. H. (1987). Lifetime prevalence of specific psychiatric disorders among Mexican Americans and non-Hispanic whites in Los Angeles. *Archives of General Psychiatry, 44,* 695–701.

Keller, M. B., & Shapiro, R. W. (1981). Major depressive disorder: Initial results from a one-year prospective naturalistic follow-up study. *Journal of Nervous and Mental Disease, 169,* 761–768.

Kendall, P. C. (1993). Cognitive-behavioural therapies with youth: Guiding theory, current status, and emerging developments. *Journal of Consulting and Clinical Psychology, 61,* 235–247.

Kendall, P. C., & Chansky, E. (1991). Considering cognition in anxiety-disordered children. *Journal of Anxiety Disorders, 5,* 167–185.

Kendall, P. C., & Ronan, K. D. (1990). Assessment of children's anxieties, fears and phobias: Cognitive-behavioral models and methods. In C. R. Reynolds & R. W. Kamphaus (Eds.), *Handbook of psychological and educational assessment of children: Vol. 2. Personality, behavior, and context* (pp. 223–244). New York: Guilford Press.

King, N. J., Ollendick, T. H., & Gullone, E. (1991). Negative affectivity in children and adolescents: Relations between anxiety and depression. *Clinical Psychology Review, 11,* 441–459.

Kuiper, N. A., Olinger, L. J., & MacDonald, M. R. (1988). Processing personal and social information: The role of vulnerability and episodic schemata in depression. In L. B. Alloy (Ed.), *Cognitive processes in depression* (pp. 289–309). New York: Guilford Press.

Last, C. G., Hersen, M., Kazdin, A., Finkestein, R., & Strauss, C. C. (1987). Comparison of DSM-III separation anxiety and overanxious disorders: Demographic characteristics and patterns of comorbidity. *Journal of the American Academy of Child and Adolescent Psychiatry, 26,* 527–531.

Lavy, E., van den Hout, M., & Arntz, A. (1993). Attentional bias and spider phobia: Conceptual and clinical issues. *Behaviour Research and Therapy, 31,* 17–24.

Lavy, E. H., van Oppen, P, & van den Hout, M. (1994). Selective processing of emotional information in obsessive compulsive disorder. *Behaviour Research and Therapy, 32,* 243–246.

Lewinsohn, P. M., Hoberman, H. M., Teri, L., & Hautzinger, M. (1985). An integrative theory of depression. In S. Reiss & R. Bootzin (Eds.), *Theoretical issues in behavior therapy* (pp. 331–359). New York: Academic Press.

MacLeod, C. (1991). Clinical anxiety and the selective encoding of threatening information. *International Review of Psychiatry, 3,* 279–292.

MacLeod, C., & Hagan, R. (1992). Individual differences in selective processing of threatening information, and emotional responses to a stressful life event. *Behaviour Research and Therapy, 30,* 151–161.

MacLeod, C., & Mathews, A. (1988). Anxiety and the allocation of attention to threat. *Quarterly Journal of Experimental Psychology, 38A,* 659–670.

MacLeod, C., & Mathews, A. (1991). Cognitive-experimental approaches to the emotional disorders. In P. R. Martin (Ed.), *Handbook of behaviour therapy and psychological science: An integrative approach.* Oxford: Pergamon Press.

MacLeod, C., Mathews, A., & Tata, P. (1986). Attentional bias in emotional disorders. *Journal of Abnormal Psychology, 95,* 15–20.

MacLeod, C., & McLaughlin, K. (1995). Implicit and explicit memory bias in anxiety: A conceptual replication. *Behaviour Research and Therapy, 33,* 1–14.

MacLeod, C., & Rutherford, E. M. (1993). Anxiety and the selective processing of emotional information: Mediating roles of awareness, trait and state variables, and personal relevance of stimulus materials. *Behaviour Research and Therapy, 30,* 479–491.

MacLeod, C., Tata, P., & Mathews, A. (1987). Perception of emotionally valenced information in depression. *British Journal of Clinical Psychology, 26,* 67–68.

Martin, M., Horder, P., & Jones, G. V. (1992). Integral bias in naming of phobia-related words. *Cognition and Emotion, 6,* 479–486.

Maser, J. D., & Cloninger, C. R. (Eds.). (1990). *Comorbidity in anxiety and mood disorders.* Washington, DC: American Psychiatric Press.

Mathews, A., & MacLeod, C. (1985). Selective processing of threat cues in anxiety states. *Behaviour Research and Therapy, 23,* 563–569.

Mathews, A., & MacLeod, C. (1986). Discrimination of threat cues without awareness in anxiety states. *Journal of Abnormal Psychology, 95,* 131–138.

Mathews, A., & MacLeod, C. (1994). Cognitive approaches to emotion. *Annual Review of Psychology, 45,* 25–50.

Mattia, J. I., Heimberg, R. G., & Hope, D. A. (1993). The revised Stroop color-naming task in social phobics. *Behaviour Research and Therapy, 31,* 305–313.

McCabe, S. B., & Gotlib, I. H. (1993). Attentional processing in clinically depressed subjects: A longitudinal investigation. *Cognitive Therapy and Research, 17,* 359–377.

McCabe, S. B., & Gotlib, I. H. (1995). Selective attention and clinical depression: Performance on a deployment-of-attention task. *Journal of Abnormal Psychology, 104,* 241–245.

McNally, R. J., Amir, N., Louro, C. E., Lukach, B. M., Riemann, B. C., & Calamari, J. E. (1994). Cognitive processing of idiographic emotional information in panic disorder. *Behaviour Research and Therapy, 32,* 119–122.

Miller, S. M., Boyer, B. A., & Rodoletz, M. (1990). Anxiety in children: Nature and development. In M. Lewis & S. M. Miller (Eds.), *Handbook of developmental psychopathology* (pp. 191–207). New York: Plenum Press.

Miranda, J., Persons, J. B., & Byers, C. N. (1990). Endorsement of dysfunctional beliefs depends on current mood state. *Journal of Abnormal Psychology, 97,* 251–264.

Mogg, K., Bradley, B. P., Williams R., & Mathews, A. (1993). Subliminal processing of emotional information in anxiety and depression. *Journal of Abnormal Psychology, 102,* 304–311.

Mogg, K., Mathews, A., & Eysenck, M. W. (1992). Attentional bias to threat in clinical anxiety states. *Cognition and Emotion, 6,* 149–159.

Mogg, K., Mathews, A., & Weinman, J. (1989). Selective processing of threat cues in anxiety states: A replication. *Behaviour Research and Therapy, 27,* 317–323.

Oatley, K., & Johnson-Laird, P. (1987). Towards a cognitive theory of emotions. *Cognition and Emotion, 1,* 29–50.

Powell, M., & Hemsley, D. R. (1984). Depression: A breakdown of perceptual defense? *British Journal of Psychiatry, 145,* 358–362.

Prieto, S. L., Cole, D. A., & Tageson, C. W. (1992). Depressive self-schemas in clinic and nonclinic children. *Cognitive Therapy and Research, 16,* 521–534.

Robins, L. N., Helzer, J. E., Weissman, M. M., Orvaschel, H., Gruenberg, E., Burke, J. D., & Regier, D. A. (1984). Lifetime prevalence of specific psychiatric disorders in three sites. *Archives of General Psychiatry, 41*, 949–958.

Robins, L. N., & Regier, D. A. (Eds.). (1991). *Psychiatric disorders in America: The Epidemiologic Catchment Area Study.* New York: Free Press.

Ronan, K. R., Kendall, P. C., & Rowe, M. (1994). Negative affectivity in children: Development and validation of a Self-Statement Questionnaire. *Cognitive Therapy and Research, 18*, 509–528.

Schank, R., & Abelson, R. (1977). *Scripts, plans, goals, and understanding: An enquiry in human knowledge structures.* Hillsdale, NJ: Erlbaum.

Slife, B. D., Miura, S., Thompson, L. W., Shapiro, J. L., & Gallagher, D. (1984). Differential recall as a function of mood disorder in clinically depressed patients: Between- and within-subject differences. *Journal of Abnormal Psychology, 9*, 391–400.

Spence, S. H. (1994). Cognitive therapy with children and adolescents: From theory to practice. *Journal of Child Psychology and Psychiatry, 35*, 1191–1228.

Strauss, C. C., Last, C. G., Hersen, M., & Kazdin, A. E. (1988). Association between anxiety and depression in children and adolescents with anxiety disorders. *Journal of Abnormal Child Psychology, 16*, 57–68.

Stroop, J. R. (1938). Factors affecting speed in serial verbal reactions. *Psychological Monographs, 50*, 38–48.

Teasdale, J. D. (1988). Cognitive vulnerability to persistent depression. *Cognition and Emotion, 2*, 247–274.

Teasdale, J. D., & Dent, J. (1987). Cognitive vulnerability to depression: An investigation of two hypotheses. *British Journal of Clinical Psychology, 26*, 113–126.

Vasey, M. W. (1993). Development and cognition in childhood anxiety: The example of worry. In T. H. Ollendick & R. J. Prinz (Eds.), *Advances in clinical child psychology* (Vol. 15, pp. 1–39). New York: Plenum Press.

Vasey, M. W., Crnic, K. A., & Carter, W. G. (1994). Worry in childhood: A developmental perspective. *Cognitive Therapy and Research, 18*, 529–549.

Vredenburg, K., Flett, G. L., & Krames, L. (1993). Analogue versus clinical depression: A critical reappraisal. *Psychological Bulletin, 113*, 327–344.

Watts, F. N., McKenna, F. P., Sharrock, R., & Trezise, L. (1986). Color-naming of phobia related words. *British Journal of Psychology, 77*, 97–108.

Whitman, P. B., & Leitenberg, H. (1990). Negatively biased recall in children with self-reported symptoms of depression. *Journal of Abnormal Child Psychology, 18*, 15–27.

Williams, J. M. G., & Nulty, D. D. (1986). Construct accessibility, depression, and the emotional Stroop task: Transient mood or stable structure? *Personality and Individual Differences, 7*, 485–491.

Williams, J. M. G., Watts, F. N., MacLeod, C., & Mathews, A. (1988). *Cognitive psychology and emotional disorders.* Chichester, UK: Wiley.

Wittchen, H., Zhao, S., Kessler, R. C., & Eaton, W. W. (1994). DSM-III-R generalized anxiety disorder in the National Comorbidity Survey. *Archives of General Psychiatry, 51*, 355–364.

Zatz, S., & Chassin, L. (1983). Cognitions of test anxious children. *Journal of Consulting and Clinical Psychology, 40*, 20–25.

Attentional Functioning of Psychopathic Individuals

CURRENT EVIDENCE AND DEVELOPMENTAL IMPLICATIONS

David S. Kosson
Timothy J. Harpur

P sychopathy is a personality disorder associated with callous manipulation and exploitation of others, superficial emotion, impulsive behavior, and criminality. Psychopaths are typically studied in prisons, and it is estimated that 15–25% of prison inmates may be psychopathic (Hare, 1991). However, population prevalence estimates of 4% of males and 1% of females reflect a widespread assumption that the disorder is not limited to those whose antisocial behavior is detected or to those who break the law (e.g., Edelmann & Vivian, 1988; Millon, 1981). The social costs of psychopathy are evident in relationships between psychopathy and violence (Hare & McPherson, 1984), recidivism (Harris, Rice, & Cormier, 1991), and revocation of conditional releases (Hart, Kropp, & Hare, 1988). Moreover, treatments have not effectively modified psychopaths' antisocial behavior (Ogloff, Wong, & Greenwood, 1990).

Historically, most research on psychopaths has focused on behavioral and physiological anomalies associated with psychopathy. However, recent research and theory converge in an emphasis on cognitive and particularly attentional abilities of psychopaths. The consistency of recent findings not only demonstrates the value of studying psychopathic cognition but also highlights some especially promising hypotheses with possible treatment implications. Our goal in this chapter is to show how this research contributes to the development of a framework for understanding the psychological processes that characterize psychopaths. In addition, to begin to identify links between specific cognitive deficits in adult and child populations, we review cognitive studies of adolescent samples at heightened risk for developing psychopathy. Though a detailed map of the origins of psychopathy is premature, extant empirical findings provide preliminary guideposts for exploring etiological issues.

A major impediment to research on psychopathy has been a lack of agreement regarding the definition of this disorder. Indeed, the recent acceleration of psychopathy research appears to be a consequence of the introduction and validation of the Hare Psychopathy Checklist (PCL; Hare, 1991), a behavioral rating scale used to identify incarcerated psychopaths on the basis of interview and prison records. However, a lack of consensus regarding psychopathy remains evident in its conspicuous absence from the fourth edition of the American Psychiatric Association's *Diagnostic and Statistical Manual of Mental Disorders* (DSM-IV). Whereas antisocial personality disorder (APD) was once construed as synonymous with psychopathy, only about half of inmates with DSM-III APD also meet diagnostic criteria for psychopathy (Hare, 1991). Moreover, although APD diagnoses correlate with ratings of antisocial and impulsive behavior, they do not correlate highly with the callous exploitation of others and shallow emotional life that many consider the personality core of the psychopath (Harpur, Hare, & Hakstian, 1989). Thus, we restrict our review of adult studies to those employing PCL-identified groups.

MULTIPLE ATTENTIONAL CONSTRUCTS

Individuals' performances on different types of attentional tasks are not highly correlated. Thus, there are several varieties of attention (Parasuraman & Davies, 1984).

Several different classification systems have in common the identification of at least three major categories of attention, namely, *sustained attention, selective attention,* and *divided attention* (e.g., Davies, Jones, & Taylor, 1984; Mirsky, Anthony, Duncan, Ahearn, & Kellam, 1991), and some investigators have added a fourth, *executive functions* (e.g., Sohlberg & Mateer, 1989).

At the outset we note a caveat related to the study of attention in psychopaths. Attentional functions are affected by motivation: Individuals generally distribute attention to what is of interest or relevant to them (e.g., Kahneman, 1973). General alertness (Eriksen & Murphy, 1987) and activation or arousal (Duffy, 1962) also moderate processing efficiency. Thus, performance measures may be used to estimate ability only if participants attempt to do their best, and psychopaths' performance deficits have sometimes been attributed to a lack of motivation (Schmauk, 1970) or underarousal (Hare, 1978; Quay, 1965), factors which reduce processing capacity (Kahneman, 1973). However, recent studies suggest that psychopaths are not characterized by generalized performance deficits. In some studies, researchers have taken precautions to ensure adequate motivation, including using monetary incentives (Kosson & Newman, 1986) or fast-paced, interesting tasks (Jutai, Hare, & Connolly, 1987). In others, abnormal performance by psychopaths is limited to certain tasks or conditions (Harpur, 1991). Nevertheless, further studies of the dependence of psychopaths' cognitive deficits on particular motivational/emotional states also appears warranted (e.g., Howland & Newman, 1993).

Sustained Attention

Sustained attention refers to the maintenance of a specific perceptual/response readiness across time and is typically measured by continuous performance tasks (CPTs). Most information-processing paradigms require participants to maintain attention across time, although different tasks differ widely in the rate at which information is presented and the interval across which attention must be sustained. Thus, most studies reviewed below also provide indirect information about psychopaths' ability to maintain vigilance. However, despite the widespread use of CPTs to study childhood behavior disorders, only one published investigation addresses sustained attention in psychopaths. This lack of research is surprising given the centrality of unreliability and boredom proneness in some accounts of the disorder (Cleckley, 1976; Quay, 1965).

Raine and Venables (1988) conducted the sole published study of sustained attention in adult psychopaths. They presented stimuli at the rate of 0.67 per second (1.5-second interstimulus intervals), and 23% of stimuli were targets. Over an interval of 6–7 minutes, psychopaths (those scoring above the median on the PCL) performed as well as nonpsychopathic inmates. However, electrocortical measures sensitive to attention allocation (i.e., amplitude of the P300 event-related potential, or ERP) did differentiate the groups. Psychopaths displayed larger P300 amplitudes and longer P300 recovery times following targets. Thus, although psychopaths were not deficient at sustained attention, Raine and Venables suggested that they allocated greater attention to the processing of targets, a selective attention hypothesis to which we will return. However, any such differences were not apparent in performance. Moreover, because the task was of short duration, it is possible that sustained attention deficits would emerge over longer intervals.

Fortunately, studies of other aspects of attention address this latter possibility. Although Jutai and Hare (1983) report deteriorating performance only for psychopaths on a video game that was their primary task, most studies report no significant interactions between psychopathy and time on task. Given that task durations in these studies ranged from 10 to 60 minutes, psychopaths appear able to sustain attention over such time periods. Nevertheless, it remains possible that their actual performance in many real-world situations does not reflect this capacity for sustained attention, particularly when tasks are monotonous or individuals are not paid for good performance.

Selective Attention

Selective attention commonly refers to both the selection or inclusion of some stimuli for enhanced processing and the exclusion of other stimuli. Psychopaths' apparent unresponsiveness to important contingencies (e.g., consequences of their actions, feelings of others) has led to suggestions that they experience heightened selective attention (Hare, 1978): Psychopaths may be especially able to focus on stimuli of immediate interest (Jutai & Hare, 1983; Raine, 1989) and to ignore irrelevant or unpleasant stimuli (Hare, 1978). Alternatively, excessive responsiveness to cues for reward may reduce psychopaths' attentiveness to other cues (Newman & Kosson, 1986). The studies reviewed below corroborate selective attention differences between psychopathic and nonpsychopathic individuals. However, such differences are evident in only a subset of experimental conditions that have been examined — those in which the selection of stimuli is mediated primarily by endogenous mechanisms and possibly by the allocation of left-hemisphere-specific processing resources.

Because components of attention involved in focusing on and screening out stimuli are sometimes assessed via distinct paradigms, we consider these components in turn. Two distinct mechanisms for facilitation have been proposed. When peripheral cues are presented prior to processing targets, allocations of attention to cue locations are termed *exogenous* and are assumed to be rapid, obligatory, and independent of cue validity. When central cues provide information about target location, less rapid *endogenous* allocations of attention to cued locations occur if cues are partially valid (Müller & Rabbit, 1989).

Facilitation is traditionally assessed by comparing response latencies on validly cued trials against response latencies on neutral or invalidly cued trials. However, in light of evidence that neutral trials are relatively arousing (Jonides & Mack, 1984), some investigators instead analyze differences between performance on validly and invalidly cued trials, a measure of responsiveness to cues that does not distinguish facilitation from inhibition but avoids assumptions about neutral cues.

Three studies of psychopaths' ability to benefit from such cues indicate that psychopaths, like nonpsychopaths, respond faster when cued to a particular target location than when they are provided no information or misinformed about target location. Harpur (1991) examined psychopaths' response latencies in detecting targets preceded by peripheral cues. In one study, cues preceding targets by 50 and 150 milliseconds correctly predicted target location on 80% of trials and presumably initiated both exogenous and endogenous shifts of attention to cued locations. In a second study, peripheral cues and central cues predicted target location on 69% of trials and preceded targets by 100 milliseconds. In both cases, no group differences in responsiveness to such cues were evident.[1] Similarly, Howland, Kosson, Patterson, and Newman (1993) used peripheral cues that predicted target location 80% of the time and preceded targets by 1 second. Again, invalid–valid difference scores indicated similar overall effects of validity for both groups. In sum, psychopaths and nonpsychopaths appear to display similar benefits from cues in simple cuing paradigms.

The suggestion of psychopathic superiority at inhibiting attention to noncued locations evolved from findings of electrodermal hyporesponsiveness to aversive stimuli. Hare (1978) interprets this hyporesponsiveness as reflecting a coping style through which psychopaths attenuate the impact of unpleasant stimuli (see also Hare, 1982). Psychopaths also allocate less attention to irrelevant stimulation than do nonpsychopaths, as indexed by smaller N100 ERPs to initial irrelevant tone pips presented during attention-demanding video games (Jutai & Hare, 1983). However, these early studies provide only limited information about psychopaths' aptitude for inhibition, because these studies neither employed cues to induce shifts of attention nor examined responsiveness to potentially relevant events.

In the studies by Harpur (1991) and Howland et al. (1993), slower responses to invalidly cued targets could be interpreted as reflecting inhibition of attention to uncued locations and/or to the need to shift attention from the miscued to the correct location. Howland et al. (1993) reports that although psychopaths and nonpsychopaths displayed comparable slowing on invalidly cued (vs. neutral) trials, psychopaths responded more often with the incorrect hand when invalidly cued to the RVF. Psychopaths' increased errors following invalid RVF cues are consistent with the possibility that psychopaths suffer excessive interference following allocation of left-hemisphere-specific resources and/or preparation of right-handed responses.

Harpur's (1991) studies also contained trials involving longer cue–target intervals, providing additional evidence of psychopathy-related differences in selective attention. On these trials, 500 milliseconds after a peripheral cue (the brightening of a lateralized box), the center box brightened again, drawing subjects' attention back to the center. Under such conditions, responses were slower to subsequent target stimuli in a location first cued than in one not cued. Harpur attributed the slowing to *inhibition of return,* an obligatory inhibition of attention to prior attended locations that is stronger than the facilitation from prior attentional allocations (Posner & Cohen, 1984).

Because inhibition of return can also be assessed through the use of bilateral cue trials that provide no information about target location, Harpur included trials in which both sides were brightened initially. These trials showed that psychopaths and nonpsychopaths developed inhibition of return to similar degrees. However, on unilateral cue trials with long cue—target intervals, psychopaths displayed smaller invalid–valid response times (RTs) to imperative stimuli than those displayed by nonpsychopaths (see Figure 15.1). Assuming no differences in the magnitude of inhibition of return, psychopaths' reduced cost for invalid–valid RTs suggests greater endogenous allocation of attention to the original cued location. Enhanced responsiveness to the initial cue may have bolstered psychopaths' ability to resist distraction by the central brightened box.

Harpur's interpretation also predicts that psychopaths should be characterized by superior facilitation effects given valid cues and long cue—target intervals. Howland et al. (1993) reported no such group differences for validly cued trials. However, two differences between these studies seem to account for this discrepancy. First, Howland et al. did not use a second cue to draw attention away from the initially cued loca-

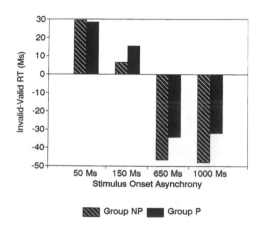

FIGURE 15.1. Difference in reaction time between invalidly and validly cued trials at each SOA for psychopaths (Group P) and nonpsychopaths (Group NP) (data from Experiment 1, Harpur, 1991).

tion: Cues were interrupted only by targets after 1 second. Thus, complete orienting (and eye movements) to the cued location could be expected for all subjects. Second, high speed–accuracy correlations reported for that study suggested that subjects were responding quite quickly, which may have reduced variance in valid trial response latencies. In light of the importance of this question and the mixed evidence to date, further studies of psychopaths' endogenous orienting are needed.

Harpur (1991) reports several additional studies examining other kinds of attentional inhibition in psychopaths. None of these provide evidence for excessive inhibition of attention. Psychopaths and nonpsychopaths displayed comparable slowing due to conflictual (i.e., Stroop) stimuli, repetition of previously ignored stimuli (i.e., negative priming), and presence of a distractor.

In sum, psychopaths perform as do nonpsychopaths when required to ignore distracting stimuli and when orienting automatically to a cued location. In contrast, they display heightened responsiveness to cues under conditions that produce endogenous allocations of attention. Psychopaths may also be prone to greater or more persistent endogenous shifts of attention and/or greater interference associated with allocation of left-hemisphere-specific resources.

Divided Attention

With training, human information processors are capable of performing even complex tasks simultaneously (e.g., Allport, Antonis, & Reynolds, 1972). Nevertheless, divided-attention performance is generally poorer than single-task performance (Moray, 1984; Welford, 1968). Of the varieties of attention addressed in this chapter, divided attention is the area least considered with respect to previous hypotheses regarding psychopaths. No classic theoretical accounts of psychopathy posit deficits in divided attention per se. Nevertheless, recent studies provide substantial evidence for specific deficits in divided attention. Moreover, such deficits appear consistent with proposed differences in endogenous allocations of attention and in the use of hemisphere-specific processing resources.

The mechanisms underlying divided attention are not entirely clear (Shaw, 1982). However, two putative processes—the ability to shift attention between stimuli, tasks, or contingencies, and the ability to distribute processing resources simultaneously among two or more stimuli, tasks, or contingencies—have been studied extensively.[2] Shifts of attention were considered above in the context of selective attention. The allocation of processing resources to an actual or anticipated stimulus is a relatively simple shift of attention. Dynamic shifts of attention from moment to moment may constitute the natural course of processing in the real world (Kahneman, 1973; Moray, 1984), and various paradigms for studying such shifts have been validated (Posner & Cohen, 1984; Reeves & Sperling, 1986).

On the other hand, when multiple stimuli of brief duration occur simultaneously, shifts of attention appear inadequate. In such situations, information processors must distribute processing resources to more than one stimulus or fail to process some stimuli. Although the prevalence of such distributions of attention in the real world is unknown, people are able to distribute attention to multiple locations, at least under some laboratory conditions (Hahn & Kramer, 1994; Hughes & Zimba, 1985). Indeed, most adults can expand/reduce the breadth of visual attention by roughly two degrees (Cohen & Ivry, 1989).

However, the study of these processes is complicated by two aspects of attention. First, most paradigms do not permit unambiguous assessments of component processes. In fact, individual differences in strategies may affect the extent to which people share versus shift attention (Shaw, 1982). Second, a variety of situational parameters may affect the likelihood and effectiveness of shifts and distributions of attention, including the number of tasks or stimuli, the rate of stimulus presentation, and the relative importance of various tasks or stimuli. Manipulations of task priority are recommended to ensure that performance differences reflect differences in processing resources versus strategy differences (Polson & Friedman, 1988).

We initially consider studies requiring responses to simultaneous stimuli, because such studies provide the clearest evidence about psychopaths' ability to distribute attention. Hare and Jutai (1988) required subjects to maintain central fixation while classifying words displayed $1.5°$ to the left or right of fixation for 80 milliseconds. Subjects pressed a button to classify the word, then reported a fixation stimulus, and finally reported the word itself. Performance on the fixation stimulus task was near ceiling with no group differences, and it is assumed that subjects invested most of their processing resources in classifying words.

This task required subjects to judge one of the following: whether a word matched a pretrial cue word, fit within a concrete semantic class (e.g., vehicle), or fit within the abstract category "living thing." If psychopaths were characterized by reduced breadth of attention, they would be expected to classify words less accurately than nonpsychopaths. Psychopaths were less accurate at classifying words but only when performing abstract semantic classification and only for words presented to the right visual field (RVF).[3] Assuming that semantic processing of RVF words was mediated primarily by left-hemisphere processing resources, Hare and Jutai (1988) suggest that psychopaths are characterized by relatively weaker left-hemisphere lateralization for complex language processing.

Hare and McPherson (1984) conducted a dichotic listening study that yielded relatively similar findings. They presented subjects with three pairs of words per trial, each consisting of a single syllable word in each ear, matched for initial letter, onset time, and acoustic length, and asked subjects to report as many of the words in each ear as possible. Psychopathic and nonpsychopathic inmates performed equally well overall, suggesting no deficit in dichotic listening or in divided attention per se. However, psychopaths displayed a smaller right-ear advantage and superior left-ear performance. Moreover, a trend toward a similar difference emerged when subjects were asked to report words from only one ear. Thus, despite differences in stimulus modalities, tasks, relative importance of concurrent stimuli, and task difficulty, results similar to those of Hare and Jutai were obtained. Psychopaths' weaker right-ear advantage was attributed to reduced cerebral specialization for language (see also Hare, Williamson, & Harpur, 1988).

Recent evidence suggesting the existence of separable pools of processing resources in the right and left cerebral hemispheres (Friedman, Polson, Dafoe, & Gaskill, 1982; Wickens, Mountford, & Schreiner, 1981) provides an alternative explanation for these group differences. Rather than reflecting reduced lateralization of cerebral function, psychopaths' performance deficits may reflect difficulty in using left-hemisphere-specific processing resources, which may be most evident in situations requiring complex processing or divided attention. The possibility of differences in right-hemisphere function in psychopaths is also suggested by the Hare and McPherson study. Indeed, evidence for right-hemisphere involvement in the control of spatial selective attention (e.g., Posner, Walker, Friedrich, & Rafal, 1984) and alerting (Tucker & Williamson, 1984) suggest fruitful avenues for further research.

We now turn our attention to paradigms designed to assess shifts of attention between tasks or stimuli. Although the complexity of these paradigms increases the difficulty of interpreting observed performance differences, the studies reviewed below contain manipulation checks, which address some alternative explanations.

Kosson and Newman (1986) paired a visual search task with a simple go/no-go auditory probe–reaction time task. The visual search required subjects to count the total number of letters from a target set provided prior to each trial across eight frames of 1.8-second duration, each presenting four letters in the corners of a computer monitor. The auditory task required subjects to depress a response button with their dominant index finger whenever they heard a low (but not high) pitched tone during visual search trials. Subjects were instructed either to attend equally to the two tasks or to attend preferentially to the visual search over the auditory task and received performance feedback either for both tasks or for only the visual task.

Among subjects tested by male experimenters, psychopaths displayed trends toward performance deficits on both tasks under equal attention conditions, and, under focusing conditions, performance advantages on the visual search primary task with no corresponding secondary task deficit.[4] Psychopaths' relative advantage on a primary task is consistent with evidence suggesting that psychopaths are sometimes overresponsive to cues. Perhaps, given a primary task, psychopaths allocate more attention or shift attention more frequently to such a task than do nonpsychopaths as predicted by an overfocusing explanation. But their adequate secondary task performance under these conditions contradicts the hypothesis that psychopaths' focus on immediate tangible goals reduces their attention to less immediate goals.

The finding of a psychopathic deficit under equally divided attention conditions is without theoretical precedent. However, because this paradigm provides the only evidence thus far regarding intermodal divided attention, it is possible that psychopaths' deficit in equally divided attention reflects deficiencies in processing resources mediating intermodal attention (vs. those mediating divided attention per se). Alternatively, because the visual task was more complex than the auditory task, equal division of attention between such disparate tasks may be unlikely. In either case, the absence of predicted trade-offs between tasks raises questions about the effectiveness of the focusing manipulation and the symmetry/asymmetry of the division of attention (Harpur & Hare, 1990).

Kosson (1996) attempts to remedy these problems and to replicate these findings using a different set of visual and auditory tasks and a different focusing manipulation. In this study, subjects categorized visual and auditory stimuli according to physical features. Visual stimuli were strings of symbols consisting of only letters, only numbers, or both letters and numbers. Auditory stimuli were sequences of four tones monotonically ascending in pitch, constant in pitch, or containing segments ascending and constant in pitch. Subjects were also required to distinguish targets from distractors on the basis of separable stimulus properties: visual targets were stimuli surrounded by horizontally elongated frames; visual distractors were stimuli surrounded by vertically elongated frames. Similarly, whereas auditory target sequences presented only low tones (less than 600 hertz), distractor sequences presented only high tones (over 1,200 hertz).

The target–distractor distinction formed the basis of the focusing manipulation: subjects were presented with twice as many visual (i.e., primary-task) targets as auditory (i.e., secondary-task) targets. Moreover, stimuli in both modalities were two-dimensional—subjects had to judge global features (shapes or overall pitch) of each stimulus as well as the nature and homogeneity of target stimulus components. Order of stimuli was counterbalanced, and both accuracy and response latency were recorded for each task. In this study, subjects performed the visual task more accurately than the auditory task and displayed expected performance trade-offs, indicating that the two tasks depended on overlapping processing resources.

Psychopaths again displayed no deficit in responding to secondary-task targets, corroborating the conclusion that focusing on an immediate tangible goal does not interfere with their responding to less relevant or less frequent target stimuli. At the same time, psychopaths more frequently made the mistake of classifying distractors — only when distractors occurred immediately following target stimuli. To the extent that subjects invest attention to classify initially occurring targets, psychopaths' relative insensitivity to the target/distractor dimension of two-dimensional stimuli is consistent with a reduced breadth of attention that has been allocated to process important signals.

Psychopathy × hand assignment interactions also indicated both performance deficits and advantages in psychopaths' responses to primary task targets immediately preceded by targets — as a function of the hand assigned to the primary task (see Figure 15.2). Among subjects completing the primary task with their right hand, psychopaths displayed a trend toward classifying such primary-task targets less accurately than nonpsychopaths. Among subjects completing the primary task with the left hand, psychopaths displayed an opposite trend toward greater accuracy on such primary-task targets. There were no differences between the groups in response latency or in classification of initially occurring targets.

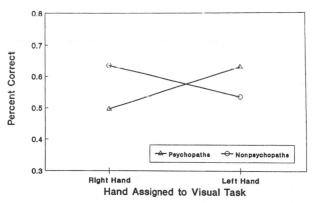

FIGURE 15.2. Primary task accuracy for targets following secondary task targets as a function of psychopathy and hand assignment. Means are covariate adjusted ($MSE = .019$). Unadjusted means (and standard deviations) for psychopaths and nonpsychopaths are 50% ($SD = 13\%$) versus 64% ($SD = 13\%$) for the primary task–right hand and 63% ($SD = 10\%$) versus 54% ($SD = 18\%$) for the primary task–left hand assignment ($MSE = .040$) (data from Kosson, 1996).

If we assume that subjects allocate attention to classify initially occurring targets and then shift attention to process subsequent targets, psychopaths' ability to shift attention appears to depend on the hand assigned to the primary-task response. In light of evidence that left- and right-hemisphere-specific processing resources can mediate attention to the component tasks of some dual-task situations (e.g., Dimond, 1972; Friedman et al., 1982) and that each hemisphere-specific resource is capable of carrying out the processing required by simple visual and auditory tasks, Kosson (1996) suggests that consistent use of one hand for most responses primes the hemisphere-specific processing resources contralateral to that hand (see also Robertson & North, 1993) and increases the likelihood that such hemisphere-specific resources will mediate performance on the primary task assigned to the contralateral hand (especially for second-occurring targets; see Kosson, 1996).

Thus, left-hemisphere processing resources were likely to mediate primary-task performance when the right hand responded to primary-task targets, especially for second-occurring primary-task targets on dual-target trials. Right-hemisphere resources were likely to mediate primary-task performance when the left hand performed such responses, especially for second-occurring primary task targets on dual-target trials. Psychopaths' poorer accuracy for second-occurring primary task targets (with the right hand) suggests greater susceptibility of left-hemisphere-specific processing to disruption by a concurrent target. By contrast, psychopaths' superior accuracy in classifying second-occurring primary task targets with the left hand suggests greater aptitude of right-hemisphere-specific processing resources under such conditions.[5]

Although poorer efficiency of left-hemisphere-specific resources is similar to reduced lateralization of function, these explanations provide different implications: the former emphasizes shifting attention deficits in situations that do not involve linguistic processing. The involvement of left-hemisphere resources in allocations of attention to the RVF (Harter & Anllo-Vento, 1991) may explain psychopaths' failure to interrupt responses to targets expected in the RVF (Howland et al., 1993); psychopaths may have difficulty interrupting left-hemisphere-based attentional allocations. This account also provides a plausible explanation for the divided-attention deficit reported by Kosson and Newman (1986). Because their subjects responded to both tasks with their dominant hand, most subjects probably used their right hands (and left-hemisphere resources) for both tasks.

One additional study of divided attention is worth noting. Jutai, Hare, and Connolly (1987) administered a video game primary task paired with an oddball discrimination secondary task. Subjects used both hands to position a plane and "shoot" enemy planes, while occasionally responding with a right-handed button press when they heard the less frequent of two tones. Unfortunately, because performance was near ceiling on the secondary task (above 90% for both groups) and no decrement from single-task to dual-task performance was observed, the absence of a deficit for psychopaths in this study does not rule out a deficit on more demanding tasks. Even so, psychopaths displayed larger late positivity than non-psychopaths in their ERPs following task stimuli at both central and left-hemisphere sites, suggesting greater processing effort by psychopaths associated with diminished left-hemisphere processing capacity (cf. Raine, 1989). Thus, results of divided-attention studies provide accumulating evidence of left-hemisphere-related processing deficits in psychopaths.

Executive Functions

A variety of higher-level cognitive processes are often grouped together as executive functions. Although many of these overlap with the neuro-psychological domain of frontal functions, the categories are not identical (Stuss & Benson, 1984). Indeed, neuropsychological hypotheses for psychopaths are numerous and reviewed elsewhere (Hart, Forth, & Hare, 1990; Miller, 1987; Smith, Arnett, & Newman, 1992). We restrict our discussion to one aspect of attention included in both categories: inter-level shifts of attention.

In contrast to shifts of attention from one of two tasks or locations to another, interlevel shifts of attention refer to shifts from one level of processing to a different or higher level. For example, the ability to respond to information by revising a strategy, considering a different perspective, or modifying goal-directed behavior reflects responsiveness to environmental input and is one of the hallmarks of flexibility. There are fewer measures of interlevel than of intralevel shifts, and most research on this ability has relied on a single tool, the Wisconsin Card Sort Test (WCST; Milner, 1964).

The WCST requires subjects to sort cards on the basis of one dimension (at a time) of the four-dimensional stimuli on each card. Once ten cards are classified correctly, the examiner changes the dimension according to which feedback is provided. Flexibility is assessed by the number of sorting rules learned and the number of perseverative errors following a rule change. Hare (1984) reported no deficit for psychopaths on the WCST or other tests of frontal function. By contrast, Howland and Newman (1993) reported that psychopaths were deficient on this task when they received concrete rewards and punishments for correct and incorrect answers on each trial but not in the absence of such reinforcers, suggesting that some of psychopaths' cognitive deficits are manifest chiefly when they are highly motivated.[6]

Though not directly informative regarding psychopaths' ability to shift attention from one level to another, substantial evidence indicates that psychopaths are frequently unresponsive to cues to modify their behavior. Indeed, psychopaths' inability to inhibit specific responses paired with punishment is probably their most widely replicated performance deficit (e.g., Lykken, 1957; Schmauk, 1970). Evidence suggesting that such deficits depend upon the presence of concrete reinforcers and the number and salience of reward-and-punishment contingencies (Newman & Kosson, 1986; Newman, Patterson, & Kosson, 1987) bolsters Howland and Newman's argument that psychopaths evince such deficits only in situations that induce high levels of motivation. Similarly, that psychopaths' overresponding to distractors in Kosson (1996) was a function of the allocation of attention to immediately preceding targets suggests that psychopaths' difficulty modulating goal-directed behavior is related to factors affecting their momentary attentional allocations.

More generally, contemporary explanations of failures in response inhibition highlight attention as a key component of passive avoidance deficits. Gray's (1982) model of behavioral inhibition links unresponsiveness to punishment cues to failures in a system that allocates attention to ongoing behavior and current environmental conditions. Similarly, Patterson and Newman's (1993) four-stage model of passive avoidance learning deficits posits multiple stages at which attentional differences may lead to passive avoidance errors. Disinhibited individuals may display more frequent or intense approach response sets in reward contexts and may therefore allocate more attention to goal-relevant cues. Given signals for punishment that produce arousal, disinhibited individuals may fail to interrupt goal-directed behavior sufficiently to process these signals. Finally, if they fail to pause, disinhibited individuals may engage in less reflection regarding links between their behavior, its consequences, and environmental signals. Patterson and Newman proposed that psychopaths fail to pause following an aversive event and therefore fail to reflect, a deficit that may be described as a failure to shift attention from goal-directed behavior to the processing of aversive signals. The possibility that psychopaths allocate excessive (endogenous) attention to goal-relevant targets is also consistent with Patterson and Newman's general model (cf. Raine, 1989).

STUDIES OF YOUNGER POPULATIONS

Preliminary evidence suggests that a syndrome like psychopathy, although not yet well validated, may exist prior to adulthood (Forth, Hart, & Hare, 1990; Frick, O'Brien, Wootton, & McBurnett, 1994; Harpur, 1993). Moreover, there is a substantial literature on childhood populations that resemble psychopaths in important ways. In particular, both the DSM-III and DSM-III-R distinguish a subtype of conduct disorder whose prognosis appears especially poor; it is variously labeled *unsocialized aggressive* (DSM-III) and *solitary aggressive* (DSM-III-R). Studies of this subtype provide speculative but exciting information regarding cognitive developmental antecedents of psychopathy.

No studies of attention have been reported to date based on PCL-identified groups. Indeed, the criteria used to identify psychopathic adolescents in studies reviewed below may be criticized for an overreliance on antisocial behavior and a relative neglect of the affective or interpersonal core of psychopathy (Harpur et al., 1989). Nevertheless, these studies yield data that are consistent with the conclusions of studies of psychopathic adults.

The only study of sustained attention in psychopathic delinquents is reported by Orris (1969), who identified subjects via Quay and Peterson's (1964, cited in Orris, 1969) self-report questionnaire. He presented one stimulus per second and one signal approximately every 2 minutes (i.e., less than 1% of the signals were relevant) for 2 blocks of 100 minutes each. Under these conditions, psychopathic delinquents began the second block of trials detecting fewer signals than other subgroups did and demonstrated consistently poorer performance over the entire block of trials. Because the psychopathic group's performance declined no faster than other groups', the data suggest a generalized deficit attributable to poor motivation or underarousal rather than a sustained attention deficit per se. On the other hand, because data from the first 100 trials were not reported, the possibility of differences during these trials remains uncertain. In any case, the absence of sustained attention deficits is consistent with the one study (Raine & Venables, 1988) reported for adults.

There are no studies of selective attention and only one study of divided attention in an adolescent sample (Raine, O'Brien, Smiley, Scerbo, & Chan, 1990). Raine et al. identified a psychopathic-like group of incarcerated adolescent males based on a cluster analysis of measures including DSM-III-R criteria for antisocial personality disorder (American Psychiatric Association, 1987), the Conduct Disorder scale of the Revised Behavior Problem Checklist (Quay & Peterson, 1987), the Self-Report Psychopathy scale (Hare, 1991), and the 17 Impulsivity scale (Eysenck, Pearson, Easting, & Allsopp, 1985). Despite the possibility that the cluster analytic method may have capitalized on chance, Raine et al. replicates Hare and McPherson's (1984) finding of unusual cerebral asymmetry in a dichotic listening task. Moreover, the task used in this study differed from the earlier version in using consonant–vowel stimuli instead of words and in presenting only one stimulus per ear per trial to minimize memory load. Thus, this replication provides independent evidence consistent with both unusual cerebral asymmetry hypotheses and with developmental continuity between adolescent and adult samples.

Finally, Newman, Widom, and Nathan (1985) assesses passive avoidance learning in psychopathic-like delinquent males. Passive avoidance, like interlevel shifts of attention, requires subjects to modify behavior in response to feedback. Psychopaths were delinquents with high scores on the Psychopathic Deviate scale of the Minnesota Multiphasic Personality Inventory (Spielberger, Kling, & O'Hagan, 1978) and low scores on the Welsh Anxiety scale (Welsh, 1956). Despite a reliance on self-report measures, findings match those obtained with adult psychopaths (Newman & Kosson, 1986). Psychopaths displayed poorer passive avoidance only in conditions in which reward and punishment contingencies competed for subjects' attention.

In sum, the few studies examining cognitive abilities of adolescents who resemble psychopaths have consistently yielded results similar to those with adult psychopaths. To date, such adolescents appear capable of adequate sustained attention but deficient in divided attention and executive function. Furthermore, one study implicates the left hemisphere as a locus for the abnormal cognitive function of such adolescents. Nevertheless, these similarities must be viewed with caution given the variety of subject selection methods and the absence of studies employing a well-validated measure of psychopathy.

Studies of Conduct Disorder

The childhood diagnostic category in DSM-III-R that most closely resembles adult psychopathy is *conduct disorder* (CD). Indeed, the solitary aggressive subtype of CD requires aggressive or violent behavior against persons in addition to a varied history of antisocial behavior. Although little evidence links CD to PCL-identified psychopathy, correlations with adolescent psychopathy (Forth et al., 1990) and with scales putatively related to psychopathy (Klinteberg, Schalling, & Magnusson, 1990) have been reported. Moreover, substantial evidence links CD to antisocial personality disorder, the DSM category related to one dimension of psychopathy (Harpur et al., 1989). In fact, childhood CD is currently necessary for the diagnosis of adult antisocial personality disorder (American Psychiatric Association, 1994). Although CD may be neither necessary (Farrington, 1991) nor sufficient (Robins, 1978) for the development of psychopathy, childhood antisocial behavior is one of the most stable predictors of adult antisocial behavior (Loeber, 1982; Robins, 1978) and the single best childhood predictor of psychopathy.[7]

We therefore briefly review empirical findings on the cognitive aptitude of children and adolescents with diagnosed CD. Most of these have addressed only sustained attention and have included groups with CD as controls in studies of attention-deficit/hyperactivity disorder (ADHD). In general, groups with CD sustain attention better than do groups with ADHD (Chee, Logan, Schachar, Lindsay, & Wachsmuth, 1989; Levy, Horn, & Dalglish, 1987; Schachar, Logan, Wachsmuth, & Chajczyk, 1988). Thus, these studies corroborate Orris's (1969) report on adolescents resembling psychopaths.

Unfortunately, there are few tests to date of selective or divided attention in boys with CD. The only study that addresses divided attention indirectly examined the performance of boys with CD on the Trail Making Test of the Halstead–Reitan Battery (Lezak, 1983). Although boys with CD performed the task more slowly than a non-CD control group (Lueger & Gill, 1990), this finding was confounded with group differences in age and IQ and is thus of limited significance.

On the other hand, several authors report deficits in executive function in CD and serious delinquency (reviewed by Moffitt, 1993). Lueger and Gill (1990) report that boys with CD, like psychopaths in some studies, performed poorer than boys without CD on the WCST, making more perseverative errors even after adjustment for IQ and age. Similarly, Krynicki (1978) reported deficits on several neuropsychological tasks for highly assaultive boys with behavior disorder unsocialized aggressive, a diagnostic precursor to CD, compared with less assaultive boys with behavior disorder. In particular, the assaultive group made more perseverative errors and displayed reduced right-handedness; Krynicki interpreted the pattern of deficits as suggesting left-hemisphere damage. Finally, Shapiro, Quay, Hogan, and Schwartz (1988) found response perseveration deficits in undersocialized aggressive CD boys similar to those of adult psychopaths, adding to the continuity between adult and child research.

CONCLUSIONS

Research findings provide a much more consistent picture of psychopathic cognition than could be expected only 10 years ago. Psychopaths do not appear deficient in their capacity to sustain attention, although little research has assessed their performance using traditional vigilance paradigms over sufficient intervals. Psychopaths are not overresponsive to cues inducing exogenous shifts of attention, nor more able than nonpsychopaths to inhibit attention to irrelevant stimuli as indexed by negative priming, inhibition of return, or interference caused by distractors.

By contrast, psychopaths may be overly responsive to cues inducing endogenous shifts of attention in some situations, an area in which further research is especially important. Such overresponsiveness may also be affected by the allocation of left-hemisphere resources or right-handed responses. Moreover, psychopaths appear to display excessively narrow attention in situations involving multiple contingencies and multi-dimensional stimuli, and their reduced breadth of attention may help to explain observed deficits in passive avoidance and interlevel shifts of attention. Alternatively, psychopaths may display a failure to shift attention from goal-directed behavior to process aversive signals (Patterson & Newman, 1993).

There is also considerable evidence that psychopaths are characterized by reduced lateralization for certain cognitive functions or by unusual strengths and weaknesses in their use of hemisphere-specific resources. Limitations in their use of left-hemisphere processsing resources provide a plausible mechanism underlying psychopaths' apparent dual-task deficits and some of their difficulties in shifting attention. In addition, psychopaths may be characterized by increased capacity with respect to the use of right-hemisphere processing resources. Such a finding could help to explain psychopaths' putative adeptness at "sizing up" situations and/or manipulating people some of the time.

The apparent links identified between adult psychopathy, adolescent psychopathy, and unsocialized aggressive conduct disorder also suggest an important new direction for future research. If the cognitive deficits (and advantages) that characterize psychopaths are evident in childhood, then these processing anomalies may be employed as convergent indices in the validation of developmental precursors of psychopathy. Of course, further research establishing the reliability of selective and divided attention differences in both child and adult samples is necessary before continuity with respect to psychopathy can be assumed. In addition, given that most conduct disordered juveniles do not grow up to be psychopaths, the etiological significance of differences in attentional function remains an independently important question. On the other hand, continuity between adult PCL-defined psychopathy and younger populations identified primarily on the basis of antisocial behavior raises the possibility that the processing deficits identified in adolescent populations may predict only the dimension of psychopathy related to impulsive antisocial behavior and antisocial personality disorder rather than psychopathy per se.

NOTES

1. Although central cues are thought to mediate selection of stimuli via endogenous mechanisms, interstimulus intervals of 100 milliseconds may be too brief to reveal psychopathic differences in such mechanisms.

2. It is worth noting that some accounts of divided attention explain performance differences in terms of allocations of multiple resource pools (Dimond, 1972; Wickens et al., 1981) instead of adequacy of specific processes.

3. Hare (1979) reports a similar study in which subjects were required to

identify words rather than classify them. At exposure durations of 80 and 40 milliseconds, psychopaths displayed no deficit in identifying words in either visual field.

4. Psychopaths tested by a female experimenter performed the primary task more poorly than all other subject groups, a finding consistent with the possibility that psychopaths allocated more attention to the female experimenter than to the experiment. However, because attention to the experimenter was not measured, Kosson and Newman (1986) emphasizes performances of the subset of subjects tested by male experimenters.

5. Kosson (1997) recently reported a replication of these findings using a divided visual field task. In this study, a group × hand assignment interaction similar to that reported by Kosson (1996) again suggested a performance deficit for psychopaths under conditions promoting reliance on left-hemisphere-specific processing resources but not under conditions promoting reliance on right-hemisphere resources. This same study also obtained additional evidence of reduced breadth of attention in psychopaths similar to that reported by Kosson (1996). The replication of findings across visual–visual and visual–auditory task combinations suggests that these findings are not a function of idiosyncratic requirements of particular tasks.

6. Studies identifying psychopathic subjects based on less well-validated measures have also obtained mixed findings on the WCST (e.g., Gorenstein, 1982; Hoffman, Hall, & Bartsch, 1987; Sutker & Allain, 1987). Two studies also examined performance on another test of frontal lobe function, the Sequential Matching Memory Test (Lezak, 1983). Findings on this measure paralleled WCST findings in both cases (Gorenstein, 1982; Hare, 1984).

7. Children with both CD and attention-deficit/hyperactivity sisorder (ADHD) may be at especially heightened risk for the development of antisocial personality disorder and psychopathy (Lilienfeld & Waldman, 1990).

REFERENCES

Allport, D. A., Antonis, B., & Reynolds, P. (1972). On the division of attention: A disproof of the single channel proposition. *Quarterly Journal of Experimental Psychology, 24,* 225–235.

American Psychiatric Association. (1987). *Diagnostic and statistical manual of mental disorders* (3rd ed., rev.). Washington, DC: Author.

American Psychiatric Association. (1994). *Diagnostic and statistical manual of mental disorders* (4th ed.). Washington, DC: Author.

Chee, P., Logan, G., Schachar, R., Lindsay, P., & Wachsmuth, R. (1989). Effects of event rate and display time on sustained attention in hyperactive, normal, and control children. *Journal of Abnormal Child Psychology, 17,* 371–391.

Cleckley, H. C. (1976). *The mask of sanity.* St. Louis, MO: Mosby.

Cohen, A., & Ivry, R. (1989). Illusory conjunctions inside and outside the focus of attention. *Journal of Experimental Psychology: Human Perception and Performance, 15,* 650–663.

Davies, D. R., Jones, D. M., & Taylor, A. (1984). Selective and sustained attention tasks: Individual and group differences. In R. Parasuraman & D. R. Davies (Eds.), *Varieties of attention* (pp. 395–447). Orlando, FL: Academic Press.

Dimond, S. J. (1972). *The double brain.* Baltimore: Williams & Wilkins.

Duffy, E. (1962). *Activation and behavior.* London: Wiley.

Edelmann, R. J., & Vivian, S. E. (1988). Further analysis of the Social Psychopathy Scale. *Personality and Individual Differences, 9,* 581–587.

Eriksen, C. W., & Murphy, T. D. (1987). Movement of attentional focus across the visual field: A critical look at the evidence. *Perception and Psychophysics, 42,* 299–305.

Eysenck, S. B. G., Pearson, P. R., Easting, G., & Allsopp, J. F. (1985). Age norms for impulsiveness, venturesomeness, and empathy in adults. *Personality and Individual Differences, 6,* 613–619.

Farrington, D. P. (1991). Antisocial personality from childhood to adulthood. *The Psychologist: Bulletin of the British Psychological Society, 4,* 389–394.

Forth, A. E., Hart, S. D., & Hare, R. D. (1990). Assessment of psychopathy in male young offenders. *Psychological Assessment: A Journal of Consulting and Clinical Psychology, 2,* 342–344.

Frick, P. J., O'Brien, B. F., Wootton, J. M., & McBurnett, K. (1994). Psychopathy and conduct problems in children. *Journal of Abnormal Psychology, 103,* 700–707.

Friedman, A., Polson, M. C., Dafoe, C. G., & Gaskill, S. J. (1982). Dividing attention within and between hemispheres: Limited capacity processing and cerebral specialization. *Journal of Experimental Psychology: Human Perception and Performance, 8,* 625–650.

Gorenstein, E. E. (1982). Frontal lobe functions in psychopaths. *Journal of Abnormal Psychology, 91,* 368–379.

Gray, J. (1982). *The neuropsychology of anxiety.* New York: Oxford University Press.

Hahn, S., & Kramer, A. (1994, May). *Distribution of attention in non-contiguous space.* Paper presented at the Festschrift honoring Charles W. Ericksen: Converging operations in the study of visual selective attention, Urbana–Champaign, IL.

Hare, R. D. (1978). Electrodermal and cardiovascular correlates of psychopathy. In R. D. Hare & D. Schalling (Eds.), *Psychopathic behaviour: Approaches to research* (pp. 107–143). Chichester, UK: Wiley.

Hare, R. D. (1979). Psychopathy and laterality of cerebral function. *Journal of Abnormal Psychology, 88,* 605–610.

Hare, R. D. (1982). Psychopathy and physiological activity during anticipation of an aversive stimulus in a distraction paradigm. *Psychophysiology, 19,* 266–271.

Hare, R. D. (1984). Performance of psychopaths on cognitive tasks related to frontal lobe function. *Journal of Abnormal Psychology, 93,* 133–140.

Hare, R. D. (1991). *The Hare Psychopathy Checklist—Revised.* North Tonawanda, NY: Multi-Health Systems.

Hare, R. D., & Jutai, J. W. (1988). Psychopathy and cerebral asymmetry in semantic processing. *Personality and Individual Differences, 9,* 329–337.

Hare, R. D., & McPherson, L. M. (1984). Psychopathy and perceptual asymmetry during verbal dichotic listening. *Journal of Abnormal Psychology, 93,* 141–149.

Hare, R. D., Williamson, S. E., & Harpur, T. J. (1988). Psychopathy and language. In T. E. Moffitt & S. A. Mednick (Eds.), *Biological contributions to crime causation* (pp. 68–92). Dordrecht, Netherlands: Nijhoff.

Harpur, T. J. (1991). *Visual attention in psychopathic criminals.* Unpublished doctoral dissertation, University of British Columbia, Vancouver.

Harpur, T. J. (1993, October). *Assessing traits characteristic of psychopathy in children and adolescents.* Paper presented at the meeting of the American Society of Criminology, Phoenix, AZ.

Harpur, T. J., & Hare, R. D. (1990). Psychopathy and attention. In J. T. Enns (Ed.), *The development of attention: Research and theory* (pp. 429–444). Amsterdam: Elsevier.

Harpur, T. J., Hare, R. D., & Hakstian, A. R. (1989). Two-factor conceptualization of psychopathy: Construct validity and assessment implications. *Psychological Assessment: A Journal of Consulting and Clinical Psychology, 1,* 6–17.

Harris, G. T., Rice, M. E., & Cormier, C. A. (1991). Psychopathy and violent recidivism. *Law and Human Behavior, 15,* 625–637.

Hart, S. D., Forth, A. E., & Hare, R. D. (1990). Performance of criminal psychopaths on selected neuropsychological tests. *Journal of Abnormal Psychology, 99,* 374–379.

Hart, S. D., Kropp, P. R., & Hare, R. D. (1988). Performance of male psychopaths following conditional release from prison. *Journal of Consulting and Clinical Psychology, 1,* 6–17.

Harter, M. R., & Anllo-Vento, L. (1991). Visual–spatial attention: Preparation and selection in children and adults. In C. H. M. Brunia, G. Mulder, & M. N. Verbaten (Eds.), *Event-related brain research (Electroencephalography and Clinical Neurophysiology,* Suppl. 42, pp. 183–194). Amsterdam: Elsevier.

Hoffman, J. J., Hall, R. W., & Bartsch, T. W. (1987). On the relative importance of "psychopathic" personality and alcoholism on neuropsychological measures of frontal lobe dysfunction. *Journal of Abnormal Psychology, 96,* 158–160.

Howland, E. W., Kosson, D. S., Patterson, C. M., & Newman, J. P. (1993). Altering a dominant response: Performance of psychopaths and low-socialization college students on a cued reaction time task. *Journal of Abnormal Psychology, 102,* 379–387.

Howland, E. W., & Newman, J. P. (1993). *The effect of incentives on Wisconsin Card Sorting Task performance in psychopaths.* Unpublished manuscript, University of Wisconsin—Madison.

Hughes, H. C., & Zimba, L. D. (1985). Spatial maps of directed visual attention. *Journal of Experimental Psychology: Human Perception and Performance, 11,* 409–430.

Jonides, J., & Mack, R. (1984). On the cost and benefit of cost and benefit. *Psychological Bulletin, 96,* 29–44.

Jutai, J. W., & Hare, R. D. (1983). Psychopathy and selective attention during performance of a complex perceptual-motor task. *Psychophysiology, 20,* 146–151.

Jutai, J. W., Hare, R. D., & Connolly, J. F. (1987). Psychopathy and event-related brain potentials (ERPS) associated with attention to speech stimuli. *Personality and Individual Differences, 8,* 175–184.

Kahneman, D. (1973). *Attention and effort.* Englewood Cliffs, NJ: Prentice-Hall.

Klinteberg, B. A., Schalling, D., & Magnusson, D. (1990). Childhood behaviour and adult personality in male and female subjects. *European Journal of Personality, 4,* 57–71.

Kosson, D. S. (1996). Psychopathy and dual-task performance under focusing conditions. *Journal of Abnormal Psychology, 105,* 391–400

Kosson, D. S. (1997). *Divided visual attention in psychopathic and nonpsychopathic offenders.* Manuscript submitted for publication.

Kosson, D. S., & Newman, J. P. (1986). Psychopathy and the allocation of attentional capacity in a divided-attention situation. *Journal of Abnormal Psychology, 95,* 257–263.

Krynicki, V. E. (1978). Cerebral dysfunction in repetitively assaultive adolescents. *Journal of Nervous and Mental Disease, 166,* 59–67.

Levy, F., Horn, K., & Dalglish, R. (1987). Relation of attention deficit and conduct disorder to vigilance and reading lag. *Australian and New Zealand Journal of Psychiatry, 21,* 242–245.

Lezak, M. D. (1983). *Neuropsychological assessment* (2nd ed.). New York: Oxford University Press.

Lilienfeld, S. O., & Waldman, I. D. (1990). The relation between childhood attention-deficit hyperactivity disorder and adult antisocial behavior reexamined: The problem of heterogeneity. *Clinical Psychology Review, 10,* 699–725.

Loeber, R. (1982). The stability of antisocial and delinquent child behavior: A review. *Child Development, 53,* 1431–1446.

Lueger, R. J., & Gill, K. J. (1990). Frontal-lobe cognitive dysfunction in conduct disorder adolescents. *Journal of Clinical Psychology, 46,* 696–705.

Lykken, D. T. (1957). A study of anxiety in the sociopathic personality. *Journal of Abnormal and Social Psychology, 55,* 6–10.

Miller, L. (1987). Neuropsychology of the aggressive psychopath: An integrative review. *Aggressive Behavior, 13,* 119–140.

Millon, T. (1981). Antisocial personality: The aggressive pattern. In *Disorders of personality: DSM-III: Axis II* (pp. 181–215). New York: Wiley.

Milner, B. (1964). Some effects of frontal lobectomy in man. In J. M. Warren, & K. Akert (Eds.), *The frontal granular cortex and behavior* (pp. 313–334). New York: McGraw-Hill.

Mirsky, A. F., Anthony, B. J., Duncan, C. C., Ahearn, M. B., & Kellam, S. G. (1991). Analysis of the elements of attention: A neuropsychological approach. *Neuropsychology Review, 2,* 109–145.

Moffit, T. E. (1993). The neuropsychology of conduct disorder. *Development and Psychopathology, 5,* 135–151.

Moray, N. (1984). Attention to dynamic visual displays in man–machine systems. In R. Parasuraman & D. R. Davies (Eds.), *Varieties of attention* (pp. 485–513). Orlando, FL: Academic Press.

Müller, H. J., & Rabbitt, P. M. A. (1989). Reflexive and voluntary orienting of visual attention: Time course of activation and resistance to interruption. *Journal of Experimental Psychology: Human Perception and Performance, 15,* 315–330.

Newman, J. P., & Kosson, D. S. (1986). Passive avoidance learning in psychopathic and nonpsychopathic offenders. *Journal of Abnormal Psychology, 95,* 257–263.

Newman, J. P., Patterson, C. M., & Kosson, D. S. (1987). Response perseveration in psychopaths. *Journal of Abnormal Psychology, 96,* 145–148.

Newman, J. P., Widom, C. S., & Nathan, S. (1985). Passive avoidance in syndromes of disinhibition: Psychopathy and extraversion. *Journal of Personality and Social Psychology, 48,* 1316–1327.

Ogloff, J. P. R., Wong, S., & Greenwood, A. (1990). Treating criminal psychopaths in a therapeutic community program. *Behavioral Sciences and the Law, 8,* 81–90.

Orris, J. B. (1969). Visual monitoring performance in three subgroups of male delinquents. *Journal of Abnormal Psychology, 74,* 227–229.

Parasuraman, R. & Davies, D. R. (Eds.). (1984). *Varieties of attention.* Orlando, FL: Academic Press.

Patterson, C. M., & Newman, J. P. (1993). Reflectivity and learning from aversive events: Toward a psychological mechanism for the syndromes of disinhibition. *Psychological Review, 100,* 716–736.

Polson, M. C., & Friedman, A. (1988). Task-sharing within and between hemispheres: A multiple-resources approach. *Human Factors, 30,* 633–643.

Posner, M. I., & Cohen, Y. (1984). Components of visual orienting. In H. Bouma & D. Bowhuis (Eds.), *Attention and performance X* (pp. 531–556). Hillsdale, NJ: Erlbaum.

Posner, M. I., Walker, J. A., Friedrich, F. J., & Rafal, R. D. (1984). Effects of parietal injury on covert orientation of attention. *Journal of Neuroscience, 4,* 1863–1874.

Quay, H. C. (1965). Psychopathic personality as pathological stimulation-seeking. *American Journal of Psychiatry, 122,* 180–183.

Quay, H. C., & Peterson, D. R. (1987). *Manual for the Revised Behavior Problem Checklist.* Miami, FL: University of Miami, Department of Psychology.

Raine, A. (1989). Evoked potentials and psychopathy. *International Journal of Psychophysiology, 8,* 1–16.

Raine, A., O'Brien, M., Smiley, N., Scerbo, A., & Chan, C. (1990). Reduced lateralization in verbal dichotic listening in adolescent psychopaths. *Journal of Abnormal Psychology, 99,* 272–277.

Raine, A., & Venables, P. H. (1988). Enhanced P3 evoked potentials and longer recovery times in psychopaths. *Psychophysiology, 25,* 30–38.

Reeves, A., & Sperling, G. (1986). Attention gating in short-term visual memory. *Psychological Review, 93,* 180–206.

Robertson, I. H., & North, N. (1993). Active and passive activation of left limbs: Influence on visual and sensory neglect. *Neuropsychologia, 31,* 293–300.

Robins, L. N. (1978). Sturdy childhood predictors of adult antisocial behaviour: Replications from longitudinal studies. *Psychological Medicine, 8,* 611–622.

Schachar, R., Logan, G., Wachsmuth, R., & Chajczyk, D. (1988). Attaining and maintaining preparation: A comparison of attention in hyperactive, normal, and disturbed control children. *Journal of Abnormal Child Psychology, 16,* 361–378.

Schmauk, F. A. (1970). Punishment, arousal, and avoidance learning in sociopaths. *Journal of Abnormal Psychology, 76,* 144–150.

Shapiro, S. K., Quay, H. C., Hogan, A. E., & Schwartz, K. P. (1988). Response perseveration and delayed responding in undersocialized aggressive conduct disorder. *Journal of Abnormal Psychology, 97,* 371–373.

Shaw, M. (1982). Attending to multiple sources of information: 1. The integration of information in decision making. *Cognitive Psychology, 14,* 353–409.

Smith, S. S., Arnett, P., & Newman, J. P. (1992). Neuropsychological differentiation of psychopathic and nonpsychopathic criminal offenders. *Personality and Individual Differences, 13,* 1233–1243.

Sohlberg, M. M., & Mateer, C. A. (1989). *Introduction to cognitive rehabilatation: Theory and practice.* New York: Guilford Press.

Spielberger, C. D., Kling, J. K., & O'Hagan, S. E. J. (1978). Dimensions of psychopathic personality: Antisocial behavior and anxiety. In R. D. Hare & D. Schalling (Eds.), *Psychopathic behaviour: Approaches to research* (pp. 23–46). New York: Wiley.

Stuss, D. T., & Benson, D. F. (1984). Neuropsychological studies of the frontal lobes. *Psychological Bulletin, 95,* 3–28.

Sutker, P. B., & Allain, A. N. (1987). Cognitive abstraction, shifting and control: Clinical sample comparisons of psychopaths and nonpsychopaths. *Journal of Abnormal Psychology, 96,* 73–75.

Tucker, D. M., & Williamson, P. A. (1984). Asymmetric neural control systems in human self-regulation. *Psychological Review, 91,* 185–215.

Welford, A. (1968). *Fundamentals of skill.* London: Methuen.

Welsh, G. S. (1956). Factor dimensions A and R. In G. S. Welsh & W. G. Dahlstrom (Eds.), *Basic readings on the MMPI in psychology and medicine* (pp. 264–281). Minneapolis: University of Minnesota Press.

Wickens, C. D., Mountford, S. J., & Schreiner, W. (1981). Multiple resources, task-hemispheric integrity, and individual differences in time-sharing. *Human Factors, 23,* 211–229.

Index

Acquired spatial neglect, 254–255
Aging, 24
    Alzheimer's disease and, 288, 309,
        310. *See also* Alzheimer's dis-
        ease cognitive development,
        289
    continuum of cognitive changes, 309
    divided attention in, 303–305,
        307–308, 310
    model system of attention, 289–291
    neural effects, 290
    neuroanatomy of visuospatial at-
        tention, 299–303
    normal visuospatial attention,
        292–293, 296, 309–310
Alcohol. *See also* Fetal alcohol ef-
        fects/syndrome
    teratogenic potential, 171
Alzheimer's disease, 24
    aging and, 288–289, 309, 310
    cognitive effects, 289
    divided attention in, 305–307,
        308, 310
    model system of attention for
        studying, 289–291
    neural deficit in, 290
    neuroanatomy of visuospatial at-
        tention, 299–303
    neurofibrillary tangles, 300, 302
    parietal lobe changes, 297, 298
    visuospatial attention in, 293,
        297–298, 309–310
Animal studies
    alcohol teratogenicity, 173,
        179–181

brain–behavior relations, 264
cocaine exposure effects, 107
limitations, 264
selective attention in nonhuman
        primates, 68–69
Antisocial personality disorders, 380
Anxiety, 24
    as adaptive mechanism, 359
    as attentional dysfunction, 350,
        370–373
    child assessment, 353–355
    clinical characteristics, 351–352
    co-occurring depression, 352, 354,
        365
    cognitive dysfunction in, 350–351
    cognitive research trends, 350
    cognitive style in children, 366–367
    color-naming tests, 361
    depression and, 351–352
    developmental theories, 357–359
    information processing selectivity
        in, 359–362, 365–366
    negative/positive affectivity in,
        352
    network theory, 356–357
    predictive utility of information
        processing style, 369–370
    prevalence, 352
    schema theory, 355–356
    stability of information processing
        biases, 367–369
    thought content in, 352–353,
        355
    thoughts of danger in, 354
    threat detection in, 360

Arousal
  in model of attention, 12–13,
    99–100, 113
  in prenatally cocaine-exposed in-
    fants, 108–110, 112–113
  in preterm infants, 103–105,
    112–113
  reactive/sustained attention, 43–44
  theoretical significance, 97
  vigilance system, 100
Artificial intelligence, 338–339
At-risk populations. *See also* Prema-
    ture infants
  attentional functioning as early in-
    dicator, 22–23
  prenatal cocaine exposure, 97–98
Attention as predictor of later func-
    tioning, 22–23
  IQ of mentally retarded, 62–63
  psychopathy predictors, 396
  selective attention to novelty, 56, 59
Attention-deficit/hyperactivity dis-
    order, 23
  age at onset, 148
  attentional functioning in, 149,
    206
  characteristics, 147
  comorbidity risk, 223
  conduct disorder and, 394–395
  etiology, 147
  as fetal alcohol syndrome out-
    come, 172
  gender differences, 222–223
  impulsivity in, 208–209
  infant assessment for, 148–149
  in infants, 152–153
  medication, 220
  with mental retardation, 205–206,
    214–224
  prevalence, 147
  problem-solving approach,
    155–159
  selective attention in, 150–152,
    207
  sustained attention in, 149–150,
    151–152, 206–207
  treatment strategies, 147–149

Attentional processes, 380. *See also*
    Selective attention; Sustained
    attention; Visual attention
  in ADHD children, 149–152
  in ADHD infants, 152–155
  alcohol dose–response effect, 181,
    186
  in anxiety disorder, 350, 359
  arousal in, 12–13, 97, 99–100, 113
  in atypical populations, conceptu-
    alizations of, 9
  autism as deficit of, 248–254
  covert orienting, 40, 76–77
  definition, 8
  divided attention, 303–308,
    385–386
  in Down syndrome infants, 123,
    125–130, 140–142
  dynamic problem-solving ap-
    proach, 155–156
  dynamic problem-solving in
    ADHD infants, 160–162
  executive function in, 235
  facilitation mechanisms, 382
  in fetal alcohol effect/syndrome,
    171–172, 174, 182–189
  infant assessment for schizophrenia
    risk, 321–322
  measurement, 15–17, 380–381
  measurement in psychopathy,
    380–381
  in mental retardation with ADHD,
    214–219
  model system for studying aging
    effects, 289–291
  motivation in, 380–381
  necessary and sufficient attributes, 9
  parenting environment effects,
    110–112, 113
  posterior–anterior systems model,
    234–235, 290–291
  in prenatally cocaine-exposed in-
    fants, 108–110, 112–113
  in preterm infants, 103–105,
    112–113
  psychological conceptualizations,
    10, 11–13, 75–76, 80

in psychopathy, 395–396
schizophrenia assessment,
     322–333, 339–340
in schizophrenia etiology, 319
scope of, 98
significance of, in psychology
     research, 8–10, 75
signs of schizophrenia, 319–320
in split-brain patients, 274–284
Autism, 23
     as affective-cognitive deficit, 233–234
     attentional–developmental model,
         254–255
     as attentional system deficit, 248–254
     disengage problem in, 251–252, 253
     executive function in, 235–248,
         253–254
     as failure of metarepresentation, 233
     information processing model, 235
     neuropsychological deficit in, 235,
         248–249
     repetitive behaviors in, 232–233
     research opportunities, 254, 255
     savants, 250–251
     social functioning in, 232
Autonomic nervous system in
     schizophrenia, 331

B

Backward masking, 329–330
Balint syndrome, 42, 270–272
Brain activity, 23–24. *See also* Neu-
     rological deficits
     in Alzheimer's disease, 297
     animal studies, 264
     attentional processes in psychopa-
         thy, 381, 383, 387, 390
     behavioral studies, 264–265
     cortical/subcortical pathways,
         32–34, 37–39, 42–43, 48,
         269–270
     in divided attention, 307–308
     early conceptualizations of atten-
         tional processes, 12, 13
     human lesion studies, 266–267,
         269–271

imaging studies, 265–266
implications of fetal alcohol ex-
     posure research, 190–191
models of perceptual development,
     14–15
neural mediation of selective atten-
     tion, 269–272
neurobiological models of visual
     development, 32–34
paradox of split-brain patients,
     274–284
research approaches to attention, 263
schizophrenia markers, 330–331
schizophrenia models, 337–339,
     340–341
split-brain studies, 267, 272–274
in visuospatial attention, 298–300
Breadth of attention tasks, 212

C

Children and adolescents
     conduct disorder, 394–395
     developmental theories of mood
         disorder, 357–359
     mood disorder assessment,
         353–355
     phobias in, 366
     prenatal alcohol exposure effects,
         183–187
     prenatally alcohol-exposed, atten-
         tional findings in, 188, 189
     psychopathy precursors, 396
     psychopathy studies, 392–394
     selective attention in mood disord-
         er, 366–367
     selective attention to novelty in
         neurologically impaired,
         63–65
Cocaine exposure, prenatal, 97–98
     arousal and attention in, 108–110,
         112–113
     biology of, 105–108
     demographics, 105
     later social functioning, 112
     parenting environment after, 110,
         111

Cognitively disordered populations.
    See also Alzheimer's disease;
    Autism; Down syndrome;
    Fetal alcohol effects/syndrome;
    Mental retardation;
    Schizophrenia
  childhood mood disorder, 366–367
  conduct disordered youths, 394–395
  executive function in psychopathy,
    391–392
  habituation performance, 127
  measurement of cognitive function-
    ing, 55–56, 138–139
  mood-disorders as cognitive dys-
    function, 350–351, 370–372
  schizophrenia models, 333, 334–336
  selective attention to visual novelty,
    55, 56, 70–71, 109, 126–127
  Standard-Transformation-Return
    assessment for infants, 132–138
  thought content in mood disor-
    ders, 352–353, 354, 355
Color-naming latencies
  in anxiety, 361
  in depression, 364
  in phobic patients, 367
  stability in mood disorders, 367–368
Competition effects, 35–37
Conduct disorders, 393, 394–395
Continuous performance tests,
    325–326, 380
Cortical/subcortical pathways,
    32–34, 37–39, 42–43, 48,
    269–270
  split-brain studies, 272–274
Cost–benefit model, 16–17
Covert orienting, 40, 76–77, 267–268
  lifespan development, 80–83, 90
  neural mediators, 269–270
  in visuospatial attention, 292

D

Dementia. *See also* Alzheimer's disease
  selective attention to novelty and,
    67–68
Depression, 24
  as adaptive mechanism, 359

anxiety and, 351–352
child assessment, 353–355
clinical characteristics, 351
clinical course, 351
co-occurring anxiety, 352, 354, 365
cognitive dysfunction in, 350–351,
    370–372
cognitive research trends, 350
cognitive style in children,
    366–367
color-naming latencies in, 364
developmental theories, 357–359
in elderly, selective attention to
    novelty and, 67–68
epidemiology, 351
gender differences, 351
information processing selectivity
    in, 359–360, 362–364,
    365–366
as memory dysfunction, 350
negative/positive affectivity in, 352
network theory, 356–357
predictive utility of information
    processing style, 369–370
schema theory, 355–356
severity, 371
stability of information processing
    biases, 367–369
thought content in, 352–353, 355
Developmental psychology
  conceptual evolution, 4–6
  consideration of social influences
    in, 5
  developmental psychopathology
    and, 3–4
  models of perceptual processes,
    13–15, 74–75, 79–80
Developmental psychopathology
  conceptual evolution, 3, 6–7
  developmental psychology and, 3–6
  evolution of attentional processes
    research, 8–9
  schema theory, 355–356
  schizophrenia course, 321–322
  schizophrenia research, 319
  seminal theorists and researchers,
    7–8
Dialectical approach, 12

Discrimination problem-solving
  by ADHD infants, 160–162
  ADHD studies, 155–159
  hypothesis generation in, 159
  in infants, 153–155
Distractors
  age effects in searching, 296
  classification tasks for psy-
    chopaths, 388–390
  in selective attention assessment in
    mental retardation, 210–212
  selective processing in anxiety,
    360–361
  target similarity in visual search,
    293–296
  in visual search performance, 77,
    83–86
Distributed systems approach, 14–15
Divided attention
  age-related changes in neuro-
    anatomy, 308
  aging effects, 303–305
  in Alzheimer's disease, 305–307, 308
  in conduct disorder, 395
  definition, 303
  functional neuroanatomy, 307–308
  mechanisms, 385–386, 393
  posterior–anterior model of func-
    tioning, 290–291
  in psychopathy, 385–391
Dopaminergic system in schizophrenia, 339
Down syndrome infants
  attention/information processing
    in, 123, 125–130, 138–142
  attentional functioning, 123,
    125–130, 138–142
  clinical features, 123
  developmental course, 123, 141–142
  habituation performance, 126, 127
  mental development assessment,
    138–142
  research challenges, 124–125, 126
  research limitations, 130–132,
    138–139
  social behaviors, 128, 129
  Standard-Transformation-Return pro-
    cedure for assessing, 136–138

E

Ecological psychology, 10
Enumeration, 78–79
  lifespan development, 86–89, 90
Event-related potentials, 265–266
  attention in psychopathy, 381, 383
  schizophrenia measures, 331
  sensory gating of P50 waves, 331
Executive function
  action of, 13
  in autism, 235–248, 253–254
  in conduct disorder, 395
  definition, 235
  mental representations in, 235
  in psychopathy, 391–392
Experiential process, 14, 74–75
Expertise theory, 79, 90
Externality effect, 45–46
Eye movements
  age-related changes in scanning,
    43–44
  brain–behavior research, 264–265
  endogenous control, 31
  exogenous control, 31
  infant visual development, 33–34
  length of fixations in habituation/
    dishabituation studies, 44–46
  in measurement of visual attention,
    31–32
  measurement of visual orienting,
    34–43, 76–77
  smooth pursuit eye tracking, 332

F

Fagan Test of Infant Intelligence,
  57–58, 62–63
Feature integration theory, 11,
  77–78, 90–91
  pop-out phenomenon, 295, 297
  serial search, 295
  target–distractor similarity in
    visual search, 294–295
Fetal alcohol effects/syndrome
  academic impairment, 176
  adolescent findings, 188, 189
  animal studies, 179–181

Fetal alcohol effects/syndrome
(*continued*)
assessment, 176–177
attentional deficits, 171–172, 176
children of alcoholic mothers,
178–179
clinical features, 175–176
dose–response relationship, 173, 186
epidemiological studies, 181–182
generalizability of deficits across
settings, 187
hyperactivity symptoms, 175–176
implications for brain–behavior
research, 190–191
lifespan development effects, 174,
175
neonate behavior, 182
neuropsychological findings,
177–178, 183–184
obstacles to research, 181–182
prevention, 193–194
remediation, 194
research development, 172–174
research opportunities, 172,
192–194
secondary disabilities, 191–192
Filtering mechanisms
in autism, 252, 253
conceptual models, 10–11
Fixation, 31
Foveation, 31
spatial limitations, 35
Freud, S., 7

G

Garmezy, N., 8
Garner, W., 16
Gender differences
ADHD in mental retardation,
222–223
depression, 351
Gibson, E. J., 12, 13–14, 15
Gibson, J. J., 10, 12
Gibson, James J., 10
Group comparison studies, 18–19
comparison group selection, 20
developmental issues, 21–22

Down syndrome infants in,
124–125
fetal alcohol effects/syndrome,
192–193
matching issues, 20–21
population definition, 19–20
requirements for effectiveness, 19
strategy, 18–19
Guided search, 295–296

H

Habituation/dishabituation, 44–46, 99
in Down syndrome infants, 126, 127
as measure of creation of mental
representations, 131
in prenatally alcohol-exposed infants, 182–183
in prenatally cocaine-exposed infants, 109
in preterm infants, 104
Hebb, D. O., 10, 14
Human associative memory,
356–357

I

Imaging technology, 265–266
human lesion studies, 266–267
Impulsivity
in ADHD, 208–209
assessment, 208
in mental retardation, 213
Individual differences
in cognitions in mood disorders,
354–355
evolution of developmentalist approach, 4–6
lifespan development, 59
in selective attention in mood disorder, 368, 370
Individuation (visual process), 78
Infant development, 22. *See also* Cocaine exposure, prenatal;
Premature infants
at-risk populations, 97–98
attentional control, 42, 48, 98–100
attentional field, 35

competition effects, 35–37
discrimination problem-solving in
    ADHD, 160–162
discrimination problem-solving
    task performance, 153–155
fetal alcohol exposure, 182–183
focusing accuracy, 46–47
habituation/dishabituation studies,
    44–46, 99
measurement of attentional
    processes, 100
neurobiological models of visual
    systems, 14–15, 32
parenting environment as develop-
    mental mediator, 110–112
scanning eye movements, 43–44
schizophrenia risk assessment,
    321–322
selective attention as predictor of
    later functioning, 56
selective attention to novelty,
    58–59, 99, 104, 109
significance of arousal, 97
Information processing
aging effects on divided attention,
    304–305
autism as deficit of, 235
conceptualization of attentional
    processes, 10–11
in Down syndrome infants,
    123–124, 125–130, 140–142
facilitation model of visual atten-
    tion, 40–41
during infancy, 58–59, 63
lifespan development, 55, 70–71
mental retardation as deficit of, 62
mood disorder models, 355–359,
    365
network theory, 356–357
predictive of emotional response to
    stress, 369–370
in prenatally alcohol-exposed in-
    fants, 183
in preterm infants, 104–105
schema theory, 355–356
schizophrenia models, 334–336
selectivity in anxiety, 360–362,
    365–366

selectivity in depression, 362–364,
    365–366
selectivity in mood disorders,
    359–360
stability of biases in mood disor-
    der, 367–369
Standard-Transformation-Return
    procedure for assessing,
    132–135
stochastic modeling, 335–336
Inhibition of return effect, 40–42
in psychopathy, 384
Inhibition of startle reflex, 330
IQ
predictive tests, 62–63
significance of low scores, 62
visual attention to novelty and, 59

J
James, William, 10, 11

K
Knight, R., 334–335

L
Lateral masking effect, 46
Learning theory, 79, 90
Lifespan development. *See also*
    Adolescents; Adults; Aging;
    Children; Elderly; Infants
attentional processes, 74–75, 89–91
covert orienting, 80–83, 90
early conceptualizations, 5
expertise theory, 79, 90
information processing and
    knowledge acquisition, 59
preference for visual novelty in
    normal development, 59–62
prenatal alcohol exposure, 174
prenatal alcohol exposure effects,
    188–189
selective attention to novelty, 55,
    70–71
speed of processing theory, 79, 90
visual enumeration, 86–89, 90
visual orienting theory, 91
visual search speed, 83–86, 90

M

Magnetic resonance imaging,
    265–266
Magnocellular visual pathway, 33
Measurement
    aging effects on divided attention,
        303–304
    alcohol dose–response effect, 186
    attentional bias in anxiety, 360–362
    in attentional process research, 15–17
    cognitive functioning in special
        populations, 55–56
    cost–benefit methodology, 16–17
    of creation of mental representa-
        tions, 131
    of eye movement in visual orient-
        ing, 34–43
    of impulsivity, 208–209
    of infant attention, 100
    infant's selective attention to
        novelty, 56
    information processing during in-
        fancy, 58–59
    motivation as mediator of atten-
        tion, 380–381
    response time as index of atten-
        tion, 17–18
    of selective attention, 207
    of sustained attention, 206–207, 380
    of visual attention, 31–32
Memory
    aging effects, 289
    in Alzheimer's disease, 289
    attentional bias in anxiety, 362
    depression as dysfunction of, 350,
        362–363, 365
    in mental retardation, 212
    in network model of mood disor-
        ders, 356–357
    in paranoid schizophrenia,
        335–336
    short-term visual, in schizophrenia,
        334–335
Mental retardation. *See also* Down
        syndrome infants
    ADHD symptoms/diagnosis in,
        205–206, 214–224
        assessment, 220–222
        attentional deficits in, 209
        breadth of attention in, 212
        gender differences, 222–223
        hyperactivity/activity level in,
            213–214
        immediate memory in, 212
        impulsivity in, 213
        information processing conceptu-
            alization of, 62
        predictive tests, 62–63
        prevalence, 215
        prevalence of attention disorders
            in, 214–215
        selective attention in, 210–212
        sustained attention in, 209–210
Methylphenidate, 220
Motivation, 380–381

N

Network theory
    of anxiety, 356–357, 358
    of depression, 356–357, 358
    developmental model of mood dis-
        order, 357–358
Neufeld, R., 335–336
Neurological deficits. *See also* Brain
        activity
    age-related changes in divided at-
        tention, 308
    aging effects in visuospatial atten-
        tion, 300–303
    in Alzheimer's disease, 289–290
    attentional functioning as early in-
        dicator, 23
    in autism, 235, 248–249
    in fetal alcohol syndrome,
        177–178, 183–184, 191, 193
    nonhuman primate research,
        68–69
    prenatal cocaine exposure,
        105–108
    in preterm infants, 101–103
    selective attention to novelty by
        adults, 65–67
    selective attention to novelty by
        children, 63–65

selective attention to novelty by prenatally cocaine-exposed infants, 109
selective attention to novelty by preterm infants, 104

O

Orthogenetic framework
developmental models of perception, 13
origins of, 4, 8
perceptual processes in, 11–12

P

Parent–child interactions, 110–112, 113
Parvocellular visual pathway, 33
Perceptual processes
attention as measure of infant functioning, 98
brain activity models, 13
cognitive model of schizophrenia, 334–335
concepts of selectivity in, 10–11
developmental models, 13–15, 74–75, 79–80
orthogenetic model, 11–12
schizophrenia assessment, 329–330
Perimetry, 35
Phobias
in children, 366
color-naming latencies, 367
Piaget, J., 5
Positron emission tomography, 265–266
Premature infants, 97–98
arousal and attention in, 103–105, 112–113
demographics, 101
developmental biology, 102–103
developmental risks, 101–102
environmental stimulation, 103
parenting environment, 111–112
Preventive interventions
fetal alcohol effects/syndrome, 193–194

information processing style as predictive of stress response, 369–370
screening for mental retardation, 63
Psychoanalytic approach, 7
Psychopathology. *See also* Developmental psychopathology
scope of research, 6–7
Psychopathy, 24
attentional processes in, 395–396
behavioral inhibition model, 392
classification of auditory–visual stimuli, 388–390
clinical characteristics, 379, 380
conduct disorder and, 394–395
cue responsiveness, 383–385, 392, 395–396
dichotic listening studies, 387
divided attention, 385–391, 393
executive functioning in, 391–392
measurement of attention in, 380–381
obstacles to research, 380
passive avoidance in, 394
predictors, 396
prevalence, 379
research trends, 379–380
selective attention, 382–385, 393
sustained attention, 381–382, 393
word classification tests, 386
in younger populations, 392–394
Pulvinar, 13

R

Reaction time crossover in schizophrenia, 323–325
Research methodology. *See also* Group comparison studies; Measurement
attention in psychopathy, 381–385
attentional functioning in schizophrenia, 322–332
brain–behavior relations, 263–267
developmental course of schizophrenia, 321

Research methodology (*continued*)
  with Down syndrome infants,
    124–125, 126, 130–132,
    138–139
  fetal alcohol exposure, 181–182
  functioning of posterior–anterior
    attentional systems, 253
  location cue paradigm, 291–292
  Standard-Transformation-Return
    procedure, 132–135
  static stimuli with infants, 126,
    131–132, 140–141
  for visuospatial studies, 291,
    293–294
Rutter, M., 8

S

Savants, 250–251
Schema theory
  of anxiety, 355–356
  of depression, 355–356
  network theory and, 358
Schizophrenia, 24
  attentional indicators, 322,
    332–333, 339–340
  auditory hallucinations, 337
  backward masking effects on per-
    ception in, 329–330
  clinical features, 318
  cognitive models, 333, 334–336,
    340–341
  continuous performance test,
    325–326, 339
  counting performance, 330
  course of, 318
  developmental risk, 321–322
  dopaminergic system in, 339
  early detection, 319
  event related potentials, 331
  excessive excitatory mechanism in,
    340
  eye-tracking deviations in, 332
  genetic risk, 322
  inhibition of startle reflex in, 330,
    339
  negative priming effect task perfor-
    mance, 330
  neural network modeling,
    338–339, 340
  paranoid, 335–336
  perceptual-cognitive tests, 329–330
  process vs. reactive, 324
  psychophysiological measures,
    330–332
  reaction time crossover, 323–325
  research opportunities, 340–341
  risk factors, 318–319
  segmental set theory, 320, 323
  signs of attentional problems, 319
  simple reaction time as indicator
    of, 322–325, 339
  skin conductance orienting
    responses, 331
  Span of Apprehension Test,
    326–329, 339
  specificity of attentional measures,
    332, 333
  stochastic modeling, 335–336
  task performance in, 319
  theoretical models of attention, 320
Segmental set theory, 320, 323
Selection-for-action mechanism, 34,
    47–48
Selective attention
  in ADHD, 150–152, 207
  in Alzheimer's disease, 289
  in anxiety, 360–362, 365–366,
    370–372
  assessment, 207
  behavioral models, 12–13
  cognitive components, 150
  conceptualization of attentional
    processes, 10–11
  covert, 267–268
  in demented/depressed elderly,
    67–68
  in depression, 362–364, 365–366,
    370–372
  dialectical model, 12
  discrimination problem-solving by
    infants, 153–155
  in Down syndrome infants,
    126–127
  lifespan development, 74–75,
    89–91

in mental retardation, 210–212
in mental retardation with ADHD, 217, 219
in mood-disordered children, 366–367
neural mediation of, 269–272
in neurologically impaired adults, 65–67
in neurologically impaired children, 63–65
in nonhuman primates, 68–69
to novelty, lifespan development of, 55, 56–58, 70–71
orthogenetic model, 11–12
as predictor of later functioning, 56, 59
in preterm infants, 103–104
in psychopathy, 382–385, 393
research approaches to brain mechanisms, 263
stability of information-processing biases, 367–369
sustained attention and, 98–99
visual crowding effect, 46
visual orienting, 34–43, 76–77, 91, 100
Sleep patterns, in alcohol-exposed neonates, 182
Smooth pursuit eye-tracking, 332
Social functioning
autism characteristics, 232–233
Down syndrome infants, 128, 129
early developmentalist research, 5–6
prenatal cocaine exposure and, 112
Span of Apprehension Test
development of, 326–327
operations, 327
research trends, 327, 328
schizophrenia assessment, 327–329
Speed of processing theory, 79, 90, 130
Standard-Transformation-Return procedure, 132–135, 141
Down syndrome infant assessment, 136–138
State regulation, in alcohol-exposed neonates, 182

Stimulus onset asynchronies, 41–42
in cued location test, 292
Stroop color conflict test, 361
Subitizing, 78–79, 86–88
Superior colliculus, 13, 15, 33, 42–43, 270
split-brain studies, 272–274
Sustained attention, 43–44, 98–99, 104
in ADHD, 149–150, 151–152, 206–207
assessment, 206–207, 380
definition, 380
as failure to lose interest, 210
in mental retardation, 209–210
in mental retardation with ADHD, 216–217, 219
in prenatally alcohol-exposed adolescents, 188
in psychopathy, 381–382, 393

T

Transactional world view, 6

V

Vigilance system. *See also* Sustained attention
in arousal, 100
in mental retardation, 209–210
prenatal alcohol exposure effects, 184, 188–189
in schizophrenia, 325
Visual attention
age-related changes in scanning eye movements, 43–44
in autism, 249–251
brain activity models, 13
covert orienting, 40, 76–77, 80–83, 267–268
endogenous control, 31
enumeration, 78–79, 86–89
exogenous control, 31
externality effect, 45–46
eye movements for visual orienting, 34–43
focusing accuracy, 46–47

Visual attention (*continued*)
  habituation/dishabituation studies,
    44–46, 99
  IQ performance and, 59
  lifespan development, 74–75,
    89–91
  measurement, 31–32
  normal process, 31
  object-based, 268–269, 270–272
  preference for novelty in normal
    development, 59–62
  preference for novelty in preterm
    infants, 104
  research needs, 49
  as selection-for-action mechanism,
    34, 47–48
  space-based, 268–270, 272,
    281–283
  temporal gap effects, 39–40
  visual search, 77–78, 83–86
Visual crowding effect, 46
Visual development
  autism as disorder of, 254–255
  infant attention, 98–100
  neurobiological models, 14–15,
    32–34
  preference for novelty in normal
    development, 59–62
  preference for novelty in preterm
    infants, 104
  scanning eye movements, 43–44, 48

Visual field
  competition effects, 35–37
  developmental changes, 35–36
  infant focusing ability, 47
Visual orienting theory, 34–43,
    76–77, 91, 100, 250
Visuospatial attention
  aging effects in neuroanatomy of,
    300–303
  in Alzheimer's disease, 293,
    297–298
  definition, 291
  feature integration theory, 295
  functional neuroanatomy in,
    298–300
  location cue paradigm, 291–292
  neural functioning in schizo-
    phrenia, 337–338
  normal aging, 292–293, 296
  parietal lobe lesions and, 297,
    298
  as serial vs. parallel process,
    295–296, 297, 298

W

Werner, H., 7–8, 11–12, 13, 15

Z

Zigler, E., 8